General Practice: Advances in Medicine

General Practice: Advances in Medicine

Editor: Zachary Ashton

AMERICAN MEDICAL PUBLISHERS
www.americanmedicalpublishers.com

AMERICAN
MEDICAL PUBLISHERS
www.americanmedicalpublishers.com

Cataloging-in-Publication Data

General practice : advances in medicine / edited by Zachary Ashton.
p. cm.
Includes bibliographical references and index.
ISBN 978-1-63927-448-2
1. Family medicine. 2. Physicians (General practice). 3. Medicine--Practice.
4. Primary care (Medicine). I. Ashton, Zachary.
R729.5.G4 H36 2022
610--dc23

American Medical Publishers,
41 Flatbush Avenue,
1st Floor, New York,
NY 11217, USA

ISBN 978-1-63927-448-2 (Hardback)

Contents

Preface

General practice is a field of medicine that focuses on providing holistic primary health care to people of all ages and sex. It aims to provide continuous and comprehensive health care to individuals as well as families. General practice aims to deliver a range of acute and chronic medical care services. It is also involved in providing preventive care such as immunization, routine check-ups and health-risk assessments. General practice is also used in conjunction with other subspecialties for the management of chronic illnesses. It plays a vital role in detecting serious diseases at an early stage and then referring the patients to specialized care. This book studies, analyzes and upholds the pillars of general practice and its utmost significance in modern times. It unfolds the innovative aspects of primary care medicine which will be crucial for the progress of this field in the future. The book is appropriate for students seeking detailed information in this area as well as for experts.

All of the data presented henceforth, was collaborated in the wake of recent advancements in the field. The aim of this book is to present the diversified developments from across the globe in a comprehensible manner. The opinions expressed in each chapter belong solely to the contributing authors. Their interpretations of the topics are the integral part of this book, which I have carefully compiled for a better understanding of the readers.

At the end, I would like to thank all those who dedicated their time and efforts for the successful completion of this book. I also wish to convey my gratitude towards my friends and family who supported me at every step.

Editor

1

'Working is out of the question': a qualitative text analysis of medical certificates of disability

Guri Aarseth[1*], Bård Natvig[1], Eivind Engebretsen[2] and Anne Kveim Lie[3]

Abstract

Background: Medical certificates influence the distribution of economic benefits in welfare states; however, the qualitative aspects of these texts remain largely unexplored. The present study is the first systematic investigation done of these texts. Our aim was to investigate how GPs select and mediate information about their patients' health and how they support their conclusions about illness, functioning and fitness for work in medical certificates.

Methods: We performed a textual analysis of thirty-three medical certificates produced by general practitioners (GP) in Norway at the request of the Norwegian Labour and Welfare Administration (NAV).The certificates were subjected to critical reading using the combined analytic methods of narratology and linguistics.

Results: Some of the medical information was unclear, ambiquous, and possibly misleading. Evaluations of functioning related to illness were scarce or absent, regardless of diagnosis, and, hence, the basis of working incapacity was unclear. Voices in the text frequently conflated, obscuring the source of speaker. In some documents, the expert's subtle use of language implied doubts about the claimant's credibility, but explicit advocacy also occurred. GPs show little insight into their patients' working lives, but rather than express uncertainty and incompetence, they may resort to making too absolute and too general statements about patients' working capacity, and fail to report thorough assessments.

Conclusions: A number of the texts in our material may not function as sufficient or reliable sources for making decisions regarding social benefits. Certificates as these may be deficient for several reasons, and textual incompetence may be one of them. Physicians in Norway receive no systematic training in professional writing. High-quality medical certificates, we believe, might be economical in the long term: it might increase the efficiency with which NAV processes cases and save costs by eliminating the need for unnecessary and expensive specialist reports. Moreover, correct and coherent medical certificates can strengthen legal protection for claimants. Eventually, reducing advocacy in these documents may contribute to a fairer evaluation of whether claimants are eligible for disability benefits or not. Therefore, we believe that professional writing skills should be validated as an important part of medical practice and should be integrated in medical schools and in further education as a discipline in its own right, preferably involving humanities professors.

Keywords: Norway, GP, Medical certificates of incapacity for work, Document analysis

* Correspondence: guri.aarseth@medisin.uio.no
[1]Department of General Practice, University of Oslo, Faculty of Medicine, Institute of Health and Society, Postboks 1130, Blindern 0318, OSLO, Norway
Full list of author information is available at the end of the article

Background

Physicians are producers of texts, although they are probably not inclined to consider themselves as such. Written reports go hand in hand with clinical work, as they have since the Hippocratic writers communicated their clinical observations in case reports. In Europe, the medical case report was refined and 'purified' during the 18th and 19th centuries, becoming a professional skill in its own right [1, 2]. In our time, society relies on medical texts to approve, testify to, and document nearly everything that can be related to 'health'. Accordingly, the amount of administrative documentary work that doctors must perform is increasing at the expense of their clinical work [3]. In doing this work, physicians are supposed to exit the mode of treating doctor and take on the role of expert, balancing the perspectives of professional sympathy and impartiality [4].

A certificate – from the Latin *certificare*, meaning to guarantee as certain or attest in an authoritative manner (Oxford English Dictionary) – verifies facts; a medical certificate, in particular, attests to the condition of a person's health. It can be used to legitimise benefits to compensate for loss of income as the result of disease, or to exempt or relieve a person from his/her normal activities. In this article we examine medical certificates written by Norwegian GPs, taking disability benefits as our point of departure. Our aim is to investigate how these physicians, when acting as experts, mediate their patients' illnesses, functioning, and fitness for work and how they report assessments made on a medical basis. Our purpose is to encourage a discussion about the role of GPs in the disability benefit scheme and address the need for a systematic incorporation of writing instruction in medical schools and in further education.

Medical certificates play a crucial role in allocating benefits in welfare states. To be legal, a medical certificate must generally be issued by authorised health personnel. The authority of the document depends on an authorised reader sharing the perception of its factual veracity [5]. A certifier must provide verifiable information; the certificate must be accurate, not misleading or flawed, and should be written based on the physician's recent, personal examination of the patient.

In Norway, according to the National Insurance Act, a medical certificate of disability must make probable the causal connection between a patient's illness, their loss of function, and their need for permanent income compensation [6]. In issuing these certificates, therefore, GPs have to navigate a problematic landscape in which persistent complaints, symptoms, and illness, with or without objective correlatives, must be subjected to the certifier's professional reasoning. GPs recognise that they have little knowledge about patients' workplaces, their functioning, or their working capacity [7–12]. In addition, formal medical knowledge may be insufficient as a basis for determining individuals' rights and eligibility for social benefits [7].

Arthur Kleinman [13] defines *illness* as the 'innately human experience of symptoms and suffering', *disease* as the practitioner's 'recasting of illness in terms of theories of disorders', and *sickness* as the understanding of a disorder (for instance tuberculosis) across a population in relation to macrosocial forces (poverty, education etc.). In contrast to this English triad, the Norwegian term *sykdom* comprises both illness and disease (in the National Insurance Act, *sykdom* also refers to injury [*skade*], impairments, and defects [*lyte*]) [14].

The ethics of issuing medical certificates differ in several respects from those of producing clinical documents. First, the information contained in a certificate is, in part, exempt from obligations to protect patient confidentiality. Second, whereas as therapists physicians are expected to always consider the best possible outcome for their patients, as experts they should act according to criteria of objectivity. In other words, physicians should provide information that is impartial, correct, verifiable, and accurate, [4], and act 'without regard to the outcome of the case' [15]. Moreover, physicians should not be passive mediators of the patient's concern and utterances, but act as a 'performer of the profession' [4].

The ethical and professional dilemmas of physicians facing the discourses of both law (including the gatekeeper function of the doctor) and medicine are treated in studies of GPs' practices of certifying sick leave [16–19]. In a questionnaire survey, Gulbrandsen et al. [20] found that it is not uncommon for Norwegian GPs to provide medical certificates strategically written in favour of the patient; however, the GPs in that study claimed that they were not twisting the facts or lying, but rather using discretion and argumentation. Other investigations have indicated that GPs may be directed by advocacy and the patient's subjective needs and wishes when issuing sickness certifications [17, 21, 22], as well as by their own personal values and attitudes [23], personality, and beliefs [24].

Direct investigation of the content of certificates is scarce, but Kiessling et al. [25] found that 90 per cent of a selection of Swedish medical certificates lacked relevant or adequate information about the patient's ability to function and capacity to work; others have shown that ambiguous statements about a patient's medical disorder are not uncommon [26]. In a previous article we presented a linguistic analysis of the same medical certificates of fitness to work which showed that certifying GPs tended to emphasise the patient or claimant principally as a passive carrier of symptoms with little or no agency [27]. The above studies indicate that ambiguities, possible biases, and a lack of relevant information may undermine the validity of decisions made on the basis of medical certificates.

In addition, officials processing disability benefits cases within the Norwegian Labour and Welfare Administration (NAV) experience that deficient or unclear information in GPs' medical certificates can lead to costly and time-consuming delays [28]. In such cases, additional information needs to be obtained; this information is increasingly (though probably unnecessarily) ordered from specialists charging significantly higher fees. Because the specialist needs to see the claimant personally and write a new note, it usually leads to an increase in the case's processing time, sometimes by several months. The delay creates temporary uncertainty for the claimant as to the outcome of the proceeding.

Compared to GPs in some other European countries, GPs in Norway play a prominent role in assessing patients' health-related inability to work [29] and, thus, are highly influential in the distribution of public resources. Their importance can be illustrated by the fact that presently 9.5 per cent (317 700) of the population between 18 and 66 years of age [30] are living on disability benefits. Altogether, the largest group of benefit recipients – 63 per cent – have been diagnosed either with diseases related to the musculoskeletal system (mainly low back pain and fibromyalgia) or with mental disorders (mainly anxiety and depression) [31, 32]. The government estimate of the total costs of working disability benefits in Norway in 2016 was 78.2 billion NOK (€8.55 billion) [33]. Decisions on disability benefits are taken by non-medical officials in the regional offices within NAV, who never meet the claimant personally and must rely entirely on textual information about that person.

In this article, using narratological and linguistic analysis, we examine a sample of texts written by GPs in their role as experts to determine how they communicate the illness, functional ability, and working capacity of people claiming disability benefits.

Methods

Data collection

Our material consists of medical certificates of incapacity for work produced by Norwegian GPs. They are, with one exception (which was written by freehand), written on a standardised form, the Medical Certificate of Disability [34]. The certificates were collected in the period March–June 2013; all of them were written between 2007 and 2013. At the time of collection, the cases had already been assessed and closed by NAV. NAV's central statistical register of assisted us in selecting 150 potential certificates within four counties in Norway.

We strategically selected individuals based on age, sex, geographic region, and diagnosis. The age range was 18–66 and at least one third belonging to one sex. One third of the certificates fell into the category of musculo-skeletal related diagnoses, one third into the category of psychiatric diagnoses, and the remaining third into the category of other disorders; thus the sample roughly reflects the distribution of diagnoses among the total population of Norwegians receiving disability benefits. The four counties were selected according to the proportion of the population receiving disability benefits: one had a relatively high proportion (>12%), two were in the median (8–12%) and one had a low proportion (<8%).

The project was approved by the Data Protection Official for Research [35], the Directorate of Labour and Welfare, and the Council of Secrecy and Research in the Ministry of Justice and Public Security. An informed consent letter, also approved by the Data Protection Official for Research, was sent to the 150 claimants via their local NAV offices. We anticipated a final number of 30–50 certificates: forty recipients of disability benefits consented to us accessing their medical certificates. Of the forty certificates, seven were excluded as they were either not about disability or not written by GPs. All the documents were anonymised with respect to the claimants. The number of different certifiers (GPs) equalled the number of certificates. The final sample is shown in Table 1. The main and additional diagnoses complied with the ICPC-2 system (International Classification of Primary Care, Second Edition).

Analysis

We apply qualitative document analysis to our empirical data, which consist of textual units formed by the GPs texts and the form text, Medical certificate for work incapacity (Table 2). Our analysis of the medical certificates draws on the discourses of narratology and formal linguistics. As subjects of analysis, documents are not 'surrogates' for reality, but are themselves social facts, exchanged as part of a social interaction [36]. Because

Table 1 Characteristics of the medical certificates of disability ($N = 33$)

Geographic region	Regional distribution	
North	12	
Northwest coast	3	
Central South	4	
Central East	14	
Male claimants	20	
Female claimants	13	
Age range of claimants	30–64 (average = median = 45)	
Diagnosis (ICPC-2)	Main:	Additional:
Musculoskeletal	20	17
Psychiatry	6	4
Others:	9	10

Table 2 Medical certificate for work incapacity

National Insurance (NAV)	
Medical certificate for work incapacity	
The physician is to send this to the local NAV office.	
0	This certificate concerns:
0.1	Assessment of work capacity at sick leave
0.2	Rehabilitation money
0.3	Disability pension
1.0	Information about the patient and employment
	Name:
	Year of birth:
	Certificate written: date
	Employer's name and address:
2	Information of diagnosis and disease
2.1	Main diagnosis
2.1.1	Code of diagnosis
2.2	Additional diagnosis
2.2.1	Code of diagnosis
2.3	Classification: ICPC-2/ICD-10
2.4	Completely incapacitated since
2.5	Story of disease, symptoms and treatment
2.6	Current clinical status (specify date). The results of relevant investigations
2.7	Should NAV consider this to be:
2.7.1.	Occupational disease? (Yes/No)
2.7.2.	If yes: date of injury
3	Plan for medical examination and treatment
3.1	Is the patient referred for
	Medical assessment (specify)?
	Medical treatment (specify)?
3.1.1	Date of referral for medical assessment. 3.1.2 Expected waiting time (weeks)
3.1.3	Date of referral for medical treatment. 3.1.4 Expected waiting time (weeks)
3.2	Plan for medical examination. Specify the planned examination and time duration.
3.3	Plan for medical treatment.Specify the planned treatments and time/duration
3.4	Re-evaluation of previous plan of examination and treatment
3.5	When should the NAV office request new medical information regarding work clarification and treatment programme?
3.6	If further treatment is not relevant, give justification
4	Proposed measures beyond medical treatment
	Are the following measures applicable, on a medical basis. Yes/No
	If *yes*, which ones? a) reference to specialist, b) transport subsidy, c) graded sick leave, d) technical aids, f) unemployment benefit, g) others – which ones? Give supplementary information.
	Are there any specific considerations to be made as to these measures?

Table 2 Medical certificate for work incapacity *(Continued)*

	If *no*, give justifications
5	Medically reasoned assessment of work ability
5.1	Describe how the patient's functionality is generally reduced because of disease.
5.2	Is the patient engaged in paid work or domestic work, a student, other?
	Specify:
	Briefly describe the type of work and the requirements:
5.3	Assessment of working capacity
	Will the patient be able to
	a) Resume the earlier work (No/Yes)? If yes: now/after treatment
	b) Take other work
5.4	a) What is it that the patient cannot do in the present work?
	b) What other possible considerations need to be taken regarding the choice of another profession/work?
6	Prognosis
	a) Is the treatment assumed to produce an improved ability to work? Yes/No
	b) Estimate the duration of the illness/injury.
	c) Estimate the duration of the functional disability.
	d) Estimate the duration of the reduced working capacity.
7	Causation
	Estimate the importance of the functional disability for the reduced working capacity.
8	Optional information
9	Co-operation/Contact
	Select those that should be contacted by the NAV office: The doctor/employer/NAV/others
10	Reservations
10.1	Is there anything in the certificate that the patient, for medical reasons, should not know? If yes, specify what the patient should not know.
11	The physician's signature, etc.
11.1	Date, the physician's name and address
11.2	The physician's signature
11.3	Telephone number

documents do not speak for themselves, they must be 'made to speak by the analyst' [36]. Hence, what we are investigating is not the patient but the documentary *depiction* of the patient, his/her illness and ability to work. Narrative analysis (as a method) investigates structures and techniques of telling, the narrator's perspective (who speaks?), and the consistency of the facts and interpretations the narrator provides. We use linguistic methods of analysis at the word and sentence levels to investigate different types of grammatical connections between sentences and their meaning.

Narratives, Barbara Smith suggests, can be defined simply as 'verbal acts consisting of someone telling someone else that something happened' [37]. The 'something happened', which Labov and Waletsky call the 'complication' of the story [38] and van Dijk calls the 'worth telling' [39], is a key concept of narrative. The 'complication' or the 'worth telling' is an essential event of the story that has an impact or changes stable situations, conditions or life trajectories. Van Dijk, for instance, emphasises events (disease, in this case) that break the established norms (e.g. of being independent and self-supported) and routines (e.g. daily doings), threaten the basic values (e.g. being healthy) and disturb the balance (e.g. abilities and mastering), plans and goals (e.g. relations, work, education) of the story's protagonist (who may be an individual with a disease).

Events may be related from different perspectives. Smith points to the inherent relativism of narrative: every narrative is a *version* of some reality, always 'constructed in accord with some set of purposes or interests' [37]. Nevertheless, as Petter Aaslestad points out, the ideal starting point of the documentary text is 'the true event', as perceived by the narrator [40]. Leaning on the narratological theories of Wayne Booth and Gérard Genette, we distinguish between the 'historic author' (the GP), the 'narrator/writer' (the telling voice in the text) and the 'implicit author' (the text's norm carrier) [41, 42]. The narrator may represent different perspectives: they may be present as the first person narrator (the 'I' of the text) who has limited knowledge of the patient, or as an all-knowing, invisible or impersonal speaker. The intentions of the historic author (the GP) may deviate from those of the narrator for several reasons [43]. Therefore, we distinguish between the GP as a treating family physician on the one hand, and as a narrator on the other. This distinction is also considered in Norwegian legal regulations [44].

The author has in mind an addressee – not a particular, identified person, but rather the author's idea of a reader, or what Wolfgang Iser terms the 'implied reader' [45]. The implied reader is anticipated in the text as a set of the addressee's competences, reactions, and values [43]. In this case of the medical certificates, the implied reader is represented by (unidentified) NAV employees, including the internal medical adviser. The latter is also an *authorised* reader who shares the knowledge and the terminology of the certifier [43].

The coherence of any given text is associated with consistency, logic, and textual unity. It also depends on the reader's willingness and ability to create meaningful relations between facts, events, and evaluations [46]. Coherence is thus a product of the text and the reader's knowledge, experience, attitudes, expectations, and cultural background [46–48]. Some narratologists may include the narrator's evaluation of facts and events as one of the main elements of a narrative, without which they regard the narrative as pointless [38].

In our analysis, we investigate the narrative thread and the linguistic markers that constitute the global 'hanging-togetherness' of the text: the diagnosis, the story of illness, the symptoms belonging to it, and the patient's ability to function and capacity to work. We use the term illness when talking about the patient's symptom complex, as claimants of disability benefits are ill or ill-functioning in the sense of having a subjective experience of being unable to work.

Results

The standard certificate form: dissociating the disease and the patient

We start with a critical review and interpretation of the form text (Table 2). As a starting point, we ask how the form deals with *disease* and *illness without disease*. On the form, information about the medical condition is requested in terms of 'diagnosis and information about the disease' (Section 2); the form breaks this information down into a 'main diagnosis' (Subsection 2.1), an 'additional diagnosis' (Subsection 2.2), a 'disease story with symptoms and treatment' (Subsection 2.5) and 'results from clinical examination and relevant tests' (Subsection 2.6). Thus far, the form reflects a model in which *disease* – composed of a set of symptoms, clinical and laboratory findings, and adequate treatment – is the main cause of dysfunction. The form reflects the idea that there is both an immediate and predictable relation between disease and dysfunction/working capacity and a medical treatment available that may improve not the patient's health but their 'functional ability' and 'working capacity'. This is shown in Subsection 5.1 and Section 6 of the form (see Table 2 for full form):

5.1 Describe how functional ability is generally reduced due to disease.

6. Prognosis:

a) Is the treatment assumed to improve working ability? Yes / No

b) Estimate the duration of the disease/injury

c) Estimate the duration of the functional disability

d) Estimate the duration of the reduced working capacity

Sections 5.1 and 6a–d assume that there is a direct relation between disease and ability to function without the *patient* being viewed as a subject with motivation, beliefs, and a will of their own. Moreover, the form does not ask for the social context (familial, educational) of the claimant, which – according to the National Insurance Act [6] – should be considered a legitimate co-factor of illness. Because an individual's experience of illness cannot be validated by 'clinical findings and relevant test results', important information about the patient and other causes of ill-health may be overlooked. In the standard form, NAV adopts a reductionist view and selects, organises, and limits the information it seeks from the GP, using terms of disease exclusively. This is also seen in Section 2.5, the heading of which – 'history of disease, symptoms, and treatment' – indicates that there is a narrative to be told. However, the story being asked for is that of the disease, not of the sick *person*.

Listing symptoms at the cost of the illness story

Probably as a reflection of the form's dissociation between the patient and their disease, there are entire certificates that mention the patient only rarely or not at all and which are almost entirely devoid of narratively organised events and their consequences. Excerpt (a), below, exemplifies how the illness story is replaced by a number of symptoms (all the excerpts are from different certificates and are labelled sequentially with letters a-j. The form questions/sections are numbered according to Table 2. Form text is in bold.)

(a) **2.5: History of disease, symptoms and treatment.** Investigated by cardiologist -12 [2012] for a tendency to arrhythmia. Allergies: suggesting wheat flour; gastrointestinal gas. Sensitivity of airways. Afflicted by tinnitus; evaluated [by] the RA [rheumatic arthritis] clinic; Natural functions: a little reflux, ventricular gas, statically: back problems for many years.

Because the list of symptoms/conditions lacks the only element that may connect them – the person to whom they belong – the information comes out fragmentarily, and in the absence of verbs, nothing *happens.* The only traces of a narrative in (a) are '-12' and 'for many years', indicating a time course. As Smith points out [37], any utterance, however small and fragmentary, can have narrative content, and 'telling about events' can be indistinguishable from stating that 'something is'. Are the conditions listed – allergies, tinnitus, back problems etc. – events of the past or are they still causing low functioning and working disability? There is nothing in the text that tells us. Listing a large number of symptoms might be the writer's attempt to comply with NAV's notion of *disease* as the legitimate basis of disability benefits. What the narrative's 'worth telling' is, however, remains unclear. A mere list without specification or evaluation does little to help up comprehend the patient's problem, and we are left with a pointless story [38]. The reader whom the text addresses will probably have difficulty interpreting the information and taking a decision; indeed, in this particular case, the disability benefits claim was rejected by the NAV.

Lack of temporal aspects of illness obscures causality

Because an illness *story* can be abbreviated, told fragmentarily, or not told at all, as shown in excerpt (a), the sequential events are often omitted. In (b), the undefined time aspect of the claimant's alcoholism and anxiety disguises a possible problematic relation between the patient's alcohol consumption and their psychiatric disorder.

(b) **2.5 History of disease, symptoms and treatment.** The patient has a long illness story of alcohol abuse. In addition, she has been struggling with anxiety problems for as many years.

The use of 'in addition', a simple transitional phrase, indicates that there is no *causal* relation between alcohol abuse and anxiety; however, a competent reader probably cannot help but pose the question: does she have anxiety problems because of alcohol abuse – or is it the other way round? The answer to this question has implications for the treatment of each of the problems. Again, the distinction between what *was* and what *is* is blurred, and the illness textually slides into a continuous, non-contextualised state of being where anxiety and alcoholism are depicted as if they were not related.

Chronicity and the doctor's chaos narrative

The medical profession is typically oriented diachronically; taking patient histories is heavily emphasised in the teaching of medical students. Throughout clinical examinations and treatment, the patient's story – as noted in their medical record – is transformed into medical discourse; but principally it remains a *story* [49]. The medical certificates in our sample, however, are mainly synchronic; it describes the patient's present symptoms and complaints as a persistent, static state of affairs. According to the sociologist Arthur Frank, disease starts with an event 'interrupt[ing] life' and in some cases slides into an 'incessant presence with no memorable past and no future worth anticipating' [50].

Medical certificates of disability typically present illness as a *status quo*, which is coherent with the purpose of the document. Furthermore, details of the patient's condition and story are often omitted. We see an example of this in excerpt (c): it starts in the present, describing the illnesses in very general terms

(c) **2.5 History of disease, symptoms, and treatment.** The patient has a complex health problem with fibromyalgia and extensive muscle pain, [...] asthma and general exhaustion.

The terms 'complex', 'extensive', and 'general' seem to replace a thorough depiction of the patient's illness story which becomes a condition with no pre-history (how was life before the illness started? How and when did the asthma influence her functioning? When – and perhaps why– did she become generally exhausted?).

Arthur Frank [50] has elaborated three empirical categories of illness narratives: first, there is the restitution narrative (the successfully ill – I was healthy, got sick, recovered); second, the quest narrative (the acceptance of illness and how to see the experience as meaningful for oneself and others); and, finally, the chaos narrative (the persistent disturbance to living caused by illness). According to Frank, the chaos narrative – as opposed to the restitution and quest narratives – is distinct in that it has 'no sequence' and 'no mediation, only immediacy' [50]. In contrast to stories in which medicine triumphs, Frank asserts, the chaos narrative is a non-plot of 'never getting better' that exposes the vulnerable, futile, and impotent sides of the profession. In excerpt (d), below, the writer describes a 59-year-old woman with chronic muscle and joint pain who has no authoritative diagnosis to explain the pain, and, consequently, has been denied disability benefits:

(d) **Diagnosis:** Low back pain L03. Pain in joints IKA L20.

2.5. History of disease, symptoms, and treatment [...] much pain and low function of the shoulder and she was referred to [polyclinic]. There, they found tendinitis. Recommended physiotherapy. The patient has consistent, chronic pain and is treated regularly without improvement of her functioning and there is no curative treatment.

2.6. Current clinical status (specify date). The results of relevant investigations. The patient comes for a talk. [...] Taking new blood tests and glucoses. Supporting talk. Follow-up of results. Try to find discharge summary from the chiropractor. Additionally, she gets a referral to the physiotherapist.

After the introduction, the narrator enters the text as a first-person narrator (although first- person pronoun is omitted), as a GP acting in present time (probably in a consultation). While the activities described here are normal activities in a family practice – the text is most likely cut and pasted from the patient's record – they are hardly *worth telling* in a medical certificate. The GP acting in the text, however empathic, does not seem to have a plan: even though therapy has proved to be without effect, the doctor continues to refer the patient to physiotherapy and recommends diverse medical checks not quoted in the excerpt (among them, another MRI). The GP in the text might accept that there is no 'diagnosis' and that further treatment and repeated MRIs will not bring more clarity. Instead, this would be a situation that has 'no mediation, only immediacy' [50]. An aimless narrative in a certificate may mirror the author's own 'chaos', the GP's experience of powerlessness when faced with illness without disease.

According to Sarah Nettleton, patients with medically unexplained symptoms (MUS) typically present illness without a clear 'plot' or 'route map', and, in addition to their ailments, suffer from not having the legitimacy of the 'sick role' [51]. Irrespective of the real illness experiences behind the documents – which we cannot know anything about – we find that some narrators take a chaos perspective, turning the patient's story into what we have chosen to call the *doctor's chaos narrative.* In the doctor's chaos narrative, the physician – implicitly or clearly – is 'stuck' with the patient, with no way out of the endless cycle of treatment that leads neither to improved health, nor even, perhaps, to welfare benefits for the patient.

Conflation of voices

In our material, we find that the voices in the texts are presented in different ways [42]. The narrator may have 'completeness of information' about the patient, being an impersonal, authorial, *all-knowing* voice, placed outside the narrative. Then there is *free indirect speech* (no quotation marks or references to the speaker) which may sometimes be inferred as the patient's voice, given the context of the narrative. Finally, the patient's voice may be explicit and rendered as *indirect speech* ('the patient claims/says that...'). The following example is from the certificate of a 50-year-old man with low back pain who has been struggling to convince the NAV official that he is unfit for work

(e) **2.6 Current clinical status (specify date). The results of relevant investigations.** A long talk with the patient [...]. For him, it is not possible to resume work because of his low back pain. Still marked by a long fight with NAV for not being believed.

5.1. Describe how the patient's functioning is generally reduced due to disease. Cannot sit or stand for long or short periods of time.

5.4. What is it that the patient cannot do in the present work? Cannot function in work, unable to withstand either physical work or sedentary work.

In excerpt (e), there are no speaking subjects or references and thus the utterances have no explicit source. The statements in sections 5.1. and 5.4 about the patient's functionality and working capacity – are they based on the author's medical observations and knowledge, 'objectivised' by the authorial voice to justify disability benefit, or are they the patient's subjective claims repeated by the narrator in free indirect speech? The conflation of voices erases the distinction between the professional evaluation and the patient's claims. By using free indirect speech, the narrator has the possibility of not committing to the utterance (which may be inferred as the patient's own voice) while at the same time making it appear 'objective' (inferred as the narrator's all-knowing voice). The effect in this case is that the narrator can be taken to implicitly promote disability benefits, but without having said it directly.

Only patients can account for their symptoms, and we find that symptoms occupy more space than the diagnosis, which only the doctor is authorised to qualify. Adapting the term *linguistic zone* used by the literary critic Mikhail Bakhtin [52], we consider *symptoms* to belong to the patient's linguistic universe, whereas *diagnosis* and medical evaluations belong to the doctor's. In our material, the number of symptoms per certificate ranges from two to fifteen, whereas the number of diagnoses is significantly less, ranging from one to five. By over-emphasising symptoms and complaints, the narrator allows the claimant's linguistic zone to spread in the text. We find that the corresponding physician's 'zone' within the texts can be displaced or weakened by the narrator's willingness to leave space for the patient's linguistic zone, which may perhaps lead the narrator to lose control of the discourse [40].

The countering voice

Sick leave certificates are often issued by GPs in response to patients' demands [21, 22, 53]. Some studies indicate that conflict or fear of conflict may underlie the decision to issue a certificate [12, 16]. Certifying permanent working disability probably involves many of the same problems, but few studies have looked at how texts made by doctors when evaluating fitness to work reflect uncertainty and possible conflict with the patient. The writer may use linguistic techniques to point to certain connections or to obscure their own opinion. The example below is from a patient applying for permanent disability benefits after years of receiving temporary benefits. The narrator summarises the patient's functioning and presents his status in a new certificate below (Certificate (f).We have *italicised* the connecting words):

(f) **Diagnosis:** Epicondylitis L93.

2.5 History of symptoms and treatment. Has been doing well in daily life, *but* not managed to resume work. He has not been working *but* has tried to occupy himself with small jobs at home. Painkillers taken occasionally — claims to have some effect — *but* still not 'healthy' enough to resume work and wants a prolongation of his disability pension. **8. Optional information.** 'He has less pain at rest *but* still has pain related to physical efforts.

With the exception of 'claims to have' in excerpt (f), which is the patient's indirect speech, the text contains *free* indirect speech; this speech is probably the patient's, as it refers to events within the private sphere to which the narrator has no direct access and to the patient's subjective experience of pain. 'But' is a concessive conjunction, which is typical of an argumentative text type; in excerpt (f) it is used systematically to counter statements [54]. We find segments of two opposing narratives, both of which stem from the patient: one referring to his private life (with some achievements) and the other repeatedly to 'work' (no achievements). It is not evident why the patient is still unable to work, and the organisation of the text with 'but' suggests doubts or disbelief about the patient's unfitness for work.

Bakhtin [55] points out that the essential quality of an utterance is its *addressiviness*: it is always directed at somebody. In the case of the medical certificates, not only is there the formal receiver of the document, but there are also *super-addressees* – potential readers who are not directly addressed but whom the writer nevertheless has in mind [55]. In excerpt (f), the writer seems to have the patient in mind as a super-addressee; he or she seems to question the patient's eligibility, but only indirectly, using free indirect style. Using free indirect style here has the double effect of seeming close to the patient while at the same time creating a professional distance [40]. Moreover, putting 'healthy' in quotation marks creates a latent irony that must be inferred by the reader, but which may weaken the claimant's case. Contrary to the narrator in excerpt (e), the narrator in excerpt (f) seems to have doubts about the patient's claims; none of the narrators, however, expresses their position directly.

Clarity and ambiguity

Clinical reports usually describe rather than explain. They address readers who have the same professional knowledge as the writer and who are able to infer connections, even in a brief and fragmentary text. In a medical certificate, however, explicit explanation is needed to make the relations between statements clear, as these relations may justify granting benefits. Connective words create meaningful relations between clauses: causal (because, so), adverse (but), temporal (then), or additive (and) words indicate that the text type is explicative, argumentative, narrative, or descriptive, respectively [54, 56]. A document may present with all text types depending on whether the writer's intention is to explain phenomena, describe facts, tell a story or evaluate/argue. A text may have formal markers showing connections between events, or it may have no markers and still clearly display such connections, as shown in the text below:

(g) **2.5. History of disease, symptoms, and treatment.** She was admitted to hospital. She had back pain, had several falls and paresis. CT showed spinal stenosis.

Even though this small text has no markers, we interpret it as recounting a series of events, a narrative. It is also implicitly *causative*: the patient was brought to hospital *because of* her symptoms which were *due to* spinal stenosis. What makes us see this text as coherent, and not as just disconnected clauses, is the co-occurrence of items (back pain – falls – paresis – spinal stenosis), which is a general tendency in texts, known as *collocation.* Accordingly, a competent lay reader will most probably grasp the causal meaning of this text even in the absence of causal conjunctions. In contrast, the additive text type in excerpt (h), below, is similar to that of (g), but unlike (g), (h) creates spurious connections of causality:

(h) **2.5. Illness story, symptoms, treatment.** Pain in the neck, numbness of hands, especially left arm and hand. MRI of the cervical spine shows a minor prolapse at the spinal level C3-C4. **2.6: Current clinical status (specify date). The results of relevant investigations:** The neck mobility is good; no objective, neurologic functional impairments of the arms and hands.

Contrary to excerpt (g), excerpt (h) uses association in a way that can be considered fraudulent. The immediate position of the sentences in relation to one another suggests that the numbness of the left hand is caused by the prolapse at the C3-C4 level of the neck as shown by an MRI. An authorised reader will know that a prolapse at the C3-C4 level of the cervical spine cannot cause general numbness of the hand and therefore will not be surprised that the personal examination of the patient is negative. However, the narrative technique used here, which draws on the reader's associative ability, is exposed: the text implicitly *suggests* connections that are faulty, even though they seem 'reasonable on the surface' [40]. The writer, however, can only be blamed for creating ambiguity, not for deliberately giving faulty information.

Assessing functionality and working capacity

A lack of information necessary to understand chains of reasoning may create the appearance of incoherence, or even of bias, for the reader. This can create problems in interpretation, especially when there is a request for causal relations between the elements. In excerpt (i), below, the writer neither describes their personal examination of the patient nor provides any other medical results of investigations:

(i) **Diagnosis:** Spondylolisthesis L4. GERD (gastro-oesophageal-reflux-syndrome) D84.

2.6 Current clinical status (specify date). The results of relevant investigations. Physical, medical problems causing pain. The patient cannot work. Working is out of the question for the patient. Permanent disease/syndrome with daily symptoms.

In this certificate, detailed medical descriptions explaining how or to what degree the spinal defect and reflux restrict the patient's bodily and practical daily functions, and how these conditions might explain his reduced working capacity, are replaced by generalisations. In some cases, as in (i), the disease-related diagnosis seems insufficient to explain a total and absolute loss of working ability and appears to serve instead as a Trojan horse of clinical 'dignity', or as a legitimate basis of disability benefits. GPs have reported having difficulty describing the impact of subjective health problems on functioning and work ability; they prefer selecting what is most concrete, organ-related, and objectively verifiable [28]. In (i), as in other certificates in our sample, there are various organ-related diagnoses, coded with 70–99 in the ICPC-2 system (International Classification of Primary Care, 2nd edition); however, none of them are accompanied by evaluations of patient functioning that might explain why the patient is unable to work. This might be because no matter the diagnosis, which itself has little to do with the patient's functional abilities, it is difficult for the doctor to assess the patient's functioning.

Breaking of the norm

The fact that 'disease' is a non-specific and relative concept, and that NAV might also consider illness as a legitimate basis for benefits – even in the absence of biomedical indicators – leaves a fair amount of room for negotiating eligibility for welfare benefits [4]. Moreover, NAV policy gives more weight to an individual's degree of impaired functioning than to the medical diagnosis itself [57]. Therefore, deliberately advocating disability pension without any indications of verified disease, illness, or reduced function threatens the narrator's reliability all the more. In excerpt (j), below, the writer explicitly disproves reduced functioning, yet still suggests that benefits should be considered:

(j) **Diagnosis:** Myalgia L18.

2.6. Current clinical status (specify date). The results of relevant investigations. One has, for more than ten years, not managed to get the patient back to work, and therefore, disability pension should be considered. **5.0 Describe how the functioning is generally reduced because of disease**. The patient claims to have myalgia, but there are no somatically reduced functional abilities.

Here, instead of providing the information requested in Section 2.6, the writer immediately introduces the realities of a failed rehabilitation. In Section 5.0, the writer denies that the patient's functioning is impaired at all. Proposing disability benefits for someone who is not really eligible puts the narrator in conflict with the basic norms of the text – and hence with the implied author (the GP), whose expert standard is expected to comply with the norms displayed in the form text. The writer's pragmatic suggestion may signify a professional resignation to a long process in which the medical problem is perhaps only of minor importance.

Discussion

In this paper, we have carried out a close, critical reading of a selection of medical certificates issued in Norway. Whereas other studies show that GPs experience certifying as challenging [8, 17], we have aimed at showing how GPs actually select and mediate information about their patients' health, functioning, and work capacity. Our text analysis indicates that GPs struggle to provide verifiable, factual information and consistent evaluations. This difficulty manifests in the texts as deficient or lacking information, incoherence (factual and evaluative), absence of professional evaluation, and ambiguity. The GPs' problems are particularly apparent in their assessments of patient functioning and working capacity regardless of diagnosis, being it subjective illness or 'organ-related' disease. The certificates display little insight into working life [8]; however, they rarely express professional uncertainty about patients' working capacity. Rather, they resort to making general statements and do not report thorough assessments of functioning. Some proved unable to structure and delimit the patient's illness story, missing the essential causes of the patient's inability to work. In most cases in our material, it was not clear to us how a particular illness had caused complete and general working disability.

Certifying GPs find the standard form problematic and partly unfit for describing the common sicknesses of our time [28, 58]. We suggest that the form is, to some extent, outdated in relation to the sicknesses and patient-oriented policy of our time and can thus be misleading as to what can in fact be verified by a physician as a cause of working disability. Certifiers seem to struggle to adapt to the form or, more precisely, to the form's implicit *assumptions* that any illness can be narrated chronologically and that 'treatment' is always needed to improve working ability. Subjective illness and chronic pain that cannot be explained by recognised biomedical criteria, and for which there is no effective treatment, create an extra burden for both the patient [51] and the treating GP acting as a certifier [28]. This sometimes results in what we have called the *doctor's chaos narrative*, reflecting the doctor's impotence when 'stuck' with the patient in a never-ending search for objective findings. In addition, our analysis identifies elements of textual 'chaos' throughout the sample texts: disconnected lists of symptoms, missing time aspects, ambiguities and conflation of voices indicating a lack of professional clarity.

The medical certificate is a particular genre of text, hovering on the border of law and medicine. Even though being a certifier engages the GP as part of 'an apparatus of social justice' [7], they show little consciousness of the ethics of the medical certificate as a juridical document. According to our analysis, GPs' 'strategic writing' [20] probably entails a variety of chosen linguistic techniques, some of which are subtle. GPs might use subtle writing in the interest of patient advocacy; however, they might also use it to express disagreement with their patients [12]. When it comes to avoiding vagueness and ambiguities, this is not merely a question of textual skills. Rather, we think that such textual failures mirror physicians' real problems with how to assess, verify and report patients' functioning and working ability. In addition, there are no specific criteria for assessing impaired functionality – guidelines are few and not mandatory and the medical information can be vague or deficient [59]. Finally, writing a deficient, inaccurate or biased certificate usually carries no negative consequences for the GP.

The mastery of textual skills in a professional genre is not self-evident and should be taught specifically. Physicians in Norway receive no systematic instruction in either medical school or subsequent training on how to produce high quality text in medical certificates. It is probable that medical certificates depend as much on the interest, writing skills, and capacity of the individual certifier as on his/her attitudes and personal values [23]. We suggest that learning in how to write medical certificates (and medical texts in general, which can all be used as juridical documentation) should be integrated as part of the professional curriculum taught in in medical schools. We assume that high quality medical certification strengthens legal protections for the claimant/the patient and reduces arbitrariness in the assessment of disability. Furthermore, we have reason to believe that providing medical certificates with sufficient and necessary information that are accurate, verifiable, and coherent is also economical. Such certificates may facilitate NAV's work with disability benefit applications, reduce the use of expensive, extra resources and shorten the processing time for disability benefits cases. In addition, the expert's impartiality and explicitness about his/her uncertainty and limited insight will probably reinforce the legitimacy and reliability of the document. Although a range of other measures is necessary to ensure that benefits are allocated fairly, we believe that GPs taking their role as certifying experts seriously according to the criteria mentioned here will contribute to a fairer evaluation of whether claimants are in fact eligible or not for disability benefits.

On the basis of our findings, it is reasonable to revise the role of GPs as certifiers of fitness for work in Norway. We suggest two possible measures: first, the GPs' role should be shared with other actors involved in evaluating patients' treatment and functioning, and the questions posed to the GPs from the NAV should be revised to fit better with the causes of reduced work ability. Second, physicians, medical students, and other health providers involved in certifying health problems should undergo specific instruction in how to write certificates, preferably taught by humanities professors. These measures may improve the quality of certifying documents, and thereby contribute to increasing efficiency and justice in the distribution of public goods.

Conclusions

Certifying GPs frequently failed to provide clear, sufficient and relevant factual information and coherent medical evaluations to justify the patient's claims of disability pension. The certificates may not function as reliable sources for making decisions regarding social benefits.

Whereas a deficient certificate has no negative consequences for the certifying GP, it may complicate NAV's treatment of the case, delay the decision and increase costs by the use of (usually unnecessary) specialists. In addition, insufficient, unclear and biased documentation may lead to wrong or unfair decisions.

Physicians in Norway receive no systematic training in professional writing. We believe that professional writing skills should be validated as an important part of medical practice and should be integrated in medical schools and in further education as a discipline in its own right, preferably involving humanities professors.

Remarks on method

Compared to our primary selection, we obtained consent to participate from more persons with musculoskeletal diagnosis and from fewer persons with psychiatric diagnosis. However, all main diagnostic categories are present in our material, and we do not think the imbalance in the diagnoses is of importance for the results.

Abbreviations

GP: General practitioner; NAV: Norwegian Administration of Labour and Welfare

Acknowledgements

The authors would like to thank statisticians in the Directorate of Labour and Welfare and the local offices of NAV that helped select and collect the medical certificates used in this study.

Funding

The study was funded by the Norwegian Research Fund for General Practice (AMFF). The funding body has not taken part in any stage of the study or in writing the manuscript.

Authors' contributions

All of the authors conceived of the study and participated in elaborating the consent letter, the study design, methods, and themes. GA carried out the data collection and the primary textual analysis and wrote the first draft. BN, AKL, EE and GA have participated in performing and refining the textual analysis and all authors have contributed to the revisions and approved the final version.

Competing interests

Second author Bård Natvig, professor of general practice, also has income as a part-time medical consultant in insurance medicine. The other authors do not report any conflicting interests.

Consent for publication

The authors made a *consent letter* which also provided information about our project and its implications to the participants. The consent letter was approved by the Norwegian Social Science Data Services (NSD)/Data Protection Official for Research (ref. 28836/ 3 /KS) and sent to all patients whom the medical certificates concerned. Only certificates of patients who, by signing and returning the consent letter had accepted participation (by permitting our access to their medical certificates) and publishing, were included.

Author details

[1]Department of General Practice, University of Oslo, Faculty of Medicine, Institute of Health and Society, Postboks 1130, Blindern 0318, OSLO, Norway. [2]Department of Health Science, University of Oslo, Faculty of Medicine, Institute of Health and Society, Postboks 1089, Blindern 0318, OSLO, Norway. [3]Departement of Community Medicine and Global Health, University of Oslo, Faculty of Medicine; Institute of Health and Society, Postboks 1130, Blindern 0318, OSLO, Norway.

References

1. Foucault M. The Birth of the Clinic. London and New York: Routledge; 1989.
2. Hurwitz B. Form and Representation in Clinical Case Reports. Lit Med. 2006; 25(2):216–40.
3. Sinsky C, Colligan L, Li L, Prgomet M, Reynolds S, Goeders L, et al. Allocation of Physician Time in Ambulatory Practice: A Time and Motion Study in 4 Specialties. Ann Intern Med. 2016. doi:10.7326/M16-0961.
4. Solli HM. Rettferdighet og objektivitet i trygdemedisinske uførhetsvurderinger. En etisk og vitenskapsfilosofisk analyse av tre uførhetsmodeller i et historisk perspektiv. Oslo: The Norwegian Medical Society. 2007.
5. Otway F. The Unreliable Narrator in Documentary. J Film Video. 2015;67(3):3–23.
6. Folketrygdloven. Rettskildene. Kapittel 12 - Uførepensjon [National Insurance Act - Disability pension]. 1997. https://www.nav.no/rettskildene/Forside/Folketrygdloven/kapittel-12-uf%C3%B8retrygd. Accessed 7 Apr 2017.
7. Dodier N. Expert medical decisions in occupational medicine: a sociological analysis of medical judgment. Sociol Health Illn. 1994;16(4):489–514.
8. Kiessling A, Arrelov B. Sickness certification as a complex professional and collaborative activity-a qualitative study. BMC Public Health. 2012. doi:10.1186/1471-2458-12-702.
9. Lofgren A, Hagberg J, Alexanderson K. What physicians want to learn about sickness certification: analyses of questionnaire data from 4019 physicians. BMC Public Health. 2010. doi:10.1186/1471-2458-10-61.
10. Shiels C, Gabbay MB. Patient, clinician, and general practice factors in long-term certified sickness. Scand J of Pub Health. 2007;35(3):250–6.
11. Swartling MS, Alexanderson KA, Wahlstrom RA. Barriers to good sickness certification – an interview study with Swedish general practitioners. Scand J of Pub Health. 2008;36(4):408–14.
12. Wynne-Jones G, Mallen CD, Main CJ, Dunn KM. What do GPs feel about sickness certification? A systematic search and narrative review. Scand J Prim Health Care. 2010;28(2):67–75.
13. Kleinman A. The Illness Narratives. Suffering, Healing & the Human Condition. United States of America: Basic Books; 1988.
14. Folketrygdloven. Folketrygdloven, Rettskildene. §8-4, første ledd - Lovens krav om arbeidsuførhet [National Insurance Act - Legal requirements of working disability]. 1993.https://www.nav.no/rettskildene/Rundskriv/8-4-arbeidsuf%C3%B8rhet. Accessed 7 Apr 2017.
15. Mæland G. Veileder i trygdemedisin. 6th ed. Oslo: Gyldendal Akademisk; 2013.
16. Engblom M, Nilsson G, Arrelöv B, Löfgren A, Skånér Y, Lindholm C, et al. Frequency and severity of problems that general practitioners experience regarding sickness certification. Scand J Prim Health Care. 2011;29(4):227–33.
17. Money A, Hussey L, Thorley K, Turner S, Agius R. Work-related sickness absence negotiations: GPs' qualitative perspectives. Br J Gen Pract. 2010. doi:10.3399/bjgp10X532350.
18. Nilsen S, Malterud K, Werner EL, Maeland S, Magnussen LH. GPs' negotiation strategies regarding sick leave for subjective health complaints. Scand J Prim Health Care. 2015. doi:10.3109/02813432.2015.1001943.
19. Winde LD, Alexanderson K, Carlsen B, Kjeldgard L, Wilteus AL, Gjesdal S. General practitioners' experiences with sickness certification: a comparison of survey data from Sweden and Norway. BMC Fam Pract. 2012. doi:10.1186/1471-2296-13-10.

20. Gulbrandsen P, Aasland OG, Førde R. Medical certificates issued to help the patient. Tidsskr for den Nor Lægefor. 2004, 124:192-4.
21. Higgins A, Porter S, O'Halloran P. General practitioners' management of the long-term sick role. Soc Sci Med. 2014. doi:10.1016/j.socscimed.2014.01.044.
22. Macdonald S, Maxwell M, Wilson P, Smith M, Whittaker W, Sutton M, et al. A powerful intervention: general practitioners'; use of sickness certification in depression. BMC Fam Pract. 2012; doi: 10.1186/1471-2296-13-82.
23. Terum LI, Nergård TB. Medisinsk skjønn og rettstryggleik. Legar som portvakter i fordelinga av offentlege goder [Medical judgement and legal security. Doctors as gatekeepers in the distrubution of public goods]. Tidsskr Nor Legefor. 1999;119(15):2192–6.
24. Nilsen S, Werner EL, Maeland S, Eriksen HR, Magnussen LH. Considerations made by the general practitioner when dealing with sick-listing of patients suffering from subjective and composite health complaints. Scand J Prim Health Care. 2011. doi:10.3109/02813432.2010.514191.
25. Kiessling A, Arrelov B, Larsson A, Henriksson P. Quality of medical certificates issued in long-term sick leave or disability in relation to patient characteristics and delivery of health care. Scand J Public Health. 2013. doi: 10.1177/1403494813477928.
26. Soderberg E, Alexanderson K. Sickness certificates as a basis for decisions regarding entitlement to sickness insurance benefits. Scand J Public Health. 2005;33(4):314–20.
27. Aarseth G, Natvig B, Engebretsen E, Maagero E, Lie AH. Writing the patient down and out: the construal of the patient in medical certificates of disability. Sociol Health Illn. 2016. doi:10.1111/1467-9566.12481.
28. Lima IAÅ, Nicolaisen H. Helse og legeerklæring i arbeidsevnevurderingen. Arbeid og velferd. 2016; 1:105-20. https://www.nav.no/no/NAV+og+samfunn/Kunnskap/Analyser+fra+NAV/Arbeid+og+velferd/Arbeid+og+velferd/arbeid-og-velferd-nr.1-2016. Accessed 7 Apr 2017.
29. OECD Library. Sickness, Disability and Work. Breaking the Barriers. A Synthesis of Findings Across OECD Countries. 2010; doi: 10.1787/9789264088856-en.
30. NAV. Utviklingen i uføretrygd per 30. juni 2016 [Development in disability benefit per June30.2016]. 2016. https://www.nav.no/no/NAV+og+samfunn/Statistikk/AAP+nedsatt+arbeidsevne+og+uforetrygd+-+statistikk/Uforetrygd/Uforetrygd+-+Statistikknotater. Accessed 7 Apr 2017.
31. NAV. Uførhetsdiagnoser statistikk [Statistics of diagnosis of disability benefit]. 2015. https://www.nav.no/no/NAV+og+samfunn/Statistikk/AAP+nedsatt+arbeidsevne+og+uforetrygd+-+statistikk/Uforetrygd/Uforetrygd+-+Statistikknotater. Accessed 7 Apr 2017.
32. Folkehelseinstituttet. Sykdomsbyrde i den norske befolkningen 1990-2013, [Disease Burden in Norway - Public Health Report 1990-2013]. 2016. https://www.fhi.no. Accessed 7 Apr 2017.
33. Arbeids- og Sosialdepartementet. Folketrygdens utgifter.Pressemelding Nr 27 [Cost development in National Insurance. Press release No 27]. 2014. https://www.regjeringen.no. Accessed 15 Jun 2016.
34. NAV. Legeerklæring ved arbeidsuførhet (form) [Medical certificate of disability] NAV 08-07.08 . Endret 03.2010. 1999.
35. NSD Data Protection Official for Research. https://www.datatilsynet.no. Accessed 18 Feb 2017.
36. Silverman D. Interpreting qualitative data. 5th ed. Los Angeles and London: Sage; 2014.
37. Smith B. Narrative Versions, Narrative Theories. Crit Inq. 1980;7(01):213–36.
38. Labov W, Waletzky J. Narrative analysis: Oral Versions of Personal Experience. In: Essays on the Verbal and Visual Arts. Edited by Helm J. Seattle: University of Washington Press; 1967: 12-44.
39. van Dijk TA. Macrostructures. New Jersey: Lawrence Earlbaum Associates; 1980.
40. Aaslestad P. The Patient as Text. The Role of the Narrator in Psychiatric Notes 1890-1990. Oxon, UK: Radcliff Publishing Ltd.; 2009.
41. Booth W. The Rhetoric of Fiction. 2.ed. Chicago and London: University of Chicago Press; 1983.
42. Genette G. Narrative discourse revisited. Ithaca, N.Y.: Cornell University Press; 1988.
43. Engebretsen E. Hva sa klienten? Oslo: J.W. Cappelens forlag AS; 2007.
44. Helse/Omsorgsdepartementet. Forskrift om krav til helsepersonells attester, erklæringer og liknende. 2008. https://lovdata.no/dokument/SF/forskrift/2008-12-18-1486. Accessed 20 Feb 2017.
45. Iser W. The Act of Reading: A Theory of Aesthetic Response. Baltimore: Johns Hopkins University Press; 1978.
46. van Dijk TA. Discourse and Context. Cambridge, UK: Cambridge University Press; 2008.
47. Thompson G. Introducing Functional Grammar. 3rd ed. Abingdon, Oxon: Routledge; 2014.
48. Fairclough N. Language and Power. 2nd ed. Pearson Education Limited: Essex, England; 2001.
49. Hunter KM. Doctors' Stories. The Narrative Structure of Medical Knowledge. New Jersey: Princeton University Press; 1991.
50. Frank A. The Wounded Storyteller. Body, Illness and Ethics. Chicago and London: The University of Chicago Press; 1995.
51. Nettleton S. 'I just want permission to be ill': Towards a sociology of medically unexplained symptoms. Soc Sci & Med. 2006;62(5):1167–78.
52. Bakhtin M. Du discourse romanesque. In: Esthétique et théorie du roman. Paris: Gallimard; 1978.
53. Foley M, Thorley K, and Denny M. 'The sick note': a qualitative study of sickness certification in general practice in Ireland. Eur J Gen Pract. 2012; doi: 10.3109/13814788.2012.672967.
54. Halliday MAK, Hasan R. Cohesion in English. London and New York: Longman; 1976.
55. Bakhtin MM. Spørsmålet om talegenrane [Speech genres and other late essays]. Oslo: Pensumtjeneste AS; 2005.
56. Hellspong L, Ledin P. Vägar genom texten. Handbok i brukstextanalys. Lund: Studentlitteratur; 1997.
57. Norges offentlige utredninger (NOU). Ny uførestønad og ny alderspensjon til uføre [A new disability benefit and a new retirement pension for receivers of disability benefit]. 2007. https://www.regjeringen.no/no/dokumenter/horing-nou-20074-ny-uforestonad-og-ny-al/id472162/. Accessed 7 April 2017.
58. Aarseth G, Natvig B, Engebretsen E, Lie AHK. Legeerklæring ved arbeidsuførhet, skjema til besvær [Medical certificates of disability, a form causing inconvenience]. Tidsskr Nor Legefor. 2014;134(1):56–61.
59. Gjersøe HM. Regulating Inflow or Outflow. A Comparison of the Work Capability Assessments in the UK and Norway. J Soc Policy. 2016;45(01):141–58.

2

Are low and high utilization related to the way GPs manage their practices?

W. A. de Graaf-Ruizendaal[1*], L. van der Hoek[1] and D. H. de Bakker[1,2^]

Abstract

Background: General practice care plays a key role in keeping healthcare effective and cost-efficient. However, variation in the utilization rates of practices may reveal variation in practice performance. Our research goal is to investigate whether the socio-demographic profile of the patients' area of residence and practice organization characteristics influence the low or high utilization of general practice care.

Methods: Data on the utilization of general practice care were derived from the electronic health records of 232 general practices participating in the NIVEL Primary Care Database for the year 2013. Census data for the year 2013 were matched with the postal code of the patients. A small area estimation (SAE) technique was used to calculate the estimated utilization rate for general practice care per practice based on the socio-demographic profile of the patients' area of residence. Subsequently, the actual utilization rates were compared to the estimated rates per practice. Linear regression analysis was used to link the differences between the actual and estimated utilization rates to practice organization characteristics.

Results: The socio-demographic profile of the patients' area of residence accounted for 25.7% of the estimated utilization rates per practice. Practice organization characteristics accounted for 19.3% of the difference between the actual utilization rates and the estimated rates. Practices had higher utilization rates than estimated when a practice was a dual practice, when it employed female GPs, when it employed other healthcare providers and/or when it offered more services related to a disease management programme.

Conclusion: We found that utilization rates of general practice care can be partially explained by the socio-demographic profile of the patients' area of residence, but also by practice organization characteristics. Insight into these factors provides both GPs and the other stakeholders involved in the organization of general practice care with information to help reflect on the utilization of care.

Keywords: Delivery of health care, Needs assessment, Regional health planning, General practice care , Utilization, SAE method

Background

General practice care plays a central role in healthcare. In the Netherlands, the general practitioner (GP) has a strong position: every resident is listed with a GP, and the GP deals with most of the health problems and coordinates the referral to specialized care [1]. Moreover, general practice care is covered by compulsory insurance and is the only health service exempt from cost sharing, which makes it accessible to everyone [2]. Many European countries regard strengthening the role of primary care, particularly general practice care, as a way to combat high healthcare costs and to meet the complex healthcare needs of the population [3–6].

Given the vital position of general practice care, it is important to study variation in utilization rates among general practices and especially the contributors to low and high utilization. Low utilization may not only indicate poor access and thus poor performance, but it could

* Correspondence: w.ruizendaal@nivel.nl
^Deceased
[1]NIVEL: Netherlands Institute for Health Service Research, PO Box 1568, 3500, BN, Utrecht, The Netherlands

also indicate efficient use of healthcare services [7]. High utilization rates may indicate both good access and good performance, as a larger part of care is handled by the GP and less is referred to other healthcare providers. However, high utilization rates may also indicate inefficient use of healthcare services.

In the literature, the concepts underuse and overuse of healthcare services are often studied [8–11]. Underuse is 'the lack of provision of necessary care' and overuse is 'the provision of care for which harms outweigh the benefits' [9, 11]. To assess underuse and overuse, it needs to be determined whether the use of care was appropriate, i.e. whether the provision of medical services was beneficial or whether it had no or little benefit [11]. However, such methods are both time-consuming and expensive [10].

In the present study, we do not focus on the appropriateness of general practice care, but rather on high or low utilization rates at general practice level. High or low utilization rates at practice level were determined by the comparison of the actual utilization rates with the estimated rates based on the socio-demographic profile of the patients' area of residence. From the literature, it is known that the socio-demographic characteristics of an area influence the use of general practice care [12]. For instance, areas with a high underprivileged index: a high percentage of the elderly living alone, children under 5 years, in single parent families, unskilled workers and unemployed adults were more likely to report a GP consultation [13].

However, differences are to be expected between the actual utilization rates of general practice care and the estimated rates based on a limited set of socio-demographic variables, because many more factors do influence healthcare utilization. We want to explore to what extent differences between the actual utilization rate and the estimated rate based on a limited set of socio-demographic variables can be related to practice organization characteristics. From the literature, it is know that service provision or general practice characteristics influence consultation rates [12]. For example, variation in frequent attendance in general practice care could for 3% be attributed to the age of the GP and the use of an appointment system [14]. Cervical smear uptake rates were substantially higher in practices with a female partner [15], and the number of partners in a practice positively influenced breast cancer screening rates [16]. Practice organization characteristics include the human resources available, specific services offered (e.g. diagnostic equipment), organization of consultation hours, participation in disease management programmes, physical accessibility of the practice and information dissemination.

In the present study, we investigated to what extent practice organization characteristics, next to socio-demographic characteristics at the four-digit postcode level, influence the utilization of general practice care. Our goal is to provide stakeholders who are involved with the organization of general practice care with useful insight into the practice organization characteristics that influence high or low utilization, to help them reflect on the organization and the utilization of general practice care.

Methods

Study design

An observational study was conducted in which for each practice the actual utilization rates of general practice care, based on medical record data, were compared with an estimated utilization rate for this practice, based on the socio-demographic profile of the patients' area of residence. Using an SAE technique, estimates were made for every four-digit postcode area in the dataset, and based on these estimates, practice estimates were calculated as a weighted average of patients' postcodes. The difference between the actual utilization rates and the estimated rates based on the socio-demographic profile of the patients' area of residence were linked to practice organization characteristics using linear regression analysis. Furthermore, practices with the largest positive difference were compared with the largest negative difference using t-tests and proportion tests.

Data

Utilization rates

Utilization rates of general practice care were derived from medical record data obtained from routine electronic health records from 240 general practices in the Netherlands participating in the NIVEL Primary Care Database for the year 2013 [17]. The database contains the utilization records, gender, age and four-digit postcodes of approximately 1 million listed patients who are representative of the Dutch population regarding gender and age. We selected general practices which had registered for a complete year and selected patients who had been registered at the same general practice for a complete year. This resulted in a dataset of 851,891 patients and 232 general practices, because 8 practices were excluded.

Practice organization characteristics

Practice characteristics were derived from the NIVEL database of health professionals (2013), which contains the characteristics of every general practice in the Netherlands ($n = 5008$) and which annually collects its data by means of surveys. Per practice, items were selected related to practice organization, such as type of practice (solo, dual, or group practice), human resources in practice (regarding GPs: number, FTE GP, age, gender, number of self-employed GPs, employed by another GP and locums, and the availability of different care providers in practice), list size (number of patients in practice) and number of patients in practice per FTE GP. Urbanization level of the practice was determined and divided into five categories from rural (less than < 500 addresses per km^2) to very strongly urbanized (more than > 2500 addresses per km^2). Subsequently, items were selected from the survey and categorized into five practice organization measures, regarding the number of medical services offered, consultation profile of the practice, physical accessibility of the practice, participation in disease management programmes, and the availability of patient information material. A higher score for a category refers to a higher occurrence of the category. The description of the measures and the items are presented in Table 1.

Socio-demographic profile of the patients' area of residence

Statistics Netherlands provided national census data at the four-digit postcode level from the year 2013 [18]. The data collected included the total population, the number of males and females in different age categories, one-person households, non-Western immigrants (at least one parent born in Africa, Latin America and/or Asia), low-income households (households with a purchasing power of less than <€9250 a year) and urbanization level of patients' area, divided into five categories. Additionally, status score was obtained from the Netherlands Institute for Social Research. Status score is an indicator of the socioeconomic status of an area [19]. The area characteristics were selected as explanatory variables of the utilization of general practice care, because they are available at the four-digit postcode level and are important determinants of healthcare use [20].

Outcome measures

The first outcome variable was the actual GP utilization rate per listed patient per practice, which was the sum of all declared consultations, such as consultations (including by email), telephone consultations, home visits and consultations involving minor surgery. The second outcome variable was the estimated GP utilization rate per listed patient per practice based on the socio-demographic profile of patients' area. The third outcome variable was the difference between the actual GP utilization rate and the estimated rate per listed patient per practice. This continuous variable was analysed as such and also defined into categories by ranking. The first 40 scores made up the category 'low utilization', in which the actual utilization rate was lower than the estimated rate. The final 40 scores made up the category 'high utilization', in which the actual utilization rate was higher than the estimated rate.

Data analyses

First, descriptive analyses were calculated to describe the sample and the explanatory variables at practice level.

Second, linear regression was used to analyse whether practice organization characteristics could explain the actual utilization rate aggregated at practice level.

Third, on the same data but now aggregated at the four-digit postcode level a linear regression model was estimated for utilization on socio-demographic characteristics of patients' area of residence. Only four-digit postcode areas with at least 100 listed patients contributed to the model. Predictions were made for all four-digit postcodes in the dataset. Subsequently, a utilization rate was calculated for each general practice as a weighted mean of the predictions of the patients' postcodes. In the model the next socio-demographic predictors were used: the percentages of male and female in seven different age categories (0–4, 5–14, 15–24, 25–39, 40–64, 65–74, 75 and older), the percentages of one-person households, non-Western immigrants, low-income households, urbanization level (which was dummy-coded) and status score.

Fourth, this estimated utilization rate per practice was compared with the actual utilization rate. Linear regression was used to analyse whether the difference could be explained by practice organization characteristics, on aggregated data at practice level. The explained variance of the linear regression models was given by R-squared.

In addition, t-tests and proportion-tests were conducted to contrast practices with the highests positive difference with those with the highest negative difference on practice characteristics.

Analyses were conducted using Stata version 14.1.

Results

Sample characteristics and practice organization measures

Table 1 presents the mean of the five practice organization measures and the percentages of the underlying items. Scheduled consultation hours, minor surgery and an emergency line are the three most frequent practice organization characteristics in general practice. Table 2 shows the distribution of the practice organization characteristics of the general practices in the sample ($n = 232$). The mean number of GPs per practice is 2.32.

Mean actual utilization rate per practice

The regression coefficients for the different practice organization characteristics on the mean actual utilization rate per practice are depicted in Table 3, F (17, 206) = 3.12; $p = 0.0001$). The results show that three practice characteristics are statistical significant positive predictors of the mean actual utilization rate, namely 'disease management programme', 'the presence of other medical providers in practice' and

Table 1 Presence of the practice organization measures and underlying items for the sample of general practices ($n = 232$)

Measures	Items	%	Mean	SD
Medical service profile	Sum score of the 9 underlying items		2.99	1.50
The practice offers the following medical services:	Deliveries	1.3		
	Pharmacy	3.9		
	Minor surgery	89.7		
	ECG equipment	50.4		
	Spirometry	81.5		
	Audiometry	44.4		
	Teleconsultation	22.4		
	Medical equipment	0.9		
	Other medical services	4.3		
Consultation profile	Sum score of the 7 underlying items		4.11	1.54
The practice offers the following consultation types:	Scheduled consultations	91.8		
	Walk–in hours	13.8		
	Call back consultations	76.7		
	Evening consultations	15.1		
	Email consultations	47.4		
	Emergency line	89.2		
	Prescription line	77.2		
Accessibility	Sum score of the 3 underlying items		1.44	0.75
The practice offers the following:	Parking for disabled people within 100 m	64.7		
	Bus stop within 300 m	78.5		
	Other accessibility services	0.4		
Disease management	Sum score of the 14 underlying items		4.18	3.25
The practice offers special consultation hours for the following diseases/categories:	Diabetes	79.3		
	Asthma	23.7		
	COPD	34.1		
	Cardiovascular diseases	62.1		
	Minor surgery	45.7		
	Pre- and post-natal care	2.2		
	Pap-smear	52.2		
	Mental healthcare	35.8		
	Geriatric care	30.2		
	Allergy/Dermatology	6.9		
	Osteoporosis	10.8		
	Immigrants	1.7		
	Travellers	25.9		
	Other special consultation hours	7.3		
Patient information material	Sum score of the 6 underlying items		3.32	1.27
The practice has the following communication channels/materials:	Leaflets	85.8		
	Leaflets in different languages	3.0		
	Website	76.7		
	Patient letters	86.6		
	Leaflet on complaint procedure	79.3		
	Other patient informational material	0.4		

Table 2 Distribution of the selected practice characteristics for the total sample of general practices ($n = 232$)

Practice characteristics	N	%
Solo practices	88	37.9
Dual practices	91	39.2
Group practices	53	22.8
Practices in rural areas	37	16.0
Practices in low urbanized areas	42	18.1
Practices in moderately urbanized areas	47	20.3
Practice in highly urbanized areas	45	19.4
Practices in very highly urbanized areas	61	26.3
Support staff per practice	N	%
Doctor's assistant	213	91.8
Practice nurse somatic disorders	85	36.6
Practice nurse mental disorders	146	62.9
Pharmacist	9	3.9
Other medical providers	25	10.8
Other non-medical providers	54	23.2
GP characteristics per practice	M	SD
GPs	2.32	1.49
FTE GP	1.62	1.12
Female GP	1.09	1.05
GPs younger than 40 years old	0.47	0.73
GPs 40–55 years old	1.18	1.10
GPs 56–65 years old	0.63	0.83
GPs 65 years or older	0.05	0.22
Self-employed GPs	1.84	1.29
GPs employed by GP	0.26	0.50
Locums	0.17	0.43

'dual practices'. The model explains 20.5% of the variation in the dependent variable.

Mean estimated utilization rate per postcode

The mean estimated utilization rate was calculated at the four-digit postcode level using linear regression analysis. The results of the linear regression analysis are given in Table 4, with the mean utilization rate as dependent variable and the socio-demographic characteristics of patients' area as independent variables, $F(21, 871) = 14.33$, $p < 0.0001$. The model explains 25.7% of the variation in the dependent variable. Seven predictors are statistical significant. The predictors 'females of 75 years and older', 'persons in a low-income household', 'low urbanized areas', 'moderately urbanized areas', 'strongly urbanized areas' and 'very strongly urbanized areas' have a positive association. The predictor 'one-person households' has a negative association with the dependent variable.

Difference between actual and postcode-based estimated utilization rate

The results of the linear regression analysis are shown in Table 5, with the difference between the actual and the estimated utilization rate as dependent variable and practice organization characteristics as independent variables, $F(17, 206) = 2.89$, $p = 0.0002$. The results show four practice characteristics with a statistical significant positive influence on the difference between the mean actual utilization rate and the mean estimated utilization rate, namely 'percentage of female GPs', 'disease management programme', 'the presence of other medical providers in practice' and 'dual practices'. The model explains 19.3% of the variation in the dependent variable.

In addition to the analysis of practice organization characteristics on the difference between the actual utilization rate and the postcode-based estimated utilization rate, we also analysed 'the postcode-based estimated utilization rate' as a predictor for the mean utilization rate per practice. The results show that on its own, the 'postcode-based estimated utilization rate' ($B = 0.93$) accounts for 9.2% of the variation in the mean utilization rate per practice.

T-tests and proportion tests on low versus high utilization practices

Table 6 illustrates the distribution of practice characteristics for the total sample of general practices and for the general practices divided into two categories: low utilization and high utilization. Table 6 also shows the results of the t-tests and the proportion-tests between the practices with the 40 highest positive and the 40 highest negative differences. Compared to practices with high utilization, practices with low utilization are significantly more often solo practices, less often dual practices, have lower numbers of GPs, female GPs, as well as GPs younger than 40 years old. They also score significantly lower on the practice organization measure 'consultation profile'.

Discussion

The present study, is a first exploration on the extent to which differences between the actual utilization rate and the estimated rate based on a limited set of socio-demographic variables can be related to practice organization characteristics. The socio-demographic profile of the patients' area of residence accounted for approximately 26% of the actual GP utilization rate at the four-digit postcode level. The investigated practice organization characteristics accounted for approximately 20% of the actual GP utilization rates. Three practice organization characteristics were statistically significant. The mean actual utilization rate per patient increased by

Table 3 Model estimates for the regression of mean actual utilization rate on practice characteristics. (Data aggregated on practice level, $n = 224$)

	B	P-value	Lower bound 95% CI	Upper bound 95% CI
Practice organization measures				
Medical service profile	0.048	0.33	−0.049	0.145
Consultation profile	0.070	0.22	−0.041	0.182
Accessibility	0.156	0.05	−0.001	0.312
Disease management	0.048[a]	0.04	0.001	0.094
Patient information material	−0.074	0.23	−0.196	0.048
Human resources in practice				
Doctor's assistant	−0.456	0.18	−1.125	0.212
Practice nurse somatic disorders	−0.265	0.07	−0.553	0.024
Practice nurse mental disorders	0.047	0.70	−0.188	0.281
Pharmacist	0.145	0.60	−0.403	0.694
Other medical providers	0.618[a]	0.00	0.298	0.938
Other non-medical providers	−0.141	0.24	−0.375	0.094
Type of practice; reference is solo practice				
Dual practices	0.283[a]	0.02	0.040	0.525
Group practices	0.141	0.32	−0.136	0.419
GP characteristics per practice				
Percentage of female GPs	0.003	0.10	−0.001	0.006
Percentage of GPs younger than 40 years	0.002	0.28	−0.002	0.006
Percentage of self-employed GPs	−0.001	0.66	−0.005	0.003
Number of patients per FTE GP	0.000	0.82	−0.000	0.000

[a]$p < 0.05$. *CI* Confidence interval, $R^2 = 20.5\%$; Adjusted $R^2 = 13.9\%$

0.6 contacts when a 'other medical provider' was present in the general practice, increased by 0.3 when the practice was a dual practice instead of a solo practice, and increased by 0.05 with every added disease management programme.

Practice organization characteristics accounted for 19% of the difference between the actual. GP utilization rates and the estimated rates based on the socio-demographic predictors. The practice characteristics mentioned above were also statistical significant here: 'the presence of other medical providers', 'dual practice' and 'the availability of a disease management programme'. Additionally, the employment of female GPs significantly increased GP utilization rates. Every extra percentage of female GPs added 0.003 to the utilization rate per patients. Together with the results of the t-tests and proportion-tests, these results indicate lower utilization rates than estimated for solo practices, with fewer GPs, female GPs, GPs younger than 40 years, and for practices which offer fewer consultation types. The actual utilization rates of these practices are lower than expected based on the socio-demographic profile of the practice population.

The present study, cannot comment on the quality of general practice care for high or low utilization practices. Huygen et al. (1992) found that patients from a doctor with an integrated practice style, which is regarded as good quality of care, have a better health and visited their doctor less frequently. Moreover, those doctors kept the referrals to a specialist to a minimum [7]. So, low utilization practices can provide good quality of care. Low utilization practices may also keep the quality of care high by the employment of more experienced GPs who need fewer follow-up consultations. The age of the GP may be seen as an indicator for experience. We found a significant lower percentage of GPs younger than 40 years in practices with low utilization. However, Kersnik found that frequent attenders were more likely to visit an experienced GP and found no differences in the age of the GP between frequent attenders and infrequent attenders. In further research, the relationship between quality of care, the experience of GPs and high or low utilization should be investigated.

Provider characteristics interact with patient characteristics to influence utilization of care [21]. One important result of our study is that a higher utilization rate is found more often in practices with a higher number of female GPs. In a Dutch study, Bensing found gender differences in practice style: female GPs spend more time

Table 4 Model estimates for the regression of mean utilization rate on sociodemographic characteristics of four-digit postcode areas (data aggregated on four-digit postcode area, $n = 893$)

	B	P-value	Lower bound 95% CI	Upper bound 95% CI
Percentage gender age categories; reference category is proportion of males 25–39 years old				
Males 0–4 years old	– 0.085	0.23	−0.225	0.055
Females 0–4 years old	0.028	0.68	−0.106	0.162
Males 5–14 years old	−0.014	0.74	−0.099	0.070
Females 5–14 years old	−0.069	0.14	−0.161	0.023
Males 15–24 years old	– 0.042	0.38	−0.135	0.052
Females 15–24 years old	−0.028	0.38	−0.092	0.035
Females 25–39 years old	0.035	0.53	−0.074	0.145
Males 40–64 years old	−0.024	0.55	−0.102	0.054
Females 40–64 years old	0.044	0.14	−0.014	0.103
Males 65–74 years old	0.053	0.35	−0.058	0.163
Females 65–74 years old	−0.064	0.24	−0.171	0.043
Males 75 years or older	0.096	0.10	−0.019	0.212
Females 75 years or older	0.080[a]	0.04	0.005	0.156
Percentage of one-person households	−0.012[a]	0.03	−0.023	– 0.001
Percentage of non-Western immigrants	0.005	0.12	−0.001	0.012
Percentage of people in low-income households	0.030[a]	0.00	0.012	0.047
Status score	0.045	0.34	−0.048	0.139
Degree of urbanization; reference category is rural				
Low urbanisation	0.387[a]	0.00	0.191	0.583
Moderately urbanised	0.302[a]	0.00	0.099	0.505
Strongly urbanised	0.381[a]	0.00	0.161	0.600
Very strongly urbanised	0.345[a]	0.02	0.059	0.631

[a]$p < 0.05$. CI=Confidence interval, $R^2 = 25.7\%$, Adjusted $R^2 = 23.9\%$

with their patients, female patients tend to choose female GPs and female GPs see more gynecologic problems and consults for family planning [22]. Also, Majeed et al. (1994) found higher cervical smear uptake rates in practices with a female partner and in larger practices. Thus, hiring female GPs will probably attract more female patients, who are more frequent attenders in general practice care for female related health problems which result in higher practice consultation rates. However, in a study of Kernsik, it was found that frequent attenders were more likely to visit a male GP. So, in future research the relationship between the use of GP care and the gender of the GP has to be further investigated.

High or low utilization of general practice care can be seen as an indicator for the accessibility of general practice care, because utilization of care is influenced by the availability and accessibility of health care services, next to health status and health related behaviour [23]. Accessibility of health care is a multidimensional concept. Elements such as geographical accessibility, availability, affordability, acceptability and accommodation can be distinguished [24–26]. A Danish study by Heje on the accessibility of general practice care found that patients experienced better accessibility in solo practices, with a short patient list and with a few employees [27]. We found that low utilization practices are more often solo practices with less FTE GP. In the study by Heje, patients may have reported better accessibility of care in these smaller solo practices because they experienced more continuous care in the doctor-patient relationship [28]. Moreover, a better perceived accessibility of care may not always lead to high utilization rates. However, we found no influence of our accessibility measure. Our accessibility measure only existed of three accessibility issues and was not based on a theoretical framework. Thus, the relationship between the accessibility measure and utilization rates should be interpreted with caution. In further research, the accessibility of low and high utilization practices should be further investigated.

To the best of our knowledge, our study is one of the first to assess low utilization or high utilization of general practice care using an SAE method, which is a relatively easy, robust and inexpensive method. Our findings indicate that high utilization was found more often in

Table 5 Model estimates for the regression of difference between the actual and estimated utilization rate on practice characteristics (data aggregated on practice level, $n = 224$)

	B	P-value	Lower bound 95% CI	Upper bound 95% CI
Practice organization measures				
Medical service profile	0.055	0.24	−0.038	0.148
Consultation profile	0.081	0.14	−0.026	0.188
Accessibility	0.107	0.16	−0.043	0.257
Disease management	0.051[a]	0.03	0.007	0.095
Patient information material	−0.052	0.38	−0.170	0.065
Human resources in practice				
Doctor's assistant	−0.500	0.13	−1.142	0.141
Practice nurse somatic disorders	−0.269	0.06	−0.546	0.008
Practice nurse mental disorders	0.000	1.00	−0.225	0.225
Pharmacist	0.183	0.49	−0.343	0.710
Other medical providers	0.463[a]	0.00	0.156	0.770
Other non-medical providers	−0.139	0.23	−0.364	0.087
Type of practice; reference is solo practice				
Dual practices	0.253[a]	0.03	0.021	0.486
Group practices	0.138	0.31	−0.129	0.404
GP characteristics per practice				
Percentage of female GPs	0.003[a]	0.04	0.0001	0.007
Percentage of GPs younger than 40 years	0.002	0.27	−0.002	0.006
Percentage of self-employed GPs	0.000	0.89	−0.004	0.004
Number of patients per FTE GP	0.000	0.42	0.000	0.000

[a]$p < 0.05$. CI=Confidence interval, $R^2 = 19.3\%$; Adjusted $R^2 = 12.6\%$

general practices that employ other medical providers and that offer a disease management programme. Our assumption is, that larger practices have more human resources and are technically better equipped to provide consultations for minor surgery or for specific diseases, resulting in higher utilization rates than solo practices. GPs in practices with high utilization rates and probably a high workload may keep their practices accessible by task shifting, task delegation, work efficiency and shorter patient time, as was concluded by Van den Berg for practices with a higher workload in the Netherlands [29, 30]. However, our study is a first exploration and future research is needed to investigate the exact influence of practice organization characteristics and their interactions.

Strengths and limitations

We would have preferred to use a crossed-effects multilevel model with practices as one source of level two variation and four-digit postcodes as the other. However, this was not feasible due to the long estimation time, because of the high number of level 2 units: 232 general practices and 893 four-digit postcode areas.

Our results are based on three large datasets of routinely registered data. One contains data on the characteristics of all the practices and GPs in the Netherlands, the other contains health record data of approximately 1 million patients who are representative of the Dutch population regarding age and gender, and the last dataset contains census data which are routinely updated by Statistics Netherlands. However, these datasets entails also limitations. GP record data may be registered with some errors. The practice characteristics are expected to be updated by the GPs yearly, however it is not known for sure whether a change in the practice organization is also being registered. Our 232 general practices are not a random sample, but comes from a historical grown register for which practices were selected. Thus, the representativity of our findings is unclear.

A strength of our study was the large number of practice characteristics, including the five practice organization measures, that we have investigated as potential factors of low or high utilization. Third, we used a powerful alternative to costly designs, i.e. the small area estimation method [31, 32]. This method has been applied in several policy areas around the

Table 6 Differences on practice organization characteristics between the 40 lowest and 40 highest scoring practices on the difference between mean actual utilization rate and the postcode-based estimate

	Total GP practices in sample ($N = 232$)		Practices with utilization lower than predicted $N = 40$		Practices with utilization higher than predicted $N = 40$		Results t-tests/pr-tests between low and high utilization practices
	Mean	*SD*	Mean	*SD*	Mean	*SD*	*P-value*
GP characteristics per practice							
GPs per practice	2.32	*1.50*	**1.73**	*0. 88*	**2.40**	*1.60*	*0.02[a]*
Female GPs per practice	1.09	*1.05*	**0.60**	*0.60*	**1.28**	*1.13*	*0.00***
GPs younger than 40 years	0.47	*0.73*	**0.20**	*0.41*	**0.53**	*0.72*	*0.02[a]*
GPs 40–55 years	1.17	*1.10*	0.98	*1.00*	1.13	*0.94*	*0.49*
GPs 56–65 years	0.63	*0.83*	0.50	*0.60*	0.63	*0.87*	*0.46*
GPs 65 years or older	0.05	*0.22*	0.05	*0.22*	0.13	*0.34*	*0.24*
Self-employed GPs per practice	1.84	*1.29*	1.38	*0.81*	1.68	*1.00*	*0.14*
GPs employed by GPs per practice	0.26	*0.51*	0.18	*0.39*	0.30	*0.61*	*0.28*
Locums per practice	0.17	*0.43*	0.18	*0.39*	0.25	*0.44*	*0.42*
Missing	0.05	–	–	–	0.17	–	–
FTE GP per practice	1.62	*1.12*	1.28	*0.70*	1.59	*1.14*	*0.15*
Practice characteristics							
List size per practice	3671	*2384*	2767	*909*	3502	*2233*	*0.06*
Utilization rate per patient	4.05	*0.75*	**3.18**	*0.35*	**5.21**	*0.63*	*0.00***
Solo practices	0.38	*0.49*	**0.60**	*0.50*	**0.30**	*0.46*	*0.00***
Dual practices	0.39	*0.49*	**0.30**	*0.46*	**0.58**	*0.50*	*0.01[a]*
Group practices	0.23	*0.42*	0.10	*0.30*	0.13	*0.34*	*0.72*
Urbanization	3.22	*1.42*	2.90	*1.50*	3.23	*1.39*	*0.32*
Practice organization measures							
Medical service profile	2.99	*1.50*	2.75	*1.43*	3.35	*1.55*	*0.08*
Consultation profile	4.11	*1.54*	**4.03**	*1.54*	**4.73**	*1.40*	*0.04[a]*
Accessibility	1.44	*0.75*	1.33	*0.80*	1.63	*0.67*	*0.07*
Disease management	4.18	*3.25*	3.75	*2.89*	5.18	*3.74*	*0.06*
Patient information material	3.32	*1.27*	3.30	*1.27*	3.53	*1.20*	*0.42*
Support staff per practice							
Doctor's assistant	0.92	*0.27*	0.90	*0.30*	0.95	*0.22*	*0.40*
Practice nurse somatic disorders	0.37	*0.48*	0.38	*0.49*	0.48	*0.51*	*0.37*
Practice nurse mental disorders	0.63	*0.48*	0.43	*0.50*	0.63	*0.49*	*0.24*
Pharmacist	0.04	*0.20*	0.03	*0.16*	0.00	*0.00*	*0.31*
Other medical providers	*0.11*	0.31	0.05	*0.22*	0.18	*0.39*	*0.08*
Other non-medical providers	0.23	*0.42*	0.25	*0.44*	0.20	*0.41*	*0.39*

[a]The score for low utilization practices is significantly different from high utilization practices; $P < 0.05$; $^{**}P < 0.01$
Bold The numbers in bold are practice characteristics which differ significantly between low and high utilization practices

world, including health. In previous research, we calculated estimates on the need for general practice care in all the local areas in the Netherlands [33].

However, the use of the SAE method also has a disadvantage. The SAE method gives the expected value for an area based on the socio-demographic predictors included in the model and not the real value for the construct. Therefore, results which are based on SAE measures are" ..usually at pains to stress that it is reporting estimates all with a degree of uncertainty and not a direct measure of the con struct of concern" [34]. This degree of uncertainty may be enhanced by the fact that the model incorporates the mean value of a socio-demographic predictor for an area, such as the percentage of low income households, while the patients belonging to a practice are a selection from this area and may in fact belong to a higher income category.

Conclusions

The contributors to the utilization of general practice care are manifold and can be found at different levels. We found contributors at the four-digit postcode level and at the general practice level. The presence of other medical providers in the practice, the presence of female GPs and the number of disease management programmes influenced the difference between the actual utilization rate and the estimated rate based on the socio-demographic profile of an area. Our findings provide stakeholders who are involved with the organization of general practice care with useful insight into the practice organization characteristics that influence high or low utilization, in order to help them reflect on the organization and utilization of general practice care.

Abbreviations

FTE GP: Full-time equivalent general practitioner; GP: General practitioner; OHCP: Other healthcare provider; SAE: Small area estimation

Acknowledgements

We acknowledge NIVEL for the collection of the data.

Funding

Financial support for this study was provided by the Dutch Ministry of Education, Culture and Science and the Dutch Ministry of Health, Welfare and Sport. Both Ministeries had no role in the design of the study and the collection, analysis, and interpretation of data and in writing the manuscript.

Authors' contributions

WAdGR and DHdB contributed to the design of this study. DHdB was responsible for the subject of this study. WAdGR was responsible for the day-to-day management and produced the first draft of the manuscript. LvdH designed the statistics of this study. LvdH and WAdGR performed the statistics of this study. All authors contributed to the write-up of this study. All authors read and approved the manuscript.

Competing interests

The authors declare that they have no competing interest.

Author details

[1]NIVEL: Netherlands Institute for Health Service Research, PO Box 1568, 3500, BN, Utrecht, The Netherlands. [2]Scientific centre for care and welfare, Tranzo, Tilburg University, PO Box 90153, 5000, LE, Tilburg, The Netherlands.

References

1. Schellevis FG, Westert GP, De Bakker DH. The actual role of general practice in the Dutch health-care system. J Public Health. 2005;13(5):265–9.
2. Van Dijk C, Verheij R, Van den Hoogen H, De Bakker D, Healthcare I. Bekostiging van de huisartsenzorg: Eindrapportage. Utrecht: NIVEL; 2009.
3. World Health Organization. The world health report 2008: primary health care now more than ever, vol. 2009. Geneva: WHO Press; 2008.
4. Starfield B. Toward international primary care reform. Can Med Assoc J. 2009;180(11):1091–2.
5. Boerma WG, Dubois C-A. Mapping primary care across Europe. Prim Care Driver's Seat. 2006:22–49.
6. Groenewegen PP, Dourgnon P, Greß S, Jurgutis A, Willems S. Strengthening weak primary care systems: steps towards stronger primary care in selected western and eastern European countries. Health Policy. 2013;113(1):170–9.
7. Huygen F, Mokkink H, Smits A, Van Son J, Meyboom W, Van Eyk J. Relationship between the working styles of general practitioners and the health status of their patients. Br J Gen Pract. 1992;42(357):141–4.
8. Emanuel EJ, Fuchs VR. The perfect storm of overutilization. JAMA. 2008; 299(23):2789–91.
9. Chassin MR. Is health care ready for six sigma quality? Milbank Q. 1998; 76(4):565–91.
10. Kale MS, Bishop TF, Federman AD, Keyhani S. Trends in the overuse of ambulatory health Care Services in the United States. JAMA. 2013; 173(2):142–8.
11. Korenstein D, Falk R, Howell EA, Bishop T, Keyhani S. Overuse of health care services in the United States: an understudied problem. Arch Intern Med. 2012;172(2):171–8.
12. Carlisle R, Johnstone S. The relationship between census-derived socio-economic variables and general practice consultation rates in three town Centre practices. Br J Gen Pract. 1998;48(435):1675–8.
13. Curtis SE. Use of survey data and small area statistics to assess the link between individual morbidity and neighbourhood deprivation. J Epidemiol Community Health. 1990;44(1):62–8.
14. Kersnik J, Svab I, Vegnuti M. Frequent attenders in general practice: quality of life, patient satisfaction, use of medical services and GP characteristics. Scand J Prim Health Care. 2001;19(3):174–7.
15. Majeed FA, Cook DG, Anderson HR, Hilton S, Bunn S, Stones C. Using patient and general practice characteristics to explain variations in cervical smear uptake rates. BMJ. 1994;308(6939):1272–6.
16. Majeed FA, Cook DG, Given-Wilson R, Vecchi P, Poloniecki J. Do general practitioners influence the uptake of breast cancer screening? J Med Screen. 1995;2(3):119–24.
17. NIVEL Primary Care Database http://www.nivel.nl/en/dossier/nivel-primary-care-database. Accessed 8 May 2014.
18. Statistics Netherlands. Census data at the four-digit postcode level. January 1th, 2013. http://statline.cbs.nl/Statweb/publication/?DM=SLNL&PA=03759ned&D1=0-14&D2=129-132&D3=0-4&D4=25-26&VW=T. Accessed 5 Apr 2014.
19. Knol F. Statusontwikkeling van wijken in Nederland 1998–2010. 2012. SES development of neighbourhoods in the Netherlands 1998–2010. 2012. https://www.scp.nl/Publicaties/Alle_publicaties/Publicaties_2012/Statusontwikkeling_van_wijken_in_Nederland_1998_2010. Accessed 6 Apr 2014.
20. Hv L, Droomers M, Westert G. Tweede Nationale studie naar ziekten en verrichtingen in de huisartspraktijk: een kwestie van verschil: verschillen in zelfgerapporteerde leefstijl, gezondheid en zorggebruik: *Second national study into diseases and contacts in general practice: a matter of difference: differences in self-reported lifestyle, health and health care use*. NIVEL: Utrecht; 2004.
21. Phillips KA, Morrison KR, Andersen R, Aday LA. Understanding the context of healthcare utilization: assessing environmental and provider-related variables in the behavioral model of utilization. Health Serv Res. 1998;33(3 Pt 1):571.
22. Bensing JM, Van Den Brink-Muinen A, De Bakker DH. Gender differences in practice style: a Dutch study of general practitioners. Med Care. 1993;31(3):219–29.
23. Andersen R, Newman JF. Societal and individual determinants of medical care utilization in the United States. The Milbank Memorial Fund quarterly. Health Soc. 1973;51:95–124.
24. Graves BA. A model for assessment of potential geographical accessibility: a case for GIS. Online J Rural Nurs Health Care. 2012;9(1):46–55.
25. Gulliford M, Morgan M: Access to health care: Routledge; 2013.
26. Peters DH, Garg A, Bloom G, Walker DG, Brieger WR, Hafizur RM. Poverty and access to health care in developing countries. Ann N Y Acad Sci. 2008; 1136(1):161–71.
27. Heje HN, Vedsted P, Sokolowski I, Olesen F. Doctor and practice characteristics associated with differences in patient evaluations of general practice. BMC Health Serv Res. 2007;7(1):46.
28. Campbell JL, Ramsay J, Green J. Practice size: impact on consultation length, workload, and patient assessment of care. Br J Gen Pract. 2001;51(469):644.
29. Van den Berg M. De werkdruk van de huisarts (The GPLs work-related pressure). Medisch Contact. 2003;58:1054–6.
30. Van den Berg M. Workload in general practice. Utrecht: NIVEL; 2010.
31. O'Donoghue C, Morrissey K, Lennon J. Spatial microsimulation modelling: a review of applications and methodological choices. Int J Microsimulation. 2014;7(1):26–75.
32. Rao JN. Small area estimation, vol. 331. Utrecht: NIVEL; 2005.
33. de Graaf-Ruizendaal WA, de Bakker DH. The construction of a decision tool to analyse local demand and local supply for GP care using a synthetic estimation model. Hum Resour Health. 2013;11(1):55.

3

Perceptions of the family physician from adolescents and their caregivers preparing to transition to adult care

Angela Xiao Han[1*], Sandy Rosalie Whitehouse[2], Steve Tsai[2], Sandy Hwang[3] and Sally Thorne[4]

Abstract

Background: Adolescents with chronic health conditions and/or disabilities (CHC/D's) often face challenges when transitioning to adult care, which leads to a higher risk of morbidity and mortality. Although it is recommended that establishing the medical home and family physician (FP) attachment prior to transfer will improve health outcomes, there is little evidence or policy surrounding the role of the FP during this transition. This study explores the described use of health services by adolescents with CHC/D's, as well as the adolescent's and caregiver's perceptions of their FP.

Methods: Participants were recruited from the British Columbia Children's Hospital, Canada and a multi-method phased approach was used. In Phase 1, 84 adolescent and caregiver pairs completed questionnaires asking what medical services they accessed for specific health needs. In Phase 2, another cohort of 21 adolescent and caregiver pairs completed the same questionnaires and were interviewed regarding their perception of their FP.

Results: 96% ($n = 81$) of adolescents with CHC/D's in phase 1 had a FP. Thirty four percent ($n = 34$) of adolescents had not seen their FP in the last 6 months. While adolescents with CHC/D mostly accessed their FP for primary health issues, they frequently also accessed specialists for prescription refills (50%, $n = 51$), mental health (29%, $n = 30$) and sexual health (16%, $n = 16$). While most adolescent/caregiver participants reported positive communication and trust in their FP, some had a poor understanding of the FP's role in coordinating care.

Conclusion: As many adolescents with CHC/D may see their FP infrequently and may not clearly understand their role, opportunities exist for strengthening primary care home attachment as well as adolescent and caregiver literacy around the potential contribution of the FP during and after transfer to adult services. Responsibility for improving care coordination for this population should be ideally shared between FPs and pediatric specialists.

Keywords: Adolescent, Chronic illness, Family physician, Medical home, Transition

Background

An estimated 15–18% of youth in North America have a chronic health condition and/or disability (CHC/D) and over 98% of these youth are expected to reach age 20, thereby requiring transition out of a familiar, family-focused pediatric care system to a dramatically different adult care system where the family physician (FP) is the primary care provider [1]. However, adolescents often feel lost in the adult care system [2]. The adult medicine culture is less attenuated to the developmental complexities of adolescents and focuses on independence, making the transition from an integrated interdisciplinary pediatric system challenging [3]. Lack of engagement with the adult system is associated with lower rates of follow-up appointments and medical compliance [2, 4] and a higher risk of mortality and morbidity [5]. While the primary care doctor has a unique opportunity to address primary health care needs and facilitate the transition process through continuity of care [1, 6–8], much of the emphasis in the transition literature (which most likely reflects clinical practice) focuses solely on specialist-to-specialist provider transition [9, 10].

Young adults have suggested a number of strategies that may facilitate effective transition including peer

* Correspondence: axhan@ualberta.ca
[1]University of Alberta, 116 St & 85 Ave, Edmonton, AB T6G 2R3, Canada

support, mentorship, and having a health care professional who has knowledge and personal understanding of their condition oversee the transfer phase [11]. This concept aligns with the "medical home" model [6]. Implementing a medical home model where health care services are accessible, family centered, continuous, comprehensive, coordinated, and compassionate improves transition preparedness [12, 13]. The patient's medical home can be defined as the place that patients feel most comfortable to discuss their health care, particularly for sensitive topics such as sexual health and mental health. It is a central hub to provide timely and coordinated care by an ongoing team of multidisciplinary caregivers, enabling best possible health outcomes [14]. There is evidence that a "shared care" model that includes patient engagement with specialists and FPs both prior to and after transfer results in better outcomes for adolescents with chronic health conditions such as diabetes [15].

In Canada, the medical home should be established at a FP's practice as they are the first point of contact and primary coordinator of care [14]. However, not all pediatric patients have a FP as some general pediatricians provide on-going primary care in certain provinces. Patients may also access walk-in clinics staffed by different FPs, or emergency departments if they do not have a FP or if their FP is not available. Once a referral is made to a specialist, patients may continue to be followed by that specialist without the involvement of a FP. Although establishing a medical home with a primary care team leads to more effective transition planning, transition protocols often fail to adequately consider the role of the FP in long term management of adolescents following transition [16]. There is little empiric evidence to guide practice or policy surrounding the role of the primary health provider during this transition [1].

The patient-FP relationship is mediated by a variety of factors including the complexity of illness, inclusive management of the patient/family at a tertiary hospital, geography and accessibility to FPs, the perceived role and importance of the FP in continuing care, and the ability to find an FP [17, 18]. Furthermore, adolescents with CHC/Ds and their families may choose walk-in clinics, community pediatricians, the internet, an alternative health provider, or a member of their subspecialty team for interim health care management between necessary specialist appointments [19]. Although these may be convenient resources, lack of continuity prevents the establishment of the medical home at the FP's office [20]. Another consideration regarding the patient-FP relationship unique to the transition period is the relationship between the adolescent and their caregiver with respect to health care management and decision-making, such as arranging appointments or seeing the physician alone during appointments. As adolescent patients transfer from pediatric family-centered care to autonomous adult care, the role of their caregiver in care coordination and management transforms. During this period, the adolescent and caregiver can be considered a decision-making unit in transition [21].

This study investigates adolescents with CHC/Ds' described use of health care services and the adolescent and caregiver's perspectives on the FP's role in health care management prior to transfer to adult services. The goal is to inform strategies to improve the continuity of care with FPs through transition and transfer. We used descriptive and qualitative methods to investigate adolescent patients' attachment with their FP by asking if they and their caregivers identified a FP, how often they saw them, and which health services they accessed for specific primary care issues. We also sought to determine the adolescent/caregiver's perceived role of FPs in regular ongoing management and sentiments surrounding trust, knowledge, and overall relationship with their FP.

Methods

This study was conducted in two phases using mixed methodology at the British Columbia Children's Hospital (BCCH) in Vancouver, Canada. Phase 1 was conducted in 2013 and involved an online questionnaire that included multiple choice and open-ended responses. Phase 2 was conducted in 2014 and included the same questionnaire, with the addition of a qualitative face-to-face interview component that was informed from the open-ended data gathered from phase 1. The University of British Columbia Research Ethics Board approved the study and informed consent was obtained from all participants.

In Phase 1, a convenience sample (n = 84) of adolescent patient/caregiver pairs were invited to participate from the in-patient wards and during subspecialty clinic appointments at the BCCH. The adolescents and caregivers completed individual, parallel online questionnaires asking if they had a FP and where they would seek medical care for specific health issues (Additional file 1 and Additional file 2). Information on demographics (age, gender, geographic region), number of hospitalizations and number of specialists involved was also collected. We defined a subset population as medically complex if two or more subspecialty clinics were involved in the adolescent's care, and/or the adolescent had at least 1 hospital admission in the past 12 months. The questionnaire asked participants about their relationship with their FP with respect to patient/provider communication, communication between providers, provider knowledge and trust. Concept domains to assess the FP's involvement in care included the perceived role of the FP in routine care, the value of the FP's role in context of multiple providers, and access to an FP. The questionnaire was developed by a team of FPs, pediatric/ adult specialists, and the Transition Steering Committee of the Shared Care Youth Transition project [8]. The questionnaire was at a grade 6 reading level and took about 15 min to complete.

For Phase 2, we recruited a further convenience sample (n = 21) of adolescent inpatients/ clinic attendees and their caregivers who identified as having a FP. In addition to completing the questionnaire from Phase 1, we interviewed these adolescents and caregiver attendees about their experiences with their FP. The individual responses were recorded in the transcriptions.

The interview questions focused on adolescents' and caregivers' perspectives of communication and role of the FP in their care (Additional file 3). The interviews were 30 min long on average and were audiotaped and transcribed. Analysis was done using a qualitative description approach [22]. We used constant comparative analysis to derive thematic patterns within the interviews [23]. Coded themes were then independently reviewed and analyzed by two members of the research team who then discussed the themes to reach consensus.

Inclusion and exclusion criteria

English speaking adolescents 14–18 years of age with a CHC/D who required transition to specialist adult care were included, with their caregivers if present. Caregivers who attended with adolescents with cognitive impairment were included even though the adolescent patient could not directly participate in the study. In phase 2, adolescents and their caregivers were excluded if they did not have a FP.

We compared the data sets from the parallel questionnaires completed independently by the adolescent patients and their caregivers and determined there was little variance between the data. However, the caregiver responses were more complete compared to the adolescent responses where questions were often left unanswered. In these cases, we determined that the caregiver represented the most competent coordinator of care and used this single data set of participants for analysis. When adolescents attended the clinic independently or when there were caregiver language barriers, the adolescent data was used for analysis. During the interviews in Phase 2, adolescents contributed equally so therefore both adolescent and caregiver responses were used for qualitative analysis. Data collected from adolescents and their caregivers in phase 1 was excluded from analysis if they indicated they did not have a FP.

Results

In Phase 1, 84 adolescent-caregiver pairs were recruited between June–August 2014 with a response rate of 90%. Three pairs indicated not having a FP and were unable to answer questions surrounding access to and relationship with an FP. These pairs were excluded from further data analysis resulting in n = 81 for phase 1. In Phase 2, 21 pairs were recruited between June–August 2015 with a response rate of 67%. The main reason for refusing to participate in the study was lack of time. Data was collected from adolescent-caregiver pairs because most visits were attended by an adolescent patient with their caregiver. However, there were four adolescents with cognitive impairment who were not able to participate, and there were ten adolescents whose caregivers did not complete the questionnaire (either not present or language barriers). A total of 102 questionnaires were analyzed representing the most responsible coordinator of care from each pair (92 caregivers and 10 adolescents). In phase 2, 17 caregiver and 19 adolescent interview responses were subjected to qualitative analysis (4 caregivers and 2 adolescents could not complete the interview due to exclusion criteria).

Demographics

The adolescents were 14–18 years old (mean 16.4 years) and 49% (n = 50) were 16–17 years old. Forty four percent (n = 45) of adolescent patients were male and 56% (n = 57) were female. Eighty three percent (n = 85) were from urban centers (within a 1 h drive of a regional hospital) (Additional file 4).

Access to family physicians

In Phase 1, 96% (n = 81) of adolescents with CHC/D reported having a FP. These adolescents were asked if they ever see their FP independently. Only 3.75% (n = 3) indicated they always saw their FP alone. Sixty three percent (n = 51) always saw their FP accompanied by a parent/ caregiver, while 28% (n = 23) occasionally saw their FP independently. Thirty eight percent (n = 39) had seen their FP two times or less over the past 2 years and 34% (n = 34) had not seen their FP in the last 6 months. A further 14% (n = 14) had not seen their FP in 12 months, and for 5% (n = 5), it was over 18 months since the last primary care visit.

Accessing other medical services

FPs, hospital specialists, internet, alternative health providers, emergency room, and walk-in clinics were accessed by adolescent study participants in the past 12 months (Additional file 4). Most participants identified that they would see their FP exclusively for primary care issues such as immunizations (74%, n = 75), cold/ flu like symptoms (68%, n = 69), injury (69%, n = 70), referrals (61%, n = 62), completion of forms (59%, n = 60). However, they were more likely to access specialists for prescription refills (50%, n = 51). While the FP was the sole source of care for 58% (n = 59) of adolescent patients for sexual health, and for 48% (n = 49) of adolescent patients for mental health, a substantial number would seek care from both FPs and specialists for sexual health (16%, n = 16) and mental health (29%, n = 30). Fifteen percent (n = 15) identified they would exclusively access the subspecialty clinic for mental health and 10% (n = 10) for sexual health. Regarding education about their medical condition, 36% (n = 37) of adolescent patients reported they would seek information from both FP and specialist, 29% (n = 30) from their specialist alone and 21% (n = 21) from their FP alone (Table 1).

Participants noted they would access other care services in addition or instead of consulting their FP or specialist (Table 2). Other services included the emergency room, walk-in clinics, alternative medicine, and the internet. The internet was selected as the primary source for education about their medical condition (31%, n = 32), sexual health (17%, n = 17) and mental health (17%, n = 17), while walk-in clinics were preferred for injuries (18%, n = 18), cold/flu like symptoms (14%, n = 14) and medication refills (10%, n = 10). In the interviews, five participants acknowledged that they obtained most of their care from walk-in clinics as their FP was not readily available, too far away, or too difficult to access. As per one caregiver: "Anything outside of his medical condition here, we would go to a walk-in clinic."

Complex patients

Fifty two percent (n = 53) of adolescents were categorized as complex based on having 2 or more subspecialty clinics involved in their care and/or at least 1 hospital admission in the past 12 months. Compared to those who were less complex, complex adolescent patients seemed more likely to see their hospital specialist rather than their FP for sexual health (16% vs. 10%) and for mental health issues (24% vs. 14%). In the interviews, 4 adolescent/caregiver pairs reported that the majority of their care was with a specialist because the main concern was the significant health issue. As one pair explained, the main health concerns were "above and beyond our family doctor's capabilities" such that "the family doctor could not handle it."

Relationship with FPs

The majority (59%, n = 60) of adolescents had the same FP for over ten years (Additional file 4). Most adolescent/caregiver participants shared the same family doctor (95%, n = 20), and agreed that their communication was generally good to excellent. They depicted communication as being conducive to sharing information (according to one adolescent, "you could talk to him about anything really") and FPs as personable (a caregiver said, "he jokes with him, which is good. It's good to make that connection.") However, the interview data also revealed communication difficulties (Table 3). One adolescent noted his FP was "pretty narrow minded sometimes" and another a caregiver reported, "sometimes we feel like they are just not listening."

When asked to reflect in Phase 2 on the role of the FP as compared to the role of the specialists, most participants (n = 15) felt more comfortable with the FP and had a sense that this was their medical home, even though they indicated the FP was "not for specific health problems or questions." They explained this by noting, "he is closer," "we see him more often" and "I've known him longer." For some participants, this sense of continuity and familiarity was a valued attribute. One adolescent explained, "sometimes I'll see him in public and I'll say hi, so definitely family doctor for me." In contrast, 4 participants indicated feeling more comfortable with specialists as they were more knowledgeable and had made a major difference to their care. In one family, the caregiver preferred the care of the specialist while the adolescent preferred his family doctor.

Table 1 Physician services participants would access for specific care needs

Care needs	FP Only		BCCH subspecialty clinic only		Both		Neither	
Total n = 102	%	n	%	n	%	n	%	n
Medication Refill	40	41	25	26	25	25	10	10
Medication Side Effect	39	40	17	17	22	22	23	23
Education about medical condition	21	21	29	30	36	37	14	14
Sexual Health	58	59	10	10	6	6	26	27
Mental Health	48	49	15	15	14	14	24	24
Forms	59	60	10	10	15	15	17	17
Referral	61	62	8	8	24	24	8	8
Injury	69	70	0	0	11	11	21	21
Cold/flu like symptoms	68	69	3	3	10	10	20	20
Immunizations	74	75	0	0	6	6	21	21

Table 2 Other services participants would access for specific care needs

Care needs	Emergency Room		Walk in Clinic		Alternative Medicine		Internet		Other	
Total n = 102	%	n	%	n	%	n	%	n	%	n
Medication Refill	6	6	10	10	2	2	0	0	4	4
Medication Side Effect	15	15	9	9	2	2	9	9	7	7
Education about medical condition	2	2	2	2	4	4	31	32	4	4
Sexual Health	1	1	2	2	4	4	17	17	10	10
Mental Health	5	5	3	3	4	4	17	17	12	12
Forms	0	0	3	3	0	0	5	5	4	4
Referral	3	3	7	7	1	1	1	1	3	3
Injury	36	37	18	18	3	3	2	2	3	3
Cold/flu like symptoms	6	6	14	14	4	4	6	6	4	4
Immunizations	1	1	8	8	2	2	1	1	13	13

Communication

With respect to communication between their specialist and FP care providers, most participants felt comfortable that necessary documentation had been sent and received. In their experience, the appropriate lab results and reports had been available in their files "most of the time." However, few had a clear understanding of whether or not this involved any direct verbal communication. Their responses were characterized by vague impressions such as "I believe they would," "I could imagine," or "I'm not really sure." One adolescent expressed, "I'm not a psychic. I don't know what they say".

Perceived knowledge of FP

When asked about the relative degree to which their health care providers were knowledgeable, most thought that while specialists and FPs had particular skillsets, the specialist possessed considerably more knowledge about their specific condition. One adolescent noted, "If the family doctor was knowledgeable enough I wouldn't be here at this hospital," and one caregiver explained, "I am most comfortable bypassing my family doctor and talking to the specialists."

Care coordination

The perspective of most of participants was that care coordination was primarily a matter of referral to specialists, and most (n = 14) felt their FP was doing this well. As one account illustrated, the participant felt the FP would not be able to fill out medical forms, but could arrange referrals, and acknowledged, "The parts he can do, he will do well." However, in two cases, specialist care was coordinated independently of the FP. In another, the adolescent felt the FP was coordinating care, but the caregiver described herself as coordinating with the specialist. Thus the idea of care coordination did not seem well understood by these families.

When explicitly questioned about their trust of the FP to manage their care, most of the participants (n = 16) agreed that their FP was trustworthy. They expressed this as "she knows the family dynamic," "she knows how I react to things," "he would tell us everything," or "she's open." However, for the remainder, there were notable hesitations, including concerns about the level of knowledge. One adolescent stated, "He isn't helpful, particularly when I am in pain."

In Phase 2, all but one participant felt that having an FP had improved their overall health, explaining this as having to do with the continuity of care and breadth of interest in factors affecting their health. "She knows him, found his problem to start with, and has medical records," "she is mostly the reason I can get better," and noting that, when seeing a specialist "all the other stuff

Table 3 Adolescents and caregivers' relationship with FP

Questions regarding relationship with FP	Not at all		Slightly		Very		Extremely	
Total n = 102	%	n	%	n	%	n	%	n
How comfortable do you and your youth feel asking questions of their FP	5	5	45	46	42	43	7	7
How likely are you and your youth to recommend your youth's FP	9	9	23	23	43	44	25	25
How knowledgeable do you and your youth feel your youth's FP is about their medical condition	8	8	45	46	38	39	8	8
How helpful is your FP at explaining your youth's medical condition	13	13	35	36	37	38	14	14
How easy is it for your youth to get to their FP's office	11	11	26	27	41	42	21	21
How easy is it to schedule urgent appointments with your youth's FP when your youth is ill	20	20	34	35	32	33	13	13

doesn't get talked about." Many aspects of care were more accessible with a FP than a specialist.

Discussion

As most of the adolescent patients arrived at subspecialty appointments with their caregiver and did not see the specialist alone during the clinic visit, we determined that during the transition-planning period (i.e. prior to transfer to adult care), caregivers were particularly influential in determining where and whom they sought for care. However, during the interviews every adolescent could describe their relationship with their FP, giving their impressions regarding care management and the role of their physicians. This finding suggests that with appropriate support and encouragement, adolescent patients could be involved in developing independent decision making for their own health care, an important component of self-management.

Most participants identified a long-term relationship with a FP, listing continuity, familiarity and proximity to be valued attributes of their FP. Overall, adolescent patients and caregivers appreciated the contributions their FPs could make and recognized the distinction between the skillset and focus of the FP and the specialist. The majority had a positive relationship with the FP, feeling they were trustworthy and improved the adolescent's overall health. Communications with their FP and between specialists and FPs were generally perceived as good, although few fully understood the intended alignment between the generalist and specialist systems. Several felt the FP's role of coordinating medical care was primarily a matter of referral to specialists.

Despite the positive recognition of the role of the FP, there was a concerning lack of regular involvement of the FP in the adolescent's medical care as determined by the number of reported patient visits in the previous two years. The most cited reason was that the FP was unavailable, too far, or too difficult to access, resulting in some participants choosing walk-in clinics for primary care. With increasing waiting times and difficulty in getting an appointment, patients are often turning to walk-in clinics. However, recently recommended practice management strategies designed to increase efficacy in the medical home model may mitigate this issue [24].

In some cases participants identified specialists as their source for primary health care, particularly when the adolescent patients had medically complex conditions (53% of our sample). These participants seem most likely to view their specialist as the exclusive care provider for concerns such as mental and sexual health. Some participants felt that the adolescent patient's medical conditions were beyond the FP's capabilities and therefore went directly to the specialist for medical concerns, establishing their medical home at the subspecialty clinic rather than with their FP. Not only is this an ineffective use of health care resources, it creates missed opportunities for establishing the FP's office as the adolescent's medical home [14]. When the specialist provides primary health care it creates a more significant handover at the time of transfer to adult specialist services. The FP who is unfamiliar with the patient needs to rapidly acquire the knowledge of a complex, chronic condition and develop a new patient/provider relationship to assume the role as the most responsible physician. Transfer to an entirely new set of providers is more likely to exacerbate the fear and resistance to transfer [25]. This is a significant concern as such adolescents are at higher risk for medical complications if lost to follow up care after transfer [5].

Given the paucity of evidence-based literature to guide practice or policy surrounding the role of the primary health provider during transition to adult services, there are some limitations in this novel study. The study was based on a small sample size, especially when narrowed down to more complex patients. A larger sample size would benefit future investigations to determine if there is a difference in the attachment to the FP between complex and non-complex adolescents, and where they establish their medical home prior to transition. Furthermore, participants were recruited via a convenience sample from multiple clinics and therefore our sample was not randomized. The data used for analysis represented the most competent coordinator of care, which was the caregiver in most cases except when the adolescent attended the clinic alone or when there were caregiver language barriers. Some questions in the youth questionnaires were left unanswered, and this may have been due to lack of knowledge or engagement with the questionnaire. Obtaining a complete and reliable set of adolescent responses for analysis would be valuable in highlighting the adolescents' use of the internet, walk-in clinics and youth clinics for medical care, particularly for sensitive topics such as mental and sexual health. Using a shorter, simplified, youth-friendly questionnaire with images designed to engage adolescents could yield such results in future studies.

Conclusions

There is limited empiric evidence to guide primary care interventions to improve transition outcomes for adolescents with CHC/D's [1]. As a result of this study, we believe that opportunities exist for strengthening the attachment adolescents with CHC/Ds have with their FP as the primary manager of care. As the FP becomes the unequivocal most responsible physician after transfer, facilitating a strong FP-patient relationship and establishing the medical home results in a more effective transition [12, 13]. Given that only 3.75% of adolescents with CHC/D's regularly see their FP alone, health care providers and caregivers should encourage adolescents to become more independent in the management of their own health care. Preparation for transition should start early in childhood [26] so that they experience a graded responsibility that facilitates their interactions with the health care system separate from that of their caregivers.

Responsibility for improving adolescent patient/caregiver health literacy and helping them understand the role of the FP in the adolescent's health management should be shared between FPs and pediatric specialists. In order to ensure continuity of care past the pediatric age, specialists have an opportunity to facilitate the relationship with their FP by encouraging adolescents to see their FP for primary health issues in between specialist visits. With support from pediatric specialists, including clear communication as to the needs of these special populations, FPs can play an integral role in improving health outcomes for adolescents with CHC/Ds during transition.

Additional files

Additional file 1: Caregiver Questionnaire Questionnaire completed by caregivers of adolescent patients.

Additional file 2: Youth Questionnaire Questionnaire completed by adolescent patients.

Additional file 3: Extension interview questions These interview questions focused on adolescents' and caregivers' perspectives of communication and role of the FP in their care.

Additional file 4: Appendix This appendix includes supplemental information regarding patient demographics, access to medical services, and relationship with the FP.

Abbreviations

CHC/D: Chronic health condition and/or disability; FP: Family physician

Acknowledgements

We thank Mary Paone as well as the On TRAC team for their involvement and support throughout this project.

Funding

Funding was provided by the Child and Family Research Institute. The CFRI funds were used for gift cards for study participants in addition to summer research student salary to support collection, analysis, and interpretation of data.

Authors' contributions

AH collected the data in phase one of the study, interpreted the data and contributed in writing the manuscript. SW initiated the conception and design of the study, played a role in data interpretation and writing the manuscript, and oversaw the project. STsai collected the data in phase two of the study, contributed to data analysis and editing of the manuscript. SH analyzed, organized and computed the overall data collected, as well as editing the manuscript. SThorne analyzed and interpreted the qualitative data and contributed in writing and editing the manuscript. All authors read and approved the final manuscript.

Consent for publication

Not applicable.

Competing interests

The authors declare that they have no competing interests.

Author details

[1]University of Alberta, 116 St & 85 Ave, Edmonton, AB T6G 2R3, Canada. [2]University of British Columbia, 2329 West Mall, Vancouver, BC V6T 1Z4, Canada. [3]Child Family Research Institute, 950 W 28th Ave, Vancouver, BC V5Z 4H4, Canada. [4]University of British Columbia School of Nursing, T201-2211 Wesbrook Mall, Vancouver, BC V6T 2B5, Canada.

References

1. Bhawra JTA, Cohen E, Moore Hepburn C, Guttmann A. Primary care interventions to improve transition of youth with chronic health conditions from paediatric to adult healthcare: a systematic review. BMJ Open. 2016; 6(5):e011871. https://doi.org/10.1136/ bmjopen-2016-71.
2. Zhou H, Roberts P, Dhaliwal S, Della P. Transitioning adolescent and young adults with chronic diseases and/or disabilities from pediatric to adult care services: an integrative review. J Clin Nurs. 2016;25(21–22):3113–30. https://doi.org/10.1111/jocn.13326.
3. Harris MA, Freeman KA, Duke DC. Transitioning from pediatric to adult health care: dropping off the face of the earth. Am J Lifestyle Med. 2011; 5(1):85–91.
4. Reid GJ, Irvine MJ, McCrindle BW, Sananes R, Ritvo PG, Siu SC, et al. Prevalence and correlates of successful transfer from pediatric to adult health care among a cohort of young adults with complex congenital heart defects. Pediatrics. 2004;113:e197–205.
5. Prestidge C, Romann A, Djurdjev O, Matsuda-Abedini M. Utility and cost of a renal transplant transition clinic. Pediatr Nephrol. 2012;27(2):295–302.
6. American Academy of Pediatrics, American Academy of family physicians, American College of Physicians, transitions clinical report authoring group, Cooley WC, Sagerman PJ. Supporting the health care transition from adolescence to adulthood in the medical home. Pediatrics. 2011;128(1):182–200.
7. McManus MA, White P, Barbour A, Downing B, Hawkins K, Quion N, et al. Pediatric to adult transition: a quality improvement model for primary care. J Adolesc Health. 2015;56(1):73–8. https://doi.org/10.1016/j.jadohealth.2014.08.006.
8. Whitehouse SR. When chronic care youth age out: transition planning. BCMJ. 2015;57(2):70–1.
9. Mennito SH, Clark JK. Transition medicine: a review of current theory and practice. South Med J. 2010;103:339–42.
10. Robertson L. When should young people with chronic rheumatic disease move from paediatric to adult-centred care? Best Pract Res Clin Rheumatol. 2006;20:387–97.
11. Reiss JG, Gibson RW, Walker LR. Health care transition: youth, family, and provider perspectives. Pediatrics. 2005;115(1):112–20.
12. Lotstein DS, McPherson M, Strickland B, Newacheck PW. Transition planning for youth with special health care needs: Results from National Survey of children with special health care needs. Pediatrics. 2005;115(6):1562–8.
13. McManus MA, Pollack LR, Cooley WC, McAllister JW, Lotstein D, Strickland B, et al. Current status of transition preparation among youth with special needs in the United States. Pediatrics. 2013;131(6):1090–7. https://doi.org/10.1542/peds.2012-3050.
14. College of Family Physicians of Canada. A vision for Canada: Fam Pract - the patient's medical home, 2011. http://www.cfpc.ca/uploadedFiles/Resources/Resource_Items/PMH_A_Vision_for_Canada.pdf Accessed 17 May, 2016.
15. Amed S, Nuernberger K, McCrea P, Reimer K, Krueger H, Aydede SK, et al. Adherence to clinical practice guidelines in the management of children, youth, and young adults with type 1 diabetes: a prospective population cohort study. J Pediatr. 2013;163(2):543–8.
16. DeBaun MR, Telfair J. Transition and sickle cell disease. Pediatrics. 2012; 130(5):926–35. https://doi.org/10.1542/peds.2011-3049.
17. Shaw TM, Delaet DE. Transition of adolescents to young adulthood for vulnerable populations. Pediatr Rev. 2010;31(12):497–504. https://doi.org/10.1542/pir.31-12-497

18. Tucker LB, Cabral DA. Transition of the adolescent patient with rheumatic disease: issues to consider. Rheum Dis Clin N Am. 2007;33:661–72. https://doi.org/10.1016/j.rdc.2007.07.005.
19. Damiano PC, Momany ET, Tyler MC, Penziner AJ, Lobas JG. Cost of outpatient medical care for children and youth with special health care needs: investigating the impact of the medical home. Pediatrics. 2006; 119(6):1187–94.
20. American Academy of Pediatrics. The medical home: medical home initiatives for children with special needs project advisory committee. Pediatrics. 2002;110(1):184–6.
21. Young RA, Marshall SK, Domene JF, Graham M, Logan C, Zaidman-Zait A, et al. Transition to adulthood as a parent-youth project: governance transfer, career promotion, and relational processes. J Couns Psych. 2008; 55(3):297–307.
22. Sandelowski M. Whatever happened to qualitative description? Res Nurs Health. 2000;23:334–40.
23. Thorne S. Interpretive description: qualitative research for applied practice. New York: Routledge; 2016.
24. Murray MM, Tantau C. Same day appointments: exploding the access paradigm. Fam Pract Manag. 2000;7(8):45–50.
25. Tuchman LK, Slap GB, Britto MT. Transition to adult care: experiences and expectations of adolescents with a chronic illness. Chind Care Health Dev. 2008;34(5):557–63.
26. Kaufman M, Pinzon J. Transition to adult care for youth with special health care needs. Position Statement, Canadian Paediatric Society. Paediatr Child Health. 2007;12:785–88.

4

The use of public performance reporting by general practitioners: a study of perceptions and referral behaviours

Khic-Houy Prang, Rachel Canaway, Marie Bismark, David Dunt and Margaret Kelaher*

Abstract

Background: Public performance reporting (PPR) of hospital data aims to improve quality of care in hospitals and to inform consumer choice. In Australia, general practitioners (GPs) are gatekeepers to secondary care with patients requiring their referral for non-emergency access. Despite their intermediary role, GPs have been generally overlooked as potential users of PPR of hospital data, with the majority of the PPR research focussing on consumers, surgeons and hospitals.

Methods: We examined the use of PPR of hospital data by GPs when referring patients to hospitals. Semi-structured interviews were conducted with 40 GPs, recruited via the Victorian Primary Care Practice-Based Research Network and GP teaching practices in Victoria, Australia. The interviews were recorded, transcribed and analysed thematically.

Results: We found that the majority of GPs did not use PPR when referring patients to hospitals. Instead, they relied mostly on informal sources of information such as their own or patients' previous experiences. Barriers that prevented GPs' use of PPR in their decision making included: lack of awareness and accessibility; perceived lack of data credibility; restrictive geographical catchments for certain hospitals; limited choices of public hospitals in regional and rural areas; and no mandatory PPR for private hospitals.

Conclusions: Our findings suggest that lack of PPR awareness prevented GPs from using it in their referral practice. As gatekeepers to secondary care, GPs are in a position to guide patients in their treatment decisions and referrals using available PPR data. We suggest that there needs to be greater involvement by GPs in the development of hospital performance and quality indicators in Australia if GPs are to make greater use of them. The indicators require further development before GPs perceive them as valid, credible, and of use for informing their referral practices.

Keywords: Public performance reporting, General practitioner, Primary care, Qualitative research

Background

Public release of performance information is widely discussed as a mechanism to improve transparency, accountability, choice, and quality of healthcare [1, 2]. Quality indicators and forms of public performance reporting (PPR) vary across different healthcare systems and countries. For example, PPR in the United States (US) includes publishing quality indicators such as mortality and complication rates in various forms - report cards, provider profiles and consumer reports [3]. In the United Kingdom (UK), ratings of individual specialists working in hospitals are publicly reported; and in many countries, data on patients' experiences of hospital care is routinely available [2]. In Australia, mandatory PPR of public hospital data was introduced in 2011, with the establishment of the National Health Performance Authority (ceased in 2016 and activities transferred to the Australian Institute of Health and Welfare [AIHW] thereafter) and the launch of the MyHospitals website [4]. Indicators reported on the MyHospitals website include staphylococcus aureus infections, time patients spent in emergency department, cancer surgery waiting times and financial performance of public hospitals. Indicators yet to be publicly reported, due

* Correspondence: mkelaher@unimelb.edu.au
Centre for Health Policy, Melbourne School of Population and Global Health, The University of Melbourne, Level 4, 207 Bouverie Street, Carlton, VIC 3010, Australia

to their associated methodological issues, include measures of mortality, unplanned readmission rates, patient experiences and access to services by type of service compared to need. Reporting to MyHospitals is mandatory for Australian public hospitals but voluntary for private hospitals. There are also other state/territory government and institution-based sources of PPR – such as the Victorian Health Services Performance website [5].

Berwick and colleagues [6] hypothesised that PPR improves quality of care through two pathways: 1) the selection pathway and 2) the quality change pathway. In the selection pathway, consumers compare PPR data and select high quality healthcare providers and services. This leads to growth of high quality providers, and contraction or exit of low quality providers. The change pathway encourages healthcare organisations to identify areas in which they underperform, leading to performance improvement, which will ultimately attract more consumers.

Although the basic conceptual framework is simple, the real-world impact of PPR on consumers' healthcare decision-making processes remains poorly understood [7]. Past research shows that patients do not often use PPR information in their healthcare decision-making [8] because they do not always perceive differences in the quality ratings of healthcare providers and services [9, 10], they do not trust the data [11] or they do not understand it [12]. Instead, many consumers expect their general practitioners (GPs, i.e. family physician, primary care physician) to recommend a medical specialist or hospital on the basis that the GP knows what is best [13, 14]. In several countries including Australia, the Netherlands and the UK, GPs are gatekeepers to secondary care with patients requiring their referral for access [15].

Australia has dual public and private healthcare sectors. All citizens have free access to a universal public system funded through the taxpayer funded Medicare scheme [16]. Voluntary private insurance reduces access fees to the private healthcare system [17]. The referral process involves a consultation with a GP to discuss medical specialist and hospital options in public or private hospitals. The GP then refers the patient to a medical specialist in an outpatient clinic at a public hospital or to a private specialist clinic at a private office, public or private hospital and the patient is placed on a waiting list for an outpatient consultation with the medical specialist. Following the consultation, the patient will be place on another waitlist for inpatient treatment if required [18]. In theory, GPs can refer a patient to any medical specialist and hospital that the patient chooses to attend. In practice, choice of medical specialist and public hospital are limited in the public system as public hospitals preferred to accept patients within their geographical catchment areas [19]. In the private system, patients can exercise choice in their medical specialist and place of care [17], although some private health insurance organisations have preferred healthcare providers to reduce out-of-pocket expenses [20]. As such, GPs play an important intermediary role in connecting patients with hospitals.

There has been little research examining whether the availability of PPR of hospital data influences GPs' referral behaviours; the majority of the PPR literature focusses on consumers and healthcare providers such as surgeons and hospitals [8, 21, 22]. Among the few studies conducted in Europe, researchers have found that GPs never or rarely used PPR information when referring patients to hospitals [14, 23–25]. Instead, GPs relied mostly on informal sources of information such as: distance to the hospital; feedback from patients and colleagues; prior experience; and personal contacts with medical specialists, departments or hospitals [14, 25, 26]. Reasons cited by GPs for not using PPR information when selecting a hospital included: lack of awareness of the existence of PPR; lack of motivation to use PPR information; uncertainty regarding how PPR data can be used as a support tool to improve patient outcomes; and concerns about the validity and reliability of the data [14, 24]. While these studies provide useful information on GPs' referral considerations and use of PPR, they employed quantitative methodologies which do not allow for a deeper understanding of the barriers and facilitators of PPR. They lack insights on how to improve PPR information and its accessibility for GPs, as well as how PPR could better inform GPs' referrals to hospitals and improve outcomes for patients. Furthermore, they were conducted in Europe, primarily in the Netherlands, so the findings might not apply to Australia given the different healthcare systems. The Netherlands has a single compulsory insurance scheme in which private health insurers and healthcare providers compete with each other for health insurance contracts and patients. Consumers have free choice of health insurer and practitioner [27].

In the PPR literature, GPs have generally been overlooked as potential users of PPR of hospital data. As gatekeepers to secondary care, GPs are responsible for discussing care options with patients and for referring patients to hospitals to receive treatment. GPs' use of PPR to guide healthcare decision-making has the potential to substantially increase the impact of PPR in meeting its objectives of increased transparency and accountability within the healthcare system, informing healthcare decision-making, and potentially improving the quality of hospital services. Given the lack of current empirical research and generalisability from the few studies conducted in this area, and the increased availability of PPR of hospitals data in Australia which can inform healthcare decision-making, there is an opportunity to review GPs' current referral processes. The aim of this study was to examine GPs' awareness and use of PPR of hospital data when referring patients to hospitals, GPs' perceptions of PPR of hospital data qualities and usefulness, and factors that facilitate or constrain GPs' use of PPR of hospital data.

Methods

Design

This study is part of a larger research program which aims to improve understanding of how PPR might improve quality of care in public and private hospitals in Australia by examining the perspectives of multiple stakeholders. Previous components of the research program included interviews with healthcare consumer advocates, providers, purchasers (public and private funders of healthcare services) [28], and senior hospital clinical administrators. This component of the research program used a qualitative approach to capture the experiences and attitudes of GP participants. We conducted semi-structured interviews with GPs using an interview guide. The interview guide was designed to elicit understanding of: the decision-making underpinning GPs' patient referral practices and the role of PPR in that process; GPs' opinions about the accessibility, comprehensibility and utility of PPR information; their perceptions of the MyHospitals website as a prominent example of PPR; and how PPR of hospital data might be improved to better suit GPs' needs [see Additional file 1]. Participants were invited to make additional comments to ensure that all topics they wished to discuss were covered.

Recruitment

Recruitment of GPs occurred in Victoria, Australia via the Victorian Primary Care Practice-Based Research Network (VicReN) and GP teaching practices in Victoria. VicReN is a collaboration between the Primary Care Research Unit, Department of General Practice at the University of Melbourne, and primary care practices around Victoria, Australia [29]. VicReN membership is voluntary, its aim is to link members with research projects to build their research capacity. An email describing the study was sent by the VicReN co-ordinator to 131 GPs. A second reminder email was sent a month after the first email. To increase participation rate, an email invitation was sent to 294 GP teaching practices in Victoria. GP teaching practices are practices in which GPs have voluntarily agreed to take medical students from the Department of General Practice at the University of Melbourne for placements. The number of GPs working in each teaching practice was not known. In total, 131 GPs from VicReN and GPs at 294 teaching practices were invited to participate. It is not known how many GPs at each teaching practice viewed the recruitment invitation, nor which recruits were from teaching practices. Each GP received two gold class movie vouchers as compensation for their time participating in the study. Recruitment ceased after four months when 40 participants had been interviewed.

Data collection

The interviews were undertaken between June and September 2016 by one researcher. Most participants were interviewed via telephone (n = 39), but one was conducted face-to-face. Interviews averaged 21 min in length (ranged from 9 to 34 min). All interviews were audio recorded with the GP's consent. A definition of PPR information was provided at the start of each interview: i.e. "information on the quality of hospitals and/or health-care providers, which is accessible to everyone".

Data analysis

Interview recordings were transcribed verbatim and imported into QSR NVivo11 for coding and storage [30]. Thematic analysis was used for identifying, analysing and reporting pattern (themes) within the data [31]. Two researchers independently analysed five interview transcripts. The resulting coding trees (theme lists) were then compared and refined through discussion between the researchers, leading to the development of an agreed coding tree. The remaining interview transcripts were then coded by one researcher, and emergent themes added as needed. For theme development and revision, similar codes were clustered together and subsequently collapsed into emergent themes. The researchers discussed the emergent themes identified from the data until consensus was reached.

Ethical considerations

Ethical approval for this study was granted by the Melbourne School of Population and Global Health Human Ethics Advisory Group, The University of Melbourne. Written consent was obtained from all GPs prior to data collection to record and use their interview data.

Results

Participants

Table 1 shows the demographic characteristics of the 40 GPs interviewed. The gender balance was fairly even (55% female), ages were spread between 30 and 69 years old, 30% were primarily overseas trained, time in practice ranged from 1 month to 43 years, some worked part-time (40%), and most worked predominantly in group practices (95%) located in metropolitan areas (87.5%). The sample were fairly representative of the GP population in Victoria except for gender (female) and location (metropolitan) which were slightly over-represented in this study [32]. The varied ages, training and years of experience of the GPs ensured that opinions were gathered from informants with a variety of experience.

Table 1 Demographic characteristic of GPs

	N (%)
Gender	
Male	18 (45%)
Female	22 (55%)
Age groups (years)	
30–39	10 (25%)
40–49	7 (17.5%)
50–59	16 (40%)
60–69	7 (17.5%)
Education & training	
Australia	28 (70%)
Overseas	12 (30%)
Work status	
Full-time	24 (60%)
Part-time	16 (40%)
Type of GP practice	
Group	38 (95%)
Solo	2 (5%)
Location of practice	
Metropolitan	35 (87.5%)
Regional/rural[a]	5 (12.5%)
Years in practice (mean)	20 (range 1 month to 43 years)
Years in practice	
0–5 years	8 (20%)
6–10 years	4 (10%)
11–15 years	2 (5%)
16–20 years	2 (5%)
21+ years	24 (60%)

[a]Regional and rural locations were combined due to the small number of cases in each location

Themes

Six main themes related to PPR were identified during analysis: (1) lack of awareness and accessibility; (2) limited utility; (3) lack of trust; (4) unintended consequences; (5) aspirations to strengthen PPR; and (6) healthcare system issues. While the themes are not entirely mutually exclusive, they are elaborated on below under the six theme headings. In doing so, a broader picture emerges of GP decision-making related to their referrals of patients to hospitals.

Lack of awareness and accessibility

The majority of GPs reported that they were not aware of any specific sources of PPR. In particular, most had not heard of the MyHospitals website. GPs did not have the time to look for PPR during their consultations nor did they have the inclination to search for it: "In my whole experience as a GP in over nearly 25 years I've never ever looked at anything like that (PPR)." (GP1). GPs also did not know where to find PPR information and considered access to it difficult:

> I wouldn't know how to access it (PPR information), that's the honest truth. Even if I was interested, it's certainly not easily available to me. I don't see it regularly. You know we get faxed through all sorts of things which we see and we acknowledge but certainly I've never come across any flyer or any advertising about how you access those reports. (GP33).

Among the few GPs that were familiar with PPR, they cited the main sources of PPR information as newspapers, the MyHospitals website, and the Department of Health and Human Services' hospital quality reports.

> When I've ever seen comparisons across hospitals it's actually been when it's been reported in the (news)paper. So if I'm reading the paper and there's something about that I will take some notes of it – but I don't seek out that information specifically. I suppose because I didn't know (it existed). I don't know why I haven't (sought it out). I think because maybe I didn't realise that the information's there, although of course it is; but also, I suppose, I don't know if it's really going to change how I refer. (GP26).

GPs' lack of awareness of PPR put focus on the information sources that they did use to inform their decision-making around patient referrals, as the following quote highlights:

> I wouldn't particularly sit and look at people's statistics or hospital statistics. (...) I'd either send them (patients) to a special unit because of the expertise available, or to a surgeon, for instance, or a physician I'd already used and had a good response from – both clinically and patient satisfaction. So I wouldn't go through statistics and look at, you know, infection rates or death rates for a consultant, orthopaedics or anything like that. (GP20).

When referring patients to public hospitals, GPs generally used their previous experiences (i.e. personal contacts with networks, colleagues, medical specialists and hospitals), their knowledge of patients' experiences and satisfaction and patients' geographical catchments area for public hospitals (i.e. distance to the hospitals).

Limited utility

Many GPs failed to see how PPR information could be utilised in their decision-making processes for public hospital referrals. It was questioned how it would be advantageous and worthwhile to "go wading into a report about public performances of public hospitals?" (GP1). Some were also concerned that such information does not account for patients' complexities such as social, geographic and economic circumstances (e.g. older patients, patients who value staying close to family, low socio-economic background, low health literacy), so it was considered of limited value to the referral process:

> I suppose one of the things is that, like everything, if you look for the hospital that's the best it may not be the easiest for the patient. It may not actually be better in the whole overall care of the patient, because of either logistics or location or cost. So you have to take more into account than just the hospital. (GP27).

Despite many GPs reporting a lack of awareness and usage of PPR, when the MyHospitals website was described to them, most considered it a valuable tool for accountability, transparency and quality improvement activities in hospitals:

> I think it (having PPR) would mean that the public hospitals were more accountable for what they were doing. It would also mean that you (would) know if one hospital was not performing adequately, or was not on par with other hospitals, you could look at why. Is it resources? Is it the patient population that lives around there? – in which case, you know, do we need to have more clinics? So I think overall it'd be beneficial (to have access to PPR data). (GP28).

Some GPs also noted that PPR may be a useful general public resource for informing and managing patients' expectations of non-urgent clinic appointment and elective surgery waiting times. However, they did not think PPR would inform public hospital choice as public hospitals preferred to accept referrals from patients who live within their geographical catchment area. These GPs did not acknowledge that in certain circumstances, referrals outside a patient geographical catchment area are possible.

> I don't see that it has a great deal of utility for a GP. I think because we're so location based you're hamstrung into using the facilities that are closest to you. (...) So even if you want to go for the best and the shiniest clinic, or whatever it is that you think your patient needs, you may be declined entry into that hospital purely based on where your patient lives. (GP26).

Lack of trust

After it was described to them, some GPs looked at the MyHospitals website during the interview, thus increasing the number of GPs who commented directly about the website. Overall, the majority of GPs questioned the integrity of PPR information – such as that found on the MyHospitals website. They were unclear about how the data were collected, how the quality indicators were calculated, and concerned about data being outdated rather than provided in real-time. They also raised concerns about its reliability and validity including issues of data falsification by hospitals:

> If I felt the complication rates were accurately reported, yes I'd take it into account but I'd have to trust how that was reported and I don't know if hospitals are accurately reporting their complication rates because it's not something surgeons like to admit to. (...) So I'd have to feel like I trusted that data before I took it on board. (GP9).

> The thing about waiting times in emergency, I know how sometimes the consultants are actually making sure the numbers look good where, in fact, they're actually just moving around patients. I don't think always good performance means that they have better patient care. I'm cynical about the numbers, because having worked in hospitals, you can work in a place that has very good numbers and things like that, but in fact the care wouldn't be as good as another place that doesn't. So I'm quite cynical about their reporting. (GP27).

Publicly reported quality indicators were also deemed to be irrelevant, lacking in meaning, and difficult to interpret as PPR was likely to be "written in language that is hard to understand and very much from a bureaucrat point of view" (GP1). For example, waiting time for elective surgery on the MyHospitals website does not take into account the time from when patients are referred by the GP to the medical specialist; rather, the published waiting time begins only when the patient has been seen by the medical specialist, thus underestimating the total waiting time. Some GPs thought that given they were having difficulties understanding the information, then it was highly likely to cause greater confusion for patients accessing the information:

> I'm a little bit concerned about that (MyHospitals) from a scaring-a-patient point of view, or from them not having an understanding of what that means, or how that's relevant to them on an individual basis. I can see that (MyHospitals) potentially creating some headaches (for patients and GPs). You know like if a patient were to look on the thing and go: "Oh, you know, hospital X has more infections" than whatever, and they might not necessarily understand where

> those infections occur or how that's relevant to them when they're going to a particular clinic. (GP36).

Despite criticisms about the indicators, some GPs said they would consider using PPR information in their future public and private hospital referrals if they thought the indicators to be relevant, specific, real-time, and trustworthy. This was said with the caveat that the use of such information would be highly dependent on whether public hospital referrals outside of patients' geographical catchment areas and mandatory PPR for private hospitals would be permitted.

Unintended consequences

GPs expressed concerns that unintended consequences may occur due to PPR. They suggested that PPR could lead to patient selection bias where hospitals or surgeons reject difficult patients whose treatment was determined as risky and could potentially increase (worsen) their complication and mortality rates:

> It [PPR] may dissuade the surgeons from taking on difficult cases because difficult cases die more often and the figures will make them look worse; so the only disadvantage of doing that is that some surgeons would just say: "You're too hard to operate on". The most life threatening cases may end up not being offered surgery. (GP23).

Some GPs perceived that short waiting times in particular hospitals might ultimately increase overall waiting times if GPs favoured referrals to that site. For example, a GP recalled that "a few years ago, Hospital X improved its waiting time for orthopaedics and the word got out and everybody sent their patients to Hospital X, and rather rapidly they got these patients from all over the place coming in" (GP7).

Some GPs were particularly concerned that PPR might also create high demand for services and increase burden in high performing hospitals, whereas low demand in lower performing hospitals might limit their opportunity to improve their processes and patient outcomes. PPR was seen as "enormously helpful (...only) if you were in a situation where there was an oversupply of services (where) people would be keen to show off that they were brilliant" (GP13). As there is not an oversupply of services, there was concern that PPR could push hospitals to manipulate their data to maintain their reputation and prevent an imbalance of patient burden across hospitals: "You obviously can't show you're significantly out of kilter with everybody else because that will produce a rush on health services" (GP13); and "If a hospital is performing badly who wants to advertise that? Who wants to publicly notify the general population about it?" (GP29). Creating fear and anxiety through publication of poor performance data among patients who might not have a choice but to use a poor performing hospital (e.g. in regional and rural areas) was of particular concern. Although it was conceded that "it's in everyone's right to know how any centre is performing per se, let it be hospital, let it be clinic, let it be public or private" (GP29).

Aspirations to strengthen PPR

Regardless of the types of PPR information currently available, GPs considered waiting times for triage, waiting times for first appointment and surgery, infection rates, complication rates, mortality rates, readmission rates, out-of-pocket costs, patients' experiences, patients' satisfaction and complaints to be important indicators that should be publicly reported. The current reporting of wait times for elective surgery were said to be "ridiculous" and in need of improvement (GP2).

The public reporting of patient experience, satisfaction and complaints information was considered particularly useful for consumers, with one GP saying it would be useful information to inform his/her own healthcare decision-making:

> I suppose what I'd be interested in, in the case of surgery, is complication rates, personal reports of patients that have received care; similar sort of things to what you do with travel when you're assessing a hotel. (...) Yes, personal experiences, saying what they have found good about the hospital, what they didn't find good about the hospital. If I was assessing that hospital for my own personal use, I would find that useful. (GP21).

GPs generally preferred information to be reported at the individual surgeon and clinical unit level instead of hospital level because the latter could mask differences among surgeons and clinical units.

> I'd like to see surgeon figures that would be the most important thing for me to see surgeon's complication rates. Information on complication rates would be really, really good. It can be done in such a way as to not make surgeons feel as if they are being scapegoated. (GP23).

However, they acknowledged that patients are unlikely to know who their surgeon will be in a public hospital, and that PPR information will also need to be case-mix adjusted for appropriate comparisons to be made. Furthermore, GPs urged for better promotion and dissemination of PPR given their lack of awareness of its existence. It was suggested that awareness could be increased via snapshot summaries of PPR data (i.e. faxed, mailed or emailed fliers from hospitals, Primary Health Networks, Royal Australian College of GPs, Australian Health Practitioner Regulation Agency, or government health departments), and a PPR website with a dedicated section targeted to GPs:

> I'm just looking at this (MyHospitals website). I work with so many different hospitals and I don't know if I'd go through and look at every hospital and then compare. I'd probably just want to know what's the access like at my local hospital compared to the next local hospital for maybe my special interest or specifically for clinics. (...) I don't really have the time with the patient load to wade through and look through all these different things, I really just want a snapshot. (GP15).

Healthcare systems issues

A number of GPs discussed PPR issues related to private hospitals and patients' limited choice of public hospitals, particularly in regional and rural areas. They remarked that PPR information would be more valuable in private hospitals than public hospitals where patients can exercise greater hospital choice:

> In the private hospital the consumer has rights, and consumers get choices and the consumer can dictate outcomes, which preferences they have. But public hospital patients don't get any of those rights. So what's the point of having a computer program that tells you "look you get better service at hospital X" if hospital X just won't take you? (GP37).

GPs were especially interested in private hospitals disclosing their specialists' fees and out-of-pocket costs. GPs also recognised that having accurate waiting times for elective surgery in public hospitals (from GPs referral to specialist to actual surgery) may be helpful in persuading patients to self-fund privately if the waiting time was deemed too long. Some GPs noted that although patients appeared to have greater choice in the private market, limited choice of surgeons and private hospitals could be imposed by private insurance organisations that have preferred healthcare providers.

In addition, GPs working in regional and rural areas recognised the lack of choice in specialists care and public hospitals. GPs noted there were only one or two public hospitals and one private hospital available in regional and rural areas:

> The other issue in the country (regional and rural areas) is availability, we only have one cardiologist that we can refer to, we only have one physician who comes to our small village, we only have one surgeon that comes so if they want to be treated in town locally without having to leave the town they've only got one surgeon or one physician. And there's no other choice. (GP23).

Discussion

Very few of the GPs that contributed to this study had heard of MyHospitals or other sources of PPR, and one had considered using MyHospitals when making patient referrals to public hospitals. These findings are consistent with past studies conducted in Europe which also found that despite the availability of PPR of hospital data, it was little utilised for hospital referrals by GPs [14, 23–25]. Despite the different healthcare systems, the similar findings are largely attributed to the lack of awareness about PPR information among GPs. A contributing factor might be that GPs, internationally, tend to have limited time within or outside of consultations to actively access and make sense of PPR Lack of perceived value in how PPR can inform healthcare decision making and improve the quality of healthcare services, as well as being unclear whether it is the GPs' responsibility to inform patients about PPR of hospital data may have prevented GPs from using it in their referrals. Our findings, that many of the interviewed GPs did not trust PPR data and did not consider it useful or easily accessible, also accounts for why GPs were not using it when referring patients for secondary care. These findings suggest lack of engagement with GPs in the design and development of PPR systems that GPs would consider trustworthy, useful and accessible. These results also indicate that across our sample of GPs, there has been poor promotion and dissemination of PPR information to this important target user group. Greater PPR resources targeted at GPs may encourage its use and lead to improvements in usability.

Referrals to hospitals, as described by our participants, are largely based on experience, including professional networks, word-of-mouth (what patients reported back to them in follow-up visits) and ease of habit. Similarly, international studies have shown that the most common factors influencing GPs' referral decisions to healthcare providers or hospitals were their own experience with the medical specialists or hospitals, feedback from patients and professional network colleagues, and distance to the hospital [14, 23–26, 33–36].

GPs' were reluctant to use PPR data because of concerns about reliability and validity, particularly related to the data being potentially unreliable, outdated and difficult to interpret. This is consistent with past studies which have shown that GPs tend to distrust PPR information as they perceived it to be invalid and unreliable due to the potential that it has been manipulated to achieve hospital targets [14, 24]. In Australia, there has been evidence of manipulation of waiting times in emergency departments and reclassification of patients on elective surgery waiting list [37]. However, it is unclear whether GPs mistrust of PPR data stem from credible evidence or a prejudice against the utility of PPR data given that the majority of GPs were not aware of the MyHospitals website. Future research is warranted to explore the mistrust of PPR data by GPs.

Although GPs did not use PPR data in their referral practice, they were aware of some of the discourse that surrounds the debate of PPR [38, 39]. GPs recognised both the potential benefits of PPR such as promoting accountability, transparency and quality improvement activities in hospitals and the potential unintended consequences of PPR such as overburden of high performing hospitals and increase waiting times which may ultimately impact service delivery, patient selection bias and a decline in public trust by inciting fear among those who may have limited choice of hospitals. These potential adverse outcomes concerns appear valid. Several reviews found some evidence that PPR may be associated with avoidance of high risk patients by doctors [21, 40] and a loss of confidence among the public [41]. Reporting of poor hospital performance may erode public trust at first; however, PPR can highlight deficiencies in healthcare delivery and drive hospital to perform better and therefore restore public confidence. GPs need to consider whether the benefits of using PPR data when referring patients to hospitals outweigh the risk of adverse outcomes. Minimising potential unintended consequences and monitoring these are important to promote trust and increase PPR usability among GPs and the public.

Healthcare systems issues such as public hospital preference for patients living within their local catchment area [42, 43] and limited choice of public hospitals for consumers in regional and rural areas were additional reasons why GPs would not use PPR information. Although these systems issues hinder the use of PPR for informing consumer choice, PPR can increase transparency and accountability, and protect patients by stimulating healthcare quality and performance improvements if hospital staff are aware that GPs and consumers are responsive to PPR information. In support, past studies showed quality improvement occurred among healthcare providers who were concerned that PPR would affect their reputation [44, 45].

Furthermore, GP's use of PPR can potentially increase the impact of PPR systems by increasing knowledge and trust about good and bad aspects of hospitals, encouraging consumer engagement in their healthcare, and choosing the better performing sites when appropriate or available. However, GPs may not have consider PPR data as part of their responsibility because they have not been educated to consider PPR and its various potential benefits when making referrals – so it remains an untapped source. Past research has shown that GPs are unclear about their role in using PPR data during consultation with patients [24]. Some GPs did not considered their responsibility to advise patients on PPR data, whereas other GPs viewed discussing PPR data with their patients during the referral process as part of their role to support decision making [46]. Future research is warranted to explore whether GPs' use of PPR data to inform hospital referrals ought to be part of their role. Assessing the comparative priorities of referral information, including hospitals proximity, familiarity and PPR data, using Delphi method or discrete choice analysis will also be helpful to ascertain the level of PPR importance.

Recommendations

This study, supported by local and international literature, illustrates that when an effective promotion and dissemination strategy for PPR, aimed at GPs, is lacking, that opportunity is lost to increase the impact of PPR. To increase awareness of PPR among GPs, PPR websites and reports should be widely publicised, published in accessible formats, easily understood and made readily available. Although we explored GPs' perceptions of their PPR needs and desired forms of delivery, it was beyond the scope of the study to comprehensively assess the design and comprehensibility of current PPR websites and reports. Future research is warranted to evaluate the appropriateness of the user interface and contents of PPR for GPs.

Involvement and collaboration with GPs is required to better target and tailor PPR to their needs to increase their accessibility and usability of PPR information. Research suggests that the routine collection and public publication of certain measures, such as patient reported experience and outcome can increase the perceived usability of the data [47, 48]. Such measures are routinely reported in England [49, 50], the Netherlands [51, 52] and the US [53, 54] as a mechanism to incorporate patient perspectives in quality improvement and to promote choice. These measures are found to be positively associated with delivery of care [55], clinical outcomes [56], clinical effectiveness and patient safety [57]. Similarly, the GPs in our study proposed inclusion of such measures which they considered to be more meaningful than those currently available.

Increasing data transparency is essential to improve its perceived trustworthiness among GPs. Educating GPs about quality indicators, PPR methodologies, and ways to discuss PPR with patients should result in more willingness by GPs to use PPR when referring patients to hospitals. Developing real-time data collection, analysis and reporting using smart management systems will facilitate the use of such data to guide decision-making. In Victoria, the establishment of an independent health information agency to analyse and share information across the health system has recently been foreshadowed [58] following a 2016 review of hospital safety and quality assurance in

Victoria [59]. The successful establishment of such an agency could enhance the perception of trust if GPs can be convinced that reported data is not being manipulated by hospital staff.

Incorporating PPR data from the public domain into electronic referral systems may also increase the use of PPR data by GPs in their referral processes. For example, in England and the Netherlands where GPs are also gatekeepers to secondary care, systems such as 'Choose and Book' and 'ZorgDomein' have been implemented to support patient choice at the point of referral [60, 61]. Both electronic referral systems include a directory of medical specialists, clinics in the hospitals and average waiting times. Technical challenges and GP resistance to the system, at least in the English experience, were identified during the implementation which limited its execution. Additional investment in IT infrastructure and remuneration for GPs by the government were required to encourage GP uptake of the system [62]. Overall, electronic referral systems have the potential to improve GPs' referral decisions by including PPR data and involving patients in the process. Mandating PPR of private hospital data in the same way as public hospital data provides necessary information to enable choice in areas where choice can be exercised [59]. Currently, only 35% of Australian private hospitals participate in PPR on the MyHospitals website, and they do not necessarily report on all of the indicators required by public providers [4]. Some private healthcare providers publish their own PPR websites to help consumers make informed decisions [e.g. [63]]. Although a positive step towards PPR, it does not assist GPs and others who want to be able to locate such information in one central place.

Limitations

The limitations related to this study should be considered when interpreting the findings. Recruitment, based on GPs members of VicReN and GP teaching practices, may have resulted in a biased sample. Given the small numbers and under-representation of GPs working in regional and rural areas, the findings are not generalisable. However, the sample of GPs, recruited via VicReN and GP teaching practices, consist primarily of GPs who are interested in research, therefore, they might be more likely to be actively engaged in learning and new knowledge, such as PPR makes available, than non-participating GPs. Given that many GPs were not aware of PPR data; their perceptions of PPR utility and data quality are likely to be limited. MyHospitals was given as the prominent example of a source of PPR and GPs perceptions of PPR may have been skewed towards that, with little comment on other sources of PPR information. Finally, a conclusion cannot be reached on what the GPs thought of PPR overall given that many GPs were unaware of specific example of it. Some GPs viewed and commented on the MyHospitals website during their interviews; their opinions were based on first impressions rather than a working knowledge of the website.

Conclusions

Given that GPs are important intermediaries between healthcare consumers and hospital care, it is of great importance that they are well informed when guiding patients in their treatment decisions and referrals to target the better performing services where possible, or to alert patients to potential quality or safety problems as indicated by PPR data. Such openness and transparency could potentially trigger quality improvement at poor performing hospitals and build patient trust and engagement with healthcare. An apparent obstacle to overcome if GPs are to better utilise PPR information is ensuring that systems of PPR are developed with collaboration from GPs to ensure that the reported performance quality indicators, formats and mediums serve their information needs. Developing systems of PPR tailored to meet the needs of various target audiences (such as GPs, consumers, hospital staff and so on) should be considered to increase the usability and impact of PPR.

Abbreviations

AIHW: Australian Institute of Health and Welfare; GP: General practitioner; PPR: Public performance reporting; UK: United Kingdom; US: United States; VicReN: Victorian Primary Care Practice-Based Research Network

Acknowledgements

We wish to thank Natalie Appleby, VicReN co-ordinator for her instrumental role in recruiting GPs. We wish to thank all the GPs for generously sharing their experiences with us.

Funding

This research was funded by Medibank Better Health Foundation. Views expressed are those of the authors and not the funding agency.

Authors' contributions

MK, DD and MB conceptualised and designed the study and obtained its funding. All authors contributed to the interview guide. KP collected the data. KP and RC analysed the data, interpreted the data and drafted the manuscript. MK, DD and MB critically reviewed and contributed to the manuscript. All authors read and approved the final manuscript.

Consent for publication

Written informed consent, including the publication of anonymised quotes, were obtained from all participants prior to data collection.

Competing interests

The authors declare that they have no competing interests.

References

1. Cacace M, Ettelt S, Brereton L, Pedersen JS, Nolte E. How health systems make available information on service providers: experience in seven countries. Rand Health Quarterly. 2011;1(1):11.
2. Rechel B, McKee M, Haas M, Marchildon GP, Bousquet F, Blümel M, et al. Public reporting on quality, waiting times and patient experience in 11 high-income countries. Health Policy. 2016;120(4):377–83.
3. Marshall MN, Shekelle PG, Davies HT, Smith PC. Public reporting on quality in the United States and the United Kingdom. Health Aff. 2003;22(3):134–48.
4. AIHW. MyHospitals 2017 [Available from: https://www.myhospitals.gov.au/. Accessed 3 Feb 2017.
5. Victoria State Government. Victorian Health Services Performance 2016 [Available from: http://performance.health.vic.gov.au/Home.aspx). Accessed 3 Feb 2017.
6. Berwick DM, James B, Coye MJ. Connections between quality measurement and improvement. Medical care. 2003;41(1):I30–8.
7. Schlesinger M, Kanouse DE, Martino SC, Shaller D, Rybowski L. Complexity, public reporting, and choice of doctors. Med Care Res Rev. 2014;71(5_suppl):38S–64S.
8. Ketelaar NA, Faber MJ, Flottorp S, Rygh LH, Deane KH, Eccles MP. Public release of performance data in changing the behaviour of healthcare consumers, professionals or organisations. Cochrane Database Syst Rev. 2011;11:CD004538. -CD
9. Damman OC, Hendriks M, Rademakers J, Spreeuwenberg P, Delnoij DMJ, Groenewegen PP. Consumers' interpretation and use of comparative information on the quality of health care: the effect of presentation approaches. Health Expect. 2012;15(2):197–211.
10. Emmert M, Schlesinger M. Hospital quality reporting in the United States: does report card design and incorporation of patient narrative comments affect hospital choice? Health Serv Res. 2017;52(3):933–58.
11. Marshall MN, Shekelle P, Leatherman S, Brook R. The public release of performance data: what do we expect to gain? A review of the evidence. JAMA. 2000;283(14):1866–74.
12. Hibbard JH, Greene J, Daniel D. What is quality anyway? Performance reports that clearly communicate to consumers the meaning of quality of care. Med Care Res Rev. 2010;67(3):275–93.
13. Victoor A, Noordman J, Sonderkamp JA, Delnoij DM, Friele RD, van Dulmen S, et al. Are patients' preferences regarding the place of treatment heard and addressed at the point of referral: an exploratory study based on observations of GP-patient consultations. BMC Fam Pract. 2013;14(1):1.
14. Doering N, Maarse H. The use of publicly available quality information when choosing a hospital or health-care provider: the role of the GP. Health Expect. 2015;18(6):2174–82.
15. Schoen C, Osborn R, Huynh PT, Doty M, Peugh J, Zapert K. On the front lines of care: primary care doctors' office systems, experiences, and views in seven countries. Health Aff. 2006;25(6):w555–w71.
16. Australian Government Department of Human Services. Medicare services 2017 [Available from: https://www.humanservices.gov.au/individuals/subjects/medicare-services. Accessed 3 Feb 2017.
17. Australian Government Private Health Insurance Ombudsman. What is covered? 2017. Available from: https://www.privatehealth.gov.au/healthinsurance/whatiscovered/. Accessed 8 Mar 2017.
18. Victoria State Government. Choosing hospitals and specialist doctors 2017 [Available from: https://www.betterhealth.vic.gov.au/health/servicesandsupport/choosing-hospitals-and-specialist-doctors. Accessed 6 July 2017.
19. Cutler H, Gu Y, Olin E. Assessing choice for public hospital patients. Centre for the Health Economy: Macquarie University; 2017.
20. BUPA. Going to hospital 2017. Available from: https://www.bupa.com.au/health-insurance/understanding-your-health-cover/going-to-hospital. Accessed 6 July 2017.
21. Chen J. Public reporting of health system performance: a rapid review of evidence on impact on patients, providers and healthcare organisations. Evidence Check. 2010;
22. Campanella P, Vukovic V, Parente P, Sulejmani A, Ricciardi W, Specchia ML. The impact of public reporting on clinical outcomes: a systematic review and meta-analysis. BMC Health Serv Res. 2016;16(1):296.
23. Ferrua M, Sicotte C, Lalloué B, Minvielle E. Comparative quality indicators for hospital choice: do general practitioners care? PLoS One. 2016;11(2):e0147296.
24. Ketelaar NA, Faber MJ, Elwyn G, Westert GP, Braspenning JC. Comparative performance information plays no role in the referral behaviour of GPs. BMC Fam Pract. 2014;15(1):1.
25. Mannion R, Goddard M. General practitioners' assessments of hospital quality and performance. Clinical Governance: An International Journal. 2004;9(1):42–7.
26. Birk HO, Henriksen LO. Which factors decided general practitioners' choice of hospital on behalf of their patients in an area with free choice of public hospital? A questionnaire study. BMC Health Serv Res. 2012;12(1):1.
27. van den Berg MJ, Kringos DS, Marks LK, Klazinga NS. The Dutch health care performance report: seven years of health care performance assessment in the Netherlands. Health Research Policy and Systems. 2014;12(1):1.
28. Canaway R, Bismark M, Dunt D, Perceived KM. Barriers to effective implementation of public reporting of hospital performance data in Australia: a qualitative study. BMC Health Serv Res. 2017;17(1):391.
29. Soós M, Temple-Smith M, Gunn J, Johnston-Ata'Ata K, Pirotta M. Establishing the Victorian primary care practice based research network. Aust Fam Physician. 2010;39(11):857.
30. QSR International Pty Ltd. NVivo qualitative data analysis software. Version. 2015;11
31. Braun V, Clarke V. Using thematic analysis in psychology. Qual Res Psychol. 2006;3(2):77–101.
32. Australian Government Department of Health. General practice. Statistics. 2015. Available from: http://www.health.gov.au/internet/main/publishing.nsf/content/general+practice+statistics-1. Accessed 24 Feb 2017.
33. Barnett ML, Keating NL, Christakis NA, O'Malley AJ, Landon BE. Reasons for choice of referral physician among primary care and specialist physicians. J Gen Intern Med. 2012;27(5):506–12.
34. Kinchen KS, Cooper LA, Levine D, Wang NY, Powe NR. Referral of patients to specialists: factors affecting choice of specialist by primary care physicians. Ann Fam Med. 2004;2(3):245–52.
35. Piterman L, Koritsas S. Part II. General practitioner–specialist referral process. Intern Med J. 2005;35(8):491–6.
36. Forrest CB, Nutting PA, Starfield B, Von Schrader S. Family physicians' referral decisions: results from the ASPN referral study. J Fam Pract. 2002;51(3):215–23.
37. Nocera A. Performance-based Hospital funding: a reform tool or an incentive for fraud? Med J Aust. 2010;192(4):222.
38. Mannion R, Braithwaite J. Unintended consequences of performance measurement in healthcare: 20 salutary lessons from the English National Health Service. Intern Med J. 2012;42(5):569–74.
39. Werner RM, Asch DA. The unintended consequences of publicly reporting quality information. JAMA. 2005;293(10):1239–44.
40. Fung CH, Lim Y-W, Mattke S, Damberg C, Shekelle PG. Systematic review: the evidence that publishing patient care performance data improves quality of care. Ann Intern Med. 2008;148(2):111–23.
41. Mannion R, Davies H, Marshall M. Impact of star performance ratings in English acute hospital trusts. Journal of Health Services Research & Policy. 2005;10(1):18–24.
42. The Royal Women's Hospital. Referrals 2017 [Available from: https://www.thewomens.org.au/health-professionals/clinical-resources/referrals/. Accessed 6 Feb 2017.
43. Alfred Health. Our local community 2017 [Available from: https://www.alfredhealth.org.au/about/patients-come-first/local-community. Accessed 6 Feb 2017.
44. Hibbard JH, Stockard J, Tusler M. It isn't just about choice: the potential of a public performance report to affect the public image of hospitals. Med Care Res Rev. 2005;62(3):358–71.
45. Hibbard JH, Stockard J, Tusler M. Hospital performance reports: impact on quality, market share, and reputation. Health Aff. 2005;24(4):1150–60.
46. Rozen R, Florin D, Hutt R. An anatomy of GP referral decisions. A qualitative study of GP's view on their role in supporting patient choice. London: The King's Fund; 2007.
47. Fasolo B, Reutskaja E, Dixon A, Boyce T. Helping patients choose: how to improve the design of comparative scorecards of hospital quality. Patient Educ Couns. 2010;78(3):344–9.
48. Hildon Z, Allwood D, Black N. Making data more meaningful: patients' views of the format and content of quality indicators comparing health care providers. Patient Educ Couns. 2012;88(2):298–304.
49. NHS Digital. Patient reported outcome measures (PROMs) 2016 [Available from: http://content.digital.nhs.uk/proms. Accessed 7 Mar 2017.
50. Weldring T, SMS S. Patient-Reported Outcomes (PROs) and patient-reported outcome measures (PROMs). Health Serv Insights. 2013;6:61–8.

51. Delnoij DM, Rademakers JJ, Groenewegen PP. The Dutch consumer quality index: an example of stakeholder involvement in indicator development. BMC Health Serv Res. 2010;10(1):88.
52. Stubbe JH, Gelsema T, Delnoij DM. The consumer quality index hip knee questionnaire measuring patients' experiences with quality of care after a total hip or knee arthroplasty. BMC Health Serv Res. 2007;7(1):60.
53. Centers for Medicare & Medicaid Services. Consumer assessment of healthcare providers & systems (CAHPS) 2016 [Available from: https://www.cms.gov/Research-Statistics-Data-and-Systems/Research/CAHPS/index.html. Accessed 7 Mar 2017.
54. Hargraves JL, Hays RD, Cleary PD. Psychometric properties of the consumer assessment of health plans study (CAHPS®) 2.0 adult Core survey. Health Serv Res. 2003;38(6p1):1509–28.
55. Elliott MN, Lehrman WG, Goldstein EH, Giordano LA, Beckett MK, Cohea CW, et al. Hospital survey shows improvements in patient experience. Health Aff. 2010;29(11):2061–7.
56. Price RA, Elliott MN, Zaslavsky AM, Hays RD, Lehrman WG, Rybowski L, et al. Examining the role of patient experience surveys in measuring health care quality. Med Care Res Rev. 2014;71(5):522–54.
57. Doyle C, Lennox L, Bell D. A systematic review of evidence on the links between patient experience and clinical safety and effectiveness. BMJ Open. 2013;3(1)
58. Victoria State Government Department of Health and Human Services. Better, safer care: Delivering a world-leading healthcare system. 2016.
59. Duckett S, Cuddihy M, Newnham H. Targeting zero: supporting the Victorian hospital system to eliminate avoidable harm and strengthen quality of care. 2016.
60. Walford S. Choose and Book. Clinical Medicine. 2006;6(5):473–6
61. Dixon A, Robertson R, Bal R. The experience of implementing choice at point of referral: a comparison of the Netherlands and England. Health Economics, Policy and Law. 2010;5(3):295–317.
62. Dixon A, Robertson R, Appleby J, Burge P, Devlin N, Magee H. Patient choice. How patients choose and how providers respond. London: The King's Fund; 2010.
63. Healthscope Hospitals. MyHealthscope - Accreditation, quality & safety 2017 [Available from: http://www.healthscopehospitals.com.au/quality/my-healthscope. Accessed 13 Mar 2017.

5

Identifying frailty in primary care: a qualitative description of family physicians' gestalt impressions of their older adult patients

Clara Korenvain[1,2†], Ida-Maisie Famiyeh[1,2†], Sheila Dunn[1,3,5], Cynthia R. Whitehead[1,3,4], Paula A. Rochon[1,3,5] and Lisa M. McCarthy[1,2,3,5*]

Abstract

Background: Many tools exist to guide family physicians' impressions about frailty status of older adults, but no single tool, instrument, or set of criteria has emerged as most useful. The role of physicians' subjective impressions in frailty decisions has not been studied. This study explores how family physicians conceptualize frailty, and the factors that they consider when making subjective decisions about patients' frailty statuses.

Methods: Descriptive qualitative study of family physicians who practice in a large urban academic family medicine center as they participated in one-on-one "think-aloud" interviews about the frailty status of their patients aged 80 years and over. Of 23 eligible family physicians, 18 shared their impressions about the frailty status of their older adult patients and the factors influencing their decisions. Interviews were audio-recorded, transcribed, and thematically analyzed.

Results: Four themes were identified, the first of which described how physicians conceptualized frailty as a spectrum and dynamic in nature, but also struggled to conceptualize it without a formal definition in place. The remaining three themes described factors considered before determining patients' frailty statuses: physical characteristics (age, weight, medical conditions), functional characteristics (physical, cognitive, social) and living conditions (level of independence, availability of supports, physical environment).

Conclusions: Family physicians viewed frailty as multifactorial, dynamic, and inclusive of functional and environmental factors. This conceptualization can be useful to make comprehensive and flexible evaluations of frailty status in conjunction with more objective frailty tools.

Keywords: Frailty, Qualitative, Primary care, Family physicians, Older adults

Background

Clinical gestalt, also referred to as a "gut feeling" or "intuition," is a reasoning method whereby healthcare practitioners actively organize clinical perceptions into a coherent whole [1]. It is a form of heuristic pattern recognition that allows efficient decision-making even with limited information [1, 2]. Gut impressions have been subdivided into feelings of alarm, which can prompt further investigation and action on the part of the provider, and reassurance in the face of an uncertain prognosis or diagnosis [2, 3]. Its usefulness has been compared to common decision rules for identifying patients with venous thromboemboli [4–6]. Some argue that gestalt can lead to systematic errors in judgment and advocate to minimize clinician reliance on this method, while others assert that it is a necessary and useful part of clinical practice [1, 2]. Enhancing understanding about gestalt in the context of frailty is important because for most family practices which lack a structured process for identifying frailty, clinicians are using gestalt to identify frailty among older adults.

* Correspondence: lisa.mccarthy@utoronto.ca
†Equal contributors
1Women's College Hospital, 76 Grenville Street, Toronto, ON, Canada
2Leslie Dan Faculty of Pharmacy, University of Toronto, 144 College Street, Toronto, ON, Canada

While frailty is widely recognized as a clinical syndrome, there is no consensus on an operational definition, nor a gold standard tool to identify or measure it. Frailty is gaining increasing attention internationally due to its association with adverse health-related outcomes [7] including functional decline, dependency, recurrent falls, fractures, poor outcomes after discharge from emergency rooms, recurrent hospitalizations, institutionalization, and death [8, 9]. It is estimated that globally, approximately 10% of community-dwelling adults aged 65 and over are frail [10].

Developing a pragmatic approach for identifying frailty within the existing constraints of primary care settings is important because family physicians are the main providers of comprehensive healthcare to increasing numbers of older adults. Multiple tools evaluating frailty have been tested in a variety of settings. They differ widely in their features (e.g. length, time to complete, phone or in-person mode of administration), domains included, and outcomes measured. No one tool has emerged as optimal for identifying frailty in primary care and it is not clear if any of the instruments will perform better than physicians' judgment.

In the context of screening for frailty, some studies suggest that clinical gestalt can be useful for predicting poor health outcomes [11, 12]. However, physicians' gestalt has not been described beyond a categorical decision with respect to a patient's frailty, or without compromising the integrity of gestalt by guiding physician notions of frailty through the research process. Understanding the themes that arise when family physicians apply gestalt to their older adults is helpful for understanding how physicians' conceptualization of frailty is similar or different from existing frailty tools. Further, this understanding contributes to discussions about the importance of investment in screening strategies that are more costly and less easily implemented within practice.

This paper reports the qualitative component of a multi-methods study called INFER-PC (**Ident**ifying **F**railty Amongst Old**er** Adults in **P**rimary **C**are), conducted between November 2014 and December 2015, which aimed to: 1) compare the usefulness of existing frailty measures to identify an appropriate screening tool for use with older adults in primary care settings, and 2) assess the relationship between family physicians' clinical impressions of frailty relative to classifications from the existing frailty measures, 3) describe factors influencing family physicians' impressions of frailty in their older adult patients. In this report, we describe themes that emerged when family physicians were asked to share their gestalt impressions about the frailty status of their patients aged 80 and over. Specifically, we were interested in how family physicians conceptualize frailty, as well as what factors they consider when making decisions about frailty status.

Methods

The study was conducted within a large family medicine clinical teaching unit that has served its more than 20,000 patients in Toronto, Canada for over 20 years. Patients are assigned to a most responsible physician but have access to many onsite interprofessional care providers including nurses, dietitians, social workers, a pharmacist and an occupational therapist. All permanent staff physicians who were registered for a minimum of 6 months as the most responsible care provider for at least one community-dwelling adult aged 80 and over were invited to participate via email. For the purposes of the study, community dwelling adults were those who lived alone, with a caregiver, or with others (including patients receiving home care services).

A qualitative research design was used for study. Analysis of linguistic data provides non-numerical answers to research questions such as *how* physicians conceptualize frailty and *what* factors they consider when assessing frailty status [13]. Since there are no previous studies exploring physicians' gestalt about frailty, a broad exploratory approach was undertaken for this study using a low-inference descriptive qualitative methodology [14].

Consenting physicians participated in individual face-to-face sessions at their workplace lasting approximately 30 min. A non-clinician research assistant with experience interviewing health care professionals and familiarity with the medical team through other research projects conducted the sessions. During the sessions, physicians were asked to review and identify from their list of patients (generated from the electronic medical record) those who satisfied (or did not satisfy) the patient inclusion criteria (i.e., who was frail). To explore clinical gestalt, a think aloud approach was used to gather physicians' views about the frailty statuses of their patients. Think-aloud is "a research method in which participants speak aloud any words in their mind as they complete a task" [15]. The process involves working from memory, which has been shown to be the most effective way to assess higher-level thinking processes [15]. In this study, physicians were given the following prompt (developed by a multidisciplinary group of research team members including a pharmacist and several physicians, see Additional file 1 Interview Guide) and asked to respond, "yes", "no", "maybe" or "I do not know": "*There are many definitions of frailty, and many factors to consider in categorizing someone as vulnerable or frail. Using your clinical judgment, which of these older patients do you consider to be frail or at-risk for frailty?*" For patients considered frail, physicians were asked to share the reason(s) if known. To maintain the integrity of the think-aloud method, physicians were not probed further after the initial prompt.

Responses to clinical gestalt questions were compiled and themes developed using a thematic analysis approach [16, 17]. Interviews with physicians were audiotaped and transcribed verbatim, de-identified, then coded inductively using conventional word processing software [17]. To develop the initial coding scheme, including broad themes and subthemes, one senior research team member (L. McCarthy, a pharmacist-researcher with experience in qualitative research) and a pharmacist/Master of Science student (I. Famiyeh – studying qualitative research) reviewed the first 10 transcripts. IF used this scheme to code the remaining transcripts. A third team member (C. Korenvain, pharmacist and Master of Science student studying qualitative research) independently reviewed all of the transcripts and participated in revising the scheme with I. Famiyeh as the analysis progressed and new themes emerged. All researchers conducting and analyzing the interviews were female.

Sample size was determined by the number of physicians who agreed to be interviewed, out of 23 that were eligible. The researchers felt that saturation of themes was achieved after analyzing all the interviews, especially since the sample was not diverse with respect to context (from a single family practice clinic) [18].

The study was approved by the Women's College Hospital Institutional Research Ethics Board, 2013-0015-B.

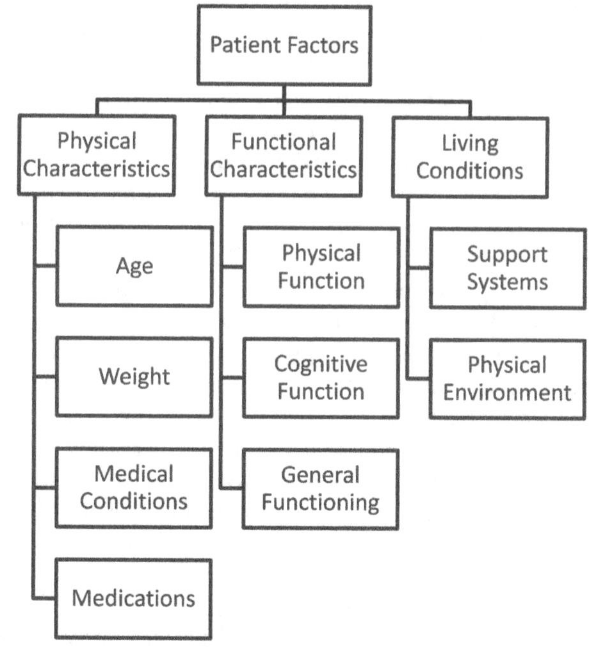

Fig. 1 Factors considered by family physicians when making decisions about frailty status

Results

Of 23 eligible physicians, 18 agreed to participate and were interviewed. Fourteen were female and the median number of years of experience as a family physician was 15 (minimum 3 years; maximum 41 years).

Emergent codes were grouped into four descriptive themes. One theme, physicians' concept of frailty (spectrum, dynamic, uncertainty), described how physicians conceptualized or defined frailty. The remaining three themes described factors that physicians considered before determining patients' frailty statuses (Fig. 1). These patient factors include: physical characteristics (age, weight, medical conditions, and medications), functional characteristics (physical, cognitive, general) and living conditions (availability of needed support systems, nature of physical environment).

Physicians' concept of frailty

Three subthemes were produced from physicians sharing their thoughts about what frailty means to them: spectrum, dynamic, and uncertainty.

Spectrum: This subtheme describes physicians' concept of frailty as being on a continuum or having different levels. One physician stated, "She's got a fair bit going on, again, there is a continuum" (Physician 3). Other physicians used unique terms to refer to different levels of frailty, such as "frailish" (Physician 4), "somewhat frail" (Physician 15), "at risk of frailty" (Physician 12), and "minimally frail" (Physician 16).

Dynamic: Physicians also described frailty in terms of how it changes in status over time. One physician talked about worsening frailty: "she [...] had a rapid decline recently and is now in palliative care home and probably going into the hospice in the next few days" (Physician 3). Sudden changes in status could occur after a single life event such as a myocardial infarction or sudden vision loss. While some physicians talked about improvement in frailty, others suggested that frailty could not always be improved: "It's not the kind of frailty that we improve on; he's getting worse no matter what..." (Physician 9).

Uncertainties: This subtheme refers to when physicians had uncertainties about the definitions of frailty or could not make a decision. One physician acknowledged the uncertainty and lack of reliability in making a decision about a patient's frailty status: "I mean it would be interesting if you guys [researchers] meet these people and have a completely different perception than I do because maybe I'm wrong you know" (Physician 15). Another physician described improvement in frailty contrary to expectations:

> "I think she may be [frail], but she's working on it...she couldn't get out of her chair very well and so I asked her that every time she went to the toilet to practice standing up and sitting down five times and she came back 2 weeks later and she said "It's a miracle" and she can actually, she's much better now

just because I got her to do a very simple exercise" (Physician 9).

Another source of uncertainty was around how much emphasis should be given to one factor versus another, "...frailty, how much is it a cognitive thing, how much is it a physical thing?" (Physician 3). Although Physician 3 considered both cognitive and physical aspects of frailty, other physicians defined it as purely a physical entity, "frailty is a physical thing... I mean I thought frailty might encompass the cognitive but in my conception of frailty it's a physical issue not a dimension in cognition" (Physician 8). There were times when physicians would consider patients as both frail and not frail. "...I would say no because she's independent but yes because she's totally blind and can't do some things" (Physician 17). One physician correlated frailty with patients' visit frequency, "I think people that haven't come in for a long time probably are frail and that's why they haven't come in...Because they are not easily able to come in cause the less frail seniors I see very often; more for social stimulation and visits, whereas the more frail find it harder to come in" (Physician 19).

Factors considered in frailty decision-making

Physical characteristics

This theme describes physical characteristics that physicians took into consideration while deciding on their patients' frailty statuses.

Age: Most physicians considered their patients' age in their frailty decisions. While most physicians considered age as a risk factor for frailty among other factors, "...he's ninety-two and he's got cardiovascular disease, congestive heart failure, degenerative disk disease of his lower back" (Physician 6), others based their decisions mainly on their patients' older age: "I would say yes...more because of age...events due to her age and her status" (Physician 11). "She must be what like ninety-two now or something? She is getting up there...Yeah I would qualify her as frail" (Physician 15). In contrast, some physicians did not consider their patients as frail despite their older age. One physician stated, "I don't think he's frail even though he's eighty-four" (Physician 1).

Weight: Seven physicians factored in their patients' weight in their thought processes and decisions about frailty. Five physicians placed emphasis on weight and considered patients who are "thin" as being frail. One physician mentioned, "if they're thin I think they're frail...I have a hard time thinking about someone who is big as being frail and I might classify someone who's thin with the same level of function as being frail" (Physician 8). For other physicians, a patient's weight was not the overriding factor, "she is incredibly frail.... she's huge but frail" (Physician 4). Likewise, another physician expressed: "...is she frail? I'm going to say no, she has COPD [Chronic Obstructive Pulmonary Disease], she's very thin, but cognitively fully intact...functions well, has good social supports" (Physician 10).

Medical Conditions: Patients' medical conditions influenced the thought processes of 15 physicians. Some physicians considered the presence of multiple medical conditions as a contributing factor to frailty: "...has multiple chronic things but still manages to function quite well but she's certainly at risk" (Physician 3). Others made a decision based on the consequences of a single medical condition: "she is incredibly frail...she has the worst gout I've ever seen and she's very disabled" (Physician 4). The presence of a specific medical condition did not always lead to the conclusion that a patient was frail, "I think...is not frail although she has had cancer..." (Physician 4).

Medications: Only one physician considered patients' number of medications in deciding about frailty: "...is frail for sure, so she's post stroke, um has many meds, cognition is okay but...her ability to function independently is probably limited but she's well supported" (Physician 10).

Functional characteristics

Subthemes about patients' functional characteristics that emerged during the physician interviews were physical, cognitive, and general function.

Physical Function: This subtheme refers to situations in which physicians considered their patients' ability to carry out physical tasks. Physical function was mainly discussed in terms of mobility. While some patients were considered to be frail due to issues with mobility, "...yes, limited ambulation and has help with all her IADLs [Instrumental Activities of Daily Living]" (Physician 2), others were not: "...I don't know if I would define her as frail, she does have mobility issues, she is a falls, a big falls risk but she lives on her own, she is fiercely independent..." (Physician 1).

Cognitive Function: Twelve physicians talked about their patients' cognitive function. For some physicians, the presence of cognitive impairment alone puts a patient at risk of frailty, "she still goes and exercises...but she's had some cognitive issues, mild cognitive stuff.... the cognitive stuff is a risk, the physical stuff she's been amazing" (Physician 3). Others listed cognition among other factors that contribute to frailty: "...is frail, so he's got mobility, cognition...he's fallen many times, and he's got, so diabetes, seizures, so like multiple conditions, poly-pharmacy, lots of side effects from drugs" (Physician 10).

General Function: This subtheme describes discussions about function that did not specifically fall under physical or cognitive function. Physicians often talked about function in terms of level of independence. Most physicians concluded that their patients were not frail because they functioned well independently, "she's actually quite independent, quite high functioning, she has a chronic underlying condition and she has arthritis, so she has some limitations from arthritic knees but she's pretty high functioning and so to me she is not particularly frail" (Physician 11). Similarly, the inability to function independently was the reason some patients were considered frail: "she's reliant on her caregivers but yeah I think she was, she I would...Define her as frail" (Physician 1). For other physicians however, patients' ability to function independently did not automatically make them non-frail: "This is a maybe, she's a maybe, she's in, in some ways she's no because she functions independently, but in some ways she's yes because she has multiple hospital admissions" (Physician 2).

Living conditions

In terms of living conditions, physicians considered patients' availability of needed support systems and the nature of their physical environment.

Availability of support systems: This subtheme refers to instances when physicians considered the presence or absence of a patient support system in their decisions about frailty. The support systems were social (family members, friends) and professional (e.g., home care). The presence of a support system was seen as a sign of robustness protecting the patient against worsening frailty: "she is frail; she copes because her husband looks after her" (Physician 14). "[The patient] is frail for sure... but she has good family support. Just her ability to function independently is probably limited but she's well supported" (Physician 10). Similarly, patients who lacked support systems were perceived to be frail, "like socially he is frail...like he just needs supports" (Physician 19). In contrast, for some physicians, the fact that a patient required support indicated his/her frailty status, "... is the frailest person I know, she has twenty-four hour care" (Physician 4).

Physical Environment: Two physicians took into consideration their patients' physical environment during their thought processes about frailty. "[She] is definitely a yes, lives in a three story house, and is extraordinarily resistant to moving...she wouldn't let me in when I went to see her because it is packed with papers I heard" (Physician 4).

Discussion

Summary

This study provides insight into the thought processes of family physicians that underlie their clinical impressions of the frailty status of their older patients. Physicians conceptualized frailty as on a spectrum and dynamic in nature, but also faced uncertainties in trying to identify frail patients or conceptualizing frailty. Physicians took a number of factors into consideration before deciding on whether or not their patients were frail, including physical characteristics (age, weight, medical conditions), functional characteristics (physical, cognitive, social) and living conditions (level of independence, availability of supports, physical environment).

Strengths and limitations

To maintain the integrity of the think-aloud approach, physicians were not probed to provide in-depth explanation during the interviews. The absence of probing could have prevented automatic thinking patterns from being verbalized [15]. This led to some physicians listing different risk factors of frailty without discussing the extent to which the factors influenced their decisions. Despite being asked to explain the reasoning behind their decisions about frailty, some physicians may have considered additional factors that were not verbalized, and would therefore only provide partial insight into their thought process. It is possible that participants only articulated the most prominent factors in their decision-making process for a particular patient case.

The study findings do not necessarily apply to all family physicians. All interviewed physicians work in a single large urban family practice clinic, limiting generalizability of findings to different contexts. The physicians in this study are mostly experienced and seemed familiar with their patients' health profiles. More experienced clinicians are more adept at pattern recognition within their area of expertise and may be more reliant on gestalt [1, 2]. Having immediate access to more information about patients through familiarity and experience with them may have increased their confidence in their decision-making about frailty.

The investigators analyzing study results (I. Famiyeh, C. Korenvain and L. McCarthy) have all practiced at the study site family practice clinic or in similar settings as pharmacists or pharmacy students, and may therefore have their own gestalt impressions of frailty. Although none of these researchers were familiar with the specific patients discussed or had close relationships with the physicians interviewed, their personal conceptualizations of frailty may have influenced the analysis. For example, CK admits that the physicians' responses have expanded her conceptualization of frailty to include a patient's environment. This finding was discovered in part because it surprised the researcher by contrasting with her own preconceived notions.

Comparison with existing literature

Physicians' conceptualization of frailty as being on a spectrum and dynamic in nature has been reported previously in the literature. As Rouge et al. state, "frailty should be considered as a dynamic and potentially reversible process and as a continuum with intermediate states that can be modified (robustness <-> frailty <-> disability)" [19]. Physicians' clinical impressions can in this way introduce flexibility into frailty screening in primary care, which a one-time or scheduled periodic assessment via objective tools may not provide.

In general, physicians did not attribute one factor to be the sole determinant of their patients' frailty statuses. They often considered other contributing factors and made a decision based on which factor they deemed most important for that patient. Risk factors for frailty that were given greater emphasis were those that appeared to affect patients' ability to function in general. For example, medical conditions that were associated with frailty were those that were disabling (gout, osteoporosis). This is consistent with some literature definitions of frailty, which state that "frailty can be thought of as a combination of factors that influence a person's physiologic state to the extent that function is greatly reduced and the person becomes more vulnerable to external stressors" [20].

Participants considered patient factors in their decisions that were beyond the scope of traditional definitions of frailty based solely on physiology [7, 21]: living conditions and functional characteristics. The incongruence between research and practitioner conceptualization of frailty has been described previously [21]. Some researchers have problematized the fact that existing frailty tools do not seem to distinguish between physiologic vulnerability and functional compromise, and do not always take into account factors outside the patient [21]. Subjective frailty determinations by US physicians highly correlated with a lack of social support noted in the patient's EMR [Electronic Medical Record] [11], which is consistent with this study's finding that physicians' gestalt impressions of frailty encompass factors beyond physiology.

Implications for research and practice

Physicians' conceptualization of frailty as dynamic and on a spectrum introduces more flexibility into frailty assessment than existing objective tools can provide. Since some participants described changes in frailty status that occurred immediately following a significant medical or psychosocial life event, clinical gestalt could prompt a re-evaluation of frailty status and the need for additional supports in an ad hoc fashion. The long-term relationships that family physicians have with patients provide opportunities for monitoring frailty status over time, and clinical gestalt can facilitate this process.

Accounting for a broad range of patient and environmental factors, as family physicians' gestalt did in this study, may prompt family physicians to link patients, who are functionally limited or living in suboptimal conditions, with supports to address these issues and thus reduce the risk of adverse health outcomes.

This study does not provide evidence to support or refute using clinical gestalt as a replacement for more objective frailty measures. Comparisons between family physicians' gestalt decisions about frailty and the results of more objective frailty tools will be reported elsewhere. However, the dynamic conceptualization of frailty by physicians allowing assessment flexibility, as well as their attention to functional and environmental factors contributing to patient vulnerability, suggests that clinical gestalt is a valuable addition to a physicians' frailty assessment toolkit.

Conclusions

This study provides insight into the factors family physicians consider when making frailty determinations in the course of their daily practices, and how they conceptualize frailty. Findings contribute to a broader discussion about effective approaches to identify and address frailty in older patients by introducing how clinical gestalt can be used to compliment frailty identification and prediction by more objective tools. Study findings could contribute to the development of future models that would acknowledge, and perhaps make use of, clinical gestalt as part of a process used by family physicians to assess and monitor frailty in their patients, to optimally support their ongoing health and safety.

Abbreviations

COPD: Chronic obstructive pulmonary disease; EMR: Electronic medical record; IADL: Instrumental activities of daily living; INFER-PC: Identifying Frailty Amongst Older Adults in Primary Care Study

Acknowledgements

The authors wish to acknowledge Sara Karlsson, research assistant at Women's College Hospital, for her contributions to this study.

Funding

This project was supported by the Canadian Institutes for Health Research (Grant: CHL 126214) (www.cihr-irsc.gc.ca). The funders had no role in designing the study, collecting, analysing or interpreting the data, the writing of the article or in the decision to submit it for publication.

Authors' contributions

LM, SD, CW, PR conceived of the study and obtained funding. LM managed data collection. IF and CK completed inductive coding of the transcripts under the supervision of LM, SD, CW, PR. IF and CK wrote the first draft of the manuscript. All authors have read and approved the final manuscript.

Authors' information

Dr. Rochon holds the Retired Teachers of Ontario (RTO/ERO) Chair in Geriatric Medicine at the University of Toronto. Dr. Whitehead holds the BMO Financial Group Chair in Health Professions Research at University Health Network.

Competing interests
The authors declare that they have no competing interests.

Author details
[1]Women's College Hospital, 76 Grenville Street, Toronto, ON, Canada. [2]Leslie Dan Faculty of Pharmacy, University of Toronto, 144 College Street, Toronto, ON, Canada. [3]Faculty of Medicine, University of Toronto, 1 King's College Circle, Toronto, ON, Canada. [4]Women's College Research Institute, 76 Grenville St, Toronto, ON M5S 1B2, Canada. [5]The Wilson Centre, University Health Network, 200 Elizabeth Street, Toronto, ON, Canada.

References

1. Cook C. Is clinical gestalt good enough? J Man Manip Ther. 2009;17(1):6–7.
2. Stolper E, Van de Wiel M, Van Royen P, Van Bokhoven M, Van der Weijden T, Dinant GJ. Gut feelings as a third track in general practitioners' diagnostic reasoning. J Gen Intern Med. 2011;26(2):197–203.
3. Stolper E, Van Royen P, Van de Wiel M, Van Bokhoven M, Houben P, Van der Weijden T, et al. Consensus on gut feelings in general practice. BMC Fam Pract. 2009;10:66.
4. Runyon MS, Richman PB, Kline JA, Group PERCS. Emergency medicine practitioner knowledge and use of decision rules for the evaluation of patients with suspected pulmonary embolism: variations by practice setting and training level. Acad Emerg Med. 2007;14(1):53–7.
5. Chunilal SD, Eikelboom JW, Attia J, Miniati M, Panju AA, Simel DL, et al. Does this patient have pulmonary embolism? JAMA. 2003;290(21):2849–58.
6. Geersing GJ, Janssen KJ, Oudega R, van Weert H, Stoffers H, Hoes A, et al. Diagnostic classification in patients with suspected deep venous thrombosis: physicians' judgement or a decision rule? Br J Gen Pract. 2010;60(579):742–8.
7. Lacas A, Rockwood K. Frailty in primary care: a review of its conceptualization and implications for practice. BMC Med. 2012;10:4.
8. Hastings SN, Purser JL, Johnson KS, Sloane RJ, Whitson HE. Frailty predicts some but not all adverse outcomes in older adults discharged from the emergency department. J Am Geriatr Soc. 2008;56(9):1651–7.
9. Borges LL, Menezes RL. Definitions and markers of frailty: a systematic review of literature. Rev Clin Gerontol. 2011;21(1):67–77.
10. Collard RM, Boter H, Schoevers RA, Oude Voshaar RC. Prevalence of frailty in community-dwelling older persons: a systematic review. J Am Geriatr Soc. 2012;60(8):1487–92.
11. Anzaldi LJ, Davison A, Boyd CM, Leff B, Kharrazi H. Comparing clinician descriptions of frailty and geriatric syndromes using electronic health records: a retrospective cohort study. BMC Geriatr. 2017;17(1):248.
12. Sutorius FL, Hoogendijk EO, Prins BA, van Hout HP. Comparison of 10 single and stepped methods to identify frail older persons in primary care: diagnostic and prognostic accuracy. BMC Fam Pract. 2016;17:102.
13. Green J, Thorogood N. Qualitative methodology and Health Research. Qualitative methods for Health Research. 2nd ed. Los Angeles: SAGE; 2009. p. 3–34.
14. Sandelowski M. Whatever happened to qualitative description? Res Nurs Health. 2000;23(4):334–40.
15. Charters E. The use of think-aloud methods in qualitative research an introduction to think-aloud methods. Brock Education. 2010;12(2):68–82.
16. Barnett-Page E, Thomas J. Methods for the synthesis of qualitative research: a critical review. BMC Med Res Methodol. 2009;9:59.
17. Braun V, Clarke V. Using thematic analysis in psychology. Qual Res Psychol. 2006;3:77–101.
18. Guest G, Bunce A, Johnson L. How many interviews are enough? Field Methods. 2006;18(1):59–82.
19. Rougé Bugat ME, Cestac P, Oustric S, Vellas B, Nourhashemi F. Detecting frailty in primary care: a major challenge for primary care physicians. J Am Med Dir Assoc. 2012;13(8):669–72.
20. Crome P, Lally F. Frailty: joining the giants. CMAJ. 2011;183(8):889–90.
21. Whitson HE, Purser JL, Cohen HJ. Frailty thy name is ... Phrailty? J Gerontol A Biol Sci Med Sci. 2007;62(7):728–30.

6

Use of a self-rating scale to monitor depression severity in recurrent GP consultations in primary care – does it really make a difference?

C. Wikberg[1], J. Westman[2], E-L. Petersson[1,3], M. E. H. Larsson[3,4], M. André[5], R. Eggertsen[1,3], J. Thorn[1,3], H. Ågren[6] and C. Björkelund[1*]

Abstract

Background: Little information is available about whether the use of self-assessment instruments in primary care affects depression course and outcome. The purpose was to evaluate whether using a depression self-rating scale in recurrent person-centred GP consultations affected depression severity, quality of life, medication use, and sick leave frequency.

Methods: Patients in the intervention group met their GP regularly at least 4 times during the 3 months intervention. In addition to treatment as usual (TAU), patients completed a self-assessment instrument (Montgomery-Asberg Depression Rating Scale) on each occasion, and then GPs used the completed instrument as the basis for a person-centred discussion of changes in depression symptoms. The control group received TAU. Frequency of visits in the TAU arm was the result of the GPs' and patients' joint assessments of care need in each case. Depression severity was measured with Beck Depression Inventory-II (BDI-II), quality of life with EQ-5D, and psychological well-being with the General Health Questionnaire-12 (GHQ-12). Data on sick leave, antidepressant and sedatives use, and care contacts were collected from electronic patient records. All variables were measured at baseline and 3, 6, and 12 months. Mean intra-individual changes were compared between the intervention and TAU group.

Results: There were no significant differences between the intervention and control group in depression severity reduction or remission rate, change in quality of life, psychological well-being, sedative prescriptions, or sick leave during the whole 12-month follow-up. However, significantly more patients in the intervention group continued antidepressants until the 6 month follow-up (86/125 vs 78/133, $p < 0.05$).

Conclusions: When GPs used a depression self-rating scale in recurrent consultations, patients more often continued antidepressant medication according to guidelines, compared to TAU patients. However, reduction of depressive symptoms, remission rate, quality of life, psychological well-being, sedative use, sick leave, and health care use 4-12 months was not significantly different from the TAU group. These findings suggest that frequent use of depression rating scales in person-centred primary care consultations has no further additional effect on patients' depression or well-being, sick leave, or health care use.

Keywords: Depression, Primary care, Self-assessment instrument, Adherence, Sick-leave, Quality-of- life

* Correspondence: cecilia.bjorkelund@allmed.gu.se
[1]Department of Primary Health Care/Public Health and Community Medicine, Institute of Medicine, Sahlgrenska Academy, University of Gothenburg, Gothenburg, Sweden
Full list of author information is available at the end of the article

Background

Depression is a leading cause of disability and affects 10 to 15% of the population of most countries in the world [1, 2]. A majority of patients with depression are treated in primary care, and approximately 75% of antidepressants are prescribed by general practitioners (GPs) [3, 4]. The usual treatment for depression in Swedish primary care, as in primary care in other countries, depends upon symptom severity. Most people treated for depression in primary care receive one or more of the following: early reassessment (watchful waiting) and symptom monitoring by their GP, cognitive behavioural therapy or other psychotherapy, and antidepressant medication [5, 6].

Depression guidelines recommend that GPs regularly use self-rating scales to evaluate and monitor symptoms in patients with depression [5, 6]. These guidelines, however, have been based largely on clinical expertise rather than on the results of randomised controlled trials [3]. Furthermore, most self-rating scales recommended for detecting and monitoring depression were designed in psychiatric care settings and have not been adapted for use in primary care [3]. Little information is thus available about whether the use of such instruments in primary care affects depression symptoms, treatment, rehabilitation, or recovery [7]. We know that using such scales for screening does not improve detection or management of depression in settings such as primary care [8]. However, we do not know whether using a self-rating scale to follow the course of depression in person-centred primary care consultations improves treatment and outcomes of depression.

The depression rating scale most commonly used in Swedish primary health care is the Montgomery-Asberg Depression Rating Scale [9]. However, its use has mainly been evaluated in psychiatric settings [9, 10]. MADRS-S is sensitive to changes in symptoms of depression and is therefore a valuable tool in person-centred consultations [10–12]. However, a qualitative study based on interviews with Swedish GPs showed that many GPs thought that MADRS-S was of limited utility in consultations [13]. It is thus still unclear whether or not future guidelines should recommend mandatory use of depression self-rating scales in primary health care.

The aim of the current study was to evaluate in a randomised control trial whether using a depression rating scale (MADRS-S) in recurrent person-centred GP consultations affected depression severity, quality of life, overall psychological well-being, antidepressant and sedative use, sick leave, and health care use in a long time perspective.

Methods

The PRI-SMA study (PRImary care Self-assessment Montgomery-Asberg) was a multicentre, controlled trial that took place at primary health care centres (PHCCs) and was randomised at the GP level. The GPs randomised to the intervention used a patient self-rating scale at recurrent monthly patient visits in addition to providing usual care. The GPs randomised to the control condition provided treatment as usual (TAU). The intervention lasted for 3 months. Adult patients who presented with a recent depressive episode (mild/moderate depression) at the PHCC were recruited to the study by the GPs.

The trial took place at 22 Swedish PHCCs between March 2010 and December 2013. All 98 PHCCs in the region were invited to participate in the intervention; 22 agreed to participate.

Randomisation of GPs at primary health care centres

All GPs took part in an information meeting about the study. All GPs also met with the study leaders when the leaders visited each participating PHCC at the time of the intervention start-up at that PHCC. Before the intervention started, the GPs at each PHCC were randomised to either intervention treatment or TAU. All GP names were written on slips of paper and mixed in a container, and an administrative employee blinded to the aim of the trial drew names. The GP whose name was first drawn was assigned to the intervention group, the GP whose name was drawn second was assigned to the control group, and so on until all names were drawn.

Study procedure

Patient recruitment took place at one PHCC at a time. During the 2 week recruitment period, a research nurse worked full-time at the PHCC to facilitate patient recruitment, collect patient data, and support PHCC staff.

Inclusion of patients

Study participants were patients aged 18 and up who visited the PHCCs and were identified and diagnosed by a GP with a new episode of mild/moderate depressive disorder [14].

During the 2 week recruitment period, all randomised GPs who met patients they suspected of having depression used the PRIME-MD diagnostic instrument to confirm or reject the diagnosis of depression in accordance with DSM-IV criteria [14]. All patients who fulfilled the diagnostic criteria for depressive disorder, i.e. mild to moderate (BDI score ≤36), were asked if they would like to participate in the study.

Inclusion criteria were: written informed consent, age ≥18 years, diagnosed with mild to moderate depressive disorder and either not prescribed antidepressant medication or had no changes in antidepressant medication during the preceding 2 months.

Exclusion criteria were: lack of written informed consent, antidepressant medication introduced or changed during the 2 months prior to baseline, diagnosed with severe depressive disorder (BDI-II >36, confirmed by diagnostic procedure by GP), diagnosed with severe mental disorder (i.e., bipolar disorder, antisocial personality disorder, psychosis, substance use disorder, or other serious mental disorder), suicidal ideation or earlier suicide attempts, did not speak or understand Swedish, and/or had cognitive disabilities that made it difficult or impossible to complete the assessment instruments, including MADRS-S.

Intervention

The intervention consisted of using a patient depression self-rating scale (MADRS-S) in recurrent monthly consultations during the 3-month intervention. Patients made 4 visits to their GPs, at which time they completed MADRS-S to monitor changes in their depressive symptoms that were then discussed in the person-centred consultation [15, 16]. MADRS-S was used as a supplement to, rather than as a substitute for, TAU.

The GPs randomised to the group that provided the intervention received four hours of guidance about how to include the results of MADRS-S in the person-centred consultation. The intervention GPs also received a video CD with the same pre-recorded information. The person-centred consultations involved patients and GPs collaborating to increase patients' ability to manage their depression. The guidance therefore included a reminder to the GPs that MADRS-S was used for the sake of the patients rather than the GPs.

Treatment as usual

The GPs randomised to the group that would provide TAU were instructed to manage patients with depression the same way they usually did (but with the addition of the diagnostic procedure in the initial consultation). In general Swedish GPs are very knowledgeable about and use of person-centred consultation methods in their daily practice of the kind described in Maguire 2002 [16].

Three months after baseline, patients in the control group were followed up in an appointment with a nurse at the PHCC.

Data collection procedure

A study nurse collected data from participants in the intervention and control groups during the first visit (baseline), at a follow-up visit to the PHCC at the end of the intervention (3 months after baseline), and by postal questionnaires 6 and 12 months after baseline (see Additional files 1 and 2).

Measures

Background variables

Background information was obtained by a questionnaire at the patients' first visit to the PHCC. Age was measured as age in years, gender as female or male. Marital status was dichotomised as single or married/cohabiting. Children living at home was dichotomised as participants who had children <18 years living at home vs. participants not having children living at home. Educational level was identified as as lower educational level (primary school or vocational school), middle educational level (high school) and higher educational level (college or university). Employment status was dichotomised as working/studying vs. unemployed/retired.

Place of birth was dichotomised as born in one of the Nordic countries vs. born outside the Nordic countries. Smoking status was categorised as "non-smokers" (participants who had not smoked during the last year), "sometimes smokers" (those who only smoked a single cigarette per week or more seldom), and "smokers" (more frequent smoking). Leisure-time physical activity was categorised as i) no or almost no physical activity during leisure time, ii) activity ≥4 hrs. per week, and iii) intensive (several times a week and vigorously).

Outcomes

Depression severity; Assessed before (at baseline) and after the intervention with the Beck Depression Inventory-II (BDI-II) and categorised as mild (BDI-II score >13-19), moderate (BDI-II score 20-28), and high moderate (BDI-II score, 29-36) [17, 18].

Remission; Identified as a BDI-II score ≤ 13 at 3-month follow up.

Quality of life; Measured with the standardised EQ-5D instrument [19, 20].

Overall psychological well-being; Assessed with the 12-item General Health Questionnaire (GHQ-12) (response scale 0-3) [21].

Prescriptions for antidepressants; Information on this measure was obtained from patients' electronic patient records (EPRs) and from responses to the patient questionnaires and dichotomised as yes (used) or no (did not use). Guidelines indicate that treatment should not be stopped before 6-12 months after recovery [5].

Prescriptions for sedatives; Information on prescriptions for sedatives was obtained from patients' electronic patient records (EPRs) and from responses to the patient questionnaires and dichotomised as yes (used) or no (did not use).

Sick leave; Information on sick leave was obtained from EPRs and responses to the patient questionnaires. Sick leave was used both as a dichotomous variable (yes or no) and as number of days of sick leave.

Health care use; This measure comprised information on number of visits to GPs, number of visits to nurses, number of visits to psychologists/psychotherapists, and total number of visits to the PHCC. Information was obtained from EPRs by study personnel and divided into the number of visits between 0 and 3 months, and 4 and 12 months.

Statistical methods

The student's t-test (paired) was used to compare mean intra-individual changes in the intervention and TAU groups. Two-sided Chi-square or Mann Whitney U-tests were used to compare frequencies. Statistical significance was set at $p < 0.05$. Logistic regression models were used to examine whether changes in the BDI-II, EQ-5D, and GHQ-12 variables from baseline to 3, 6 and 12 months follow-ups were associated with sex, age, education, antidepressant medication, and group assignment (intervention/TAU).The results are presented as odds ratios (OR) with 95% confidence intervals (CI). All analyses were performed in SPSS. All analyses were conducted on an intention to treat basis.

Power calculation

Power was calculated for the BDI-II-score outcome on the basis of empirical experience of the variation in this factor, taking into account that GPs were the unit of randomisation. The power estimate was based on the assumption of an alpha error = 0.05 and a beta error = 0.20 (power = 0.80). Given an expected effect difference of 2 units (BDI-II) over time between the intervention and TAU groups, we calculated that we would need 105 patients in each group to achieve sufficient statistical power. To safeguard for dropouts, we recruited 20% more patients than the power calculation indicated that we needed.

Ethics

The Regional Ethical Review Board in Gothenburg, Sweden approved this study (Dnr 746-09; T612-10). Prior to inclusion and after receiving oral and written information about the study, participants provided written informed consent. The trial was registered at ClinicalTrials.gov (Identifier: NCT01402206) [22].

Results

Of the 91 participating GPs, 45 were randomised into a group that provided the intervention and 46 into a group that provided TAU. The participating GPs enrolled 258 patients, and the flow of the patients through the study is shown in Fig. 1 [23]. There was no significant difference in participation rate in the patients in the intervention and control groups at the 3-, 6- or 12-months follow-ups.

Table 1 presents the background characteristics of the study population. No significant differences were found between the participants in the intervention and TAU groups at baseline.

There was a statistically significant difference between participants and drop-outs during the study concerning age (mean age 44.3 in participants, mean age 37.3 in drop-outs, $p = 0.02$), gender (male 14/62, 22.6%, female 16/166, 9.6%, $p = 0.034$), and ethnicity (born in Sweden 21/194, 10.8%, and born outside Sweden 9/32, 28.1%, $p = 0.035$)

Figures 2, 3, and 4 shows depression symptoms (BDI-II), quality of life (EQ-5D), and overall psychological well-being (GHQ-12) in intervention and TAU groups at baseline and 3, 6, and 12 months (boxplots). All patients who participated in the study, both those in the intervention and those in the TAU group, improved in

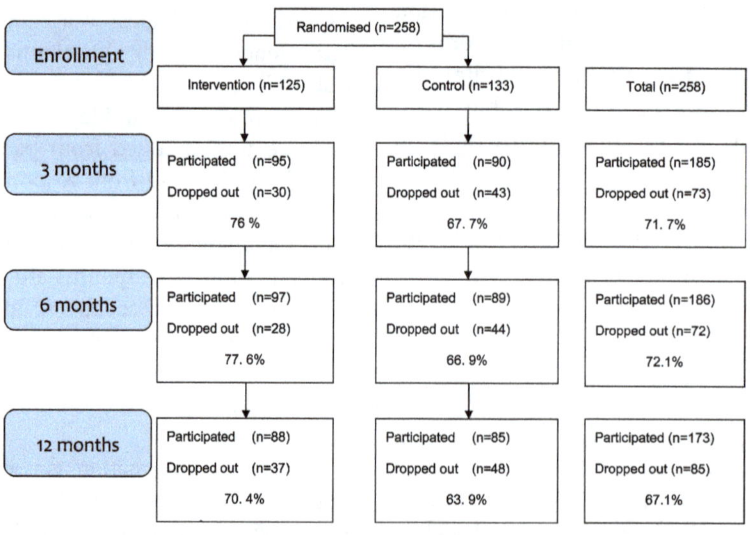

Fig. 1 PRI-SMA-Study (CONSORT Flowchart)

Table 1 Baseline characteristics of participants in the PRI-SMA trial ($n = 258$)

Characteristics	Total *n* (%)	Intervention *n* (%)	TAU[a] *n* (%)	*p*
Participants	258	125	133	
Age (years, mean)	43.48	44.84	42.19	0.2
men	76 (29.5)	31 (24.8)	45 (33.8)	
women	182 (70.5)	94 (75.2)	88 (66.2)	0.1
Marital status				
single	118 (45.7)	61 (48.8)	57 (42.9)	
married/cohabiting	140 (54.3)	64 (51.2)	76 (57.1)	
children <18 years at home	82 (43.2)	36 (40.4)	46 (45.5)	0.5
Lower educational level	34 (13.2)	17 (13.7)	17 (12.8)	
Middle educational level	115 (44.7)	61 (49.2)	54 (40.6)	
High educational level	108 (42.0)	46 (37.1)	62 (46.6)	0.3
Employment				
working/studying	181 (80.8)	90 (81.1)	91 (80.5)	
unemployed/retired	43 (19.2)	21 (18.9)	22 (19.5)	0.9
Born outside the Nordic countries	41 (16)	19 (15.3)	22 (16.7)	0.8
Smoking (yes or sometimes)	75 (29.4)	36 (29.3)	39 (29.5)	0.9
Leisure-time physical activity				
never	109 (42.1)	57 (46)	52 (39.1)	
at least 4 hrs/week	124 (48.2)	55 (44.4)	69 (51.9)	
intensive	24 (9.3)	12 (9.7)	12 (9,0)	0.5
Depression				
mild (BDI-II 12-19)	32 (13)	16 (13.6)	16 (12.4)	
moderate (BDI-II 20-28)	82 (33.2)	39 (33.1)	43 (33.3)	
high moderate (BDI-II 29-36)	68 (27.5)	35 (29.7)	33 (25.6)	0.9

[a]*TAU* treatment as usual

all three variables between baseline and 3 months but there were no significant differences in mean changes (mean of intra-individual Δ) between the groups. Improvements were substantial in both groups; at the 3-month follow-up, nearly half the patients no longer had depression (BDI <13) (49% in the intervention and 47.3% in the TAU group, $p = 0.89$). We also performed logistic regression analyses. The models showed that at the 12-month follow-up, older age was associated with improved BDI-II score (OR 1.05, CI 1.01-1.99), and a higher level of education was associated with improved EQ-5D score (OR 3.9, CI 1.77 8.73). The factors added to the model (sex, age, education, antidepressant medication, and participation in the intervention or TAU group) explained the same amount of variation in both the intervention and TAU groups. Thus, the difference between the groups remained non-significant (data not shown). No adverse events were reported from intervention or TAU group.

Table 2 shows differences between the intervention and TAU groups in the percent of patients who had prescriptions for antidepressants and sedatives. At baseline, 22% of patients in the intervention group and 32% of patients in the TAU group were on maintenance antidepressant medication. After 3 months, the proportion of patients with prescriptions for antidepressant medication was 72% in both the intervention and the TAU group. At the 6-month follow-up, the proportion of patients taking antidepressants had dropped to 69% in the intervention group and 59% in the TAU group (p = 0.007). At the 12-month follow-up, there were no significant differences in the percent of patients who had prescriptions for antidepressants or sedatives in the intervention and TAU groups (Table 2).

Table 3 shows the mean number of days of sick leave by patient group. There were no significant differences in the percentage of patients on sick leave in the intervention and TAU groups between baseline and 3 months, or 4 -12 months, or during the entire study period. The mean total duration of sick leave (days) was not significantly different between the intervention and TAU groups (Table 3).

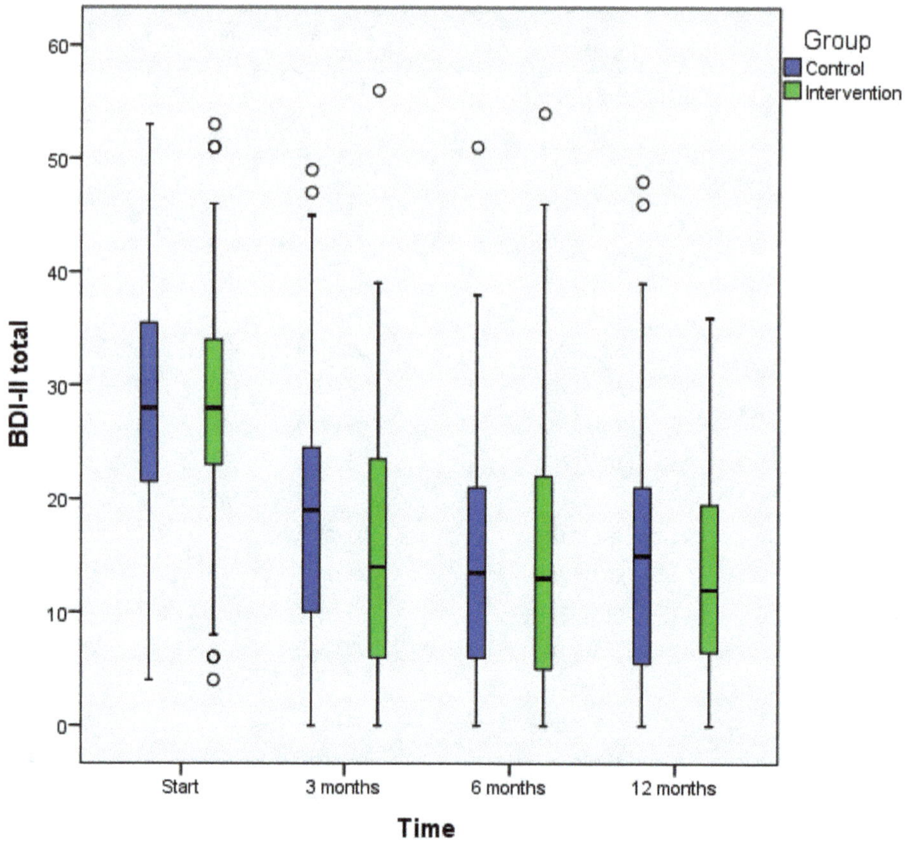

Fig. 2 Depression severity (BDI-II values) in the intervention and TAU groups. Boxplots for baseline, 3-months follow up, 6-months follow up, and 12-months follow up. The outcome variable is presented as box plot with medians, minimum and maximum values and lower and upper quartiles. Y-axis: BDI-II, X-axis: time 0, 3, 6, 12 months. Outliers (*circle*) are cases with values between 1.5 and 3 times the interquartile range (5 cases with BDI-II ≥50 in patients with difficulties in Swedish language, where complementary diagnostic procedure by the GP ended up on medium depressive disorder)

Health care use

Mean number of visits at the PHCC, including visits to GP, nurse, psychologist/therapist and total visits to PHCC, was compared between intervention and TAU groups. All information was obtained from EPRs (Table 4). We also compared the total number of visits. There were no significant differences between the intervention and TAU groups regarding these outcomes, during the total 12-month follow-up period. However, during the 0-3 month period, the TAU group made significantly more visits to psychologists/psychotherapists than the intervention group and the intervention group made significantly more total visits to the PHCC than the TAU group.

Discussion

In this RCT, which evaluated use of a depression self-rating scale in recurrent person-centred GP consultations, more patients in the intervention than control group adhered to antidepressant treatment for the recommended 6 months. However, compared to TAU, there were no significant differences between the effects on depression symptom reduction, quality of life or overall psychological well-being, sedative use, sick leave, or health care use. These findings suggest that recurrent use of depression self-assessment scales in person-centred primary care consultations does have an effect on antidepressant medication adherence, but has no further additional effects, compared to the treatment usually provided in Swedish primary care.

Strengths and weaknesses of the study

The intervention was conducted in ordinary primary care rather than advertising for participants, which would have resulted in a sample that was not representative of patients in primary health care. The study compared the intervention with a TAU group rather than using a control group that consisted of patients on a waiting list. Studies of the effects of cognitive behavioural therapy show that being on a waiting list has a nocebo effect (i.e. results in worsening depression symptoms), which in turn makes intervention effects appear

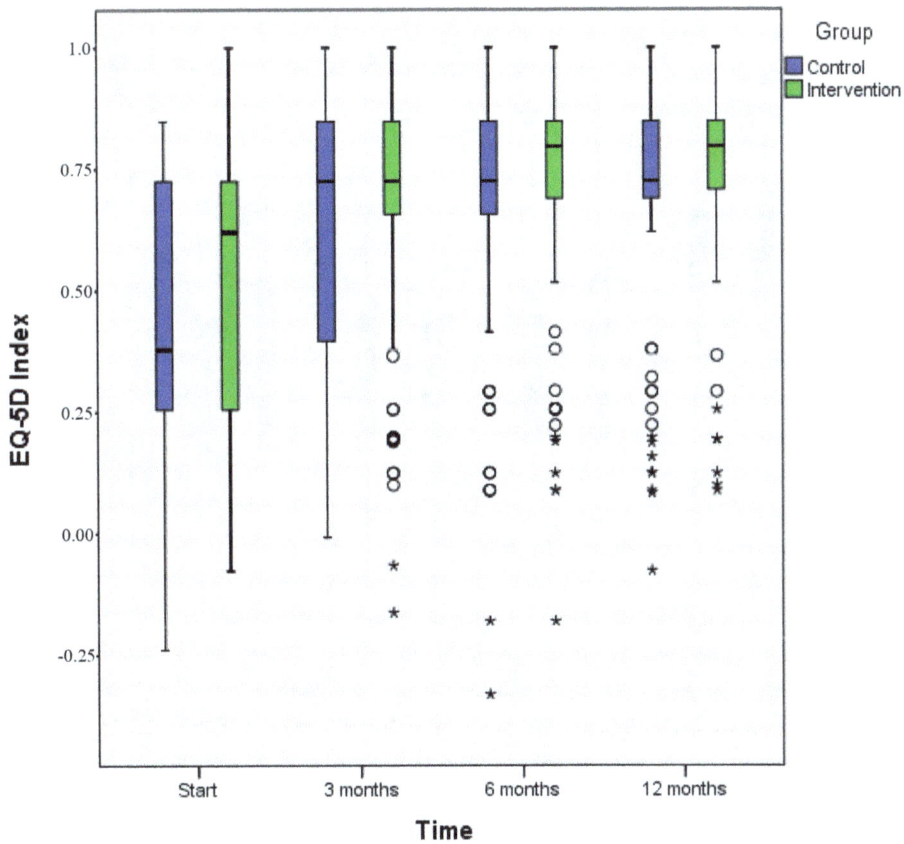

Fig. 3 Quality of life (EQ-5D values) in the intervention and TAU groups. Boxplots for baseline, 3-months follow up, 6-months follow up, and 12-months follow up. The outcome variable is presented as box plot with medians, minimum and maximum values and lower and upper quartiles. Y-axis: EQ-5D, X-axis: time 0, 3, 6, 12 months. Outliers (*circle*) are cases with values between 1.5 and 3 times the interquartile range, extremes (*star*) are cases with values more than 3 times the interquartile range

larger than they really are [24, 25]. We had access to all patients' EPRs, a good source of information on prescriptions, sick leave, and health care use. In the current study, we had the opportunity to observe the course of depression symptoms, perceived quality of life, sick leave, and health care use for a full year after baseline. Another major strength is that a research nurse was stationed at each PHCC during the recruitment period. The nurse collected baseline data, gathered oral and written consent, and supported the staff at the site, functions that primary care personnel stress are important to make it easier to combine clinical work and research [26].We were well aware of the possible obstacles to conducting a RCT at a PHCC as described by Richter and Roy-Byrne [27, 28].

We randomised at the GP level. Randomisation at the patient level would have necessitated changing doctor for some patients, or GPs trained in the intervention would have provided the intervention to some patients but treatment as usual to others, increasing the possibility of contamination. We chose not to randomise at the PHCC level, as regional and socioeconomic differences between areas served by the PHCCs might have affected the results.

Another limitation was absence of a blinded control arm. The control GPs were aware that their colleagues at the same PHCC were providing the intervention, and this might have affected treatment as usual, even if they were requested to continue patient care as usual. This possible bias would support the notion of randomisation at PHCC level, but this would in turn increase the risk of e.g. selection effects. Another limitation is that the intervention of recurrent use of self-rating scales also included regular GP visits, and it is not possible to separate possible effects of the regular GP visits from effects of the patient's frequent self-rating monitoring. However, during the 3-month intervention, patients in the TAU arm made only 0.85 fewer visits to their GPs than patients in the intervention arm. The frequency of visits in the TAU arm was the result of the GPs' and patients' joint assessments of care needs in each case. That frequency of patient visits did not differ markedly in the TAU arm is likely attributable to the current wide-spread emphasis on person-centred care in Swedish primary care.

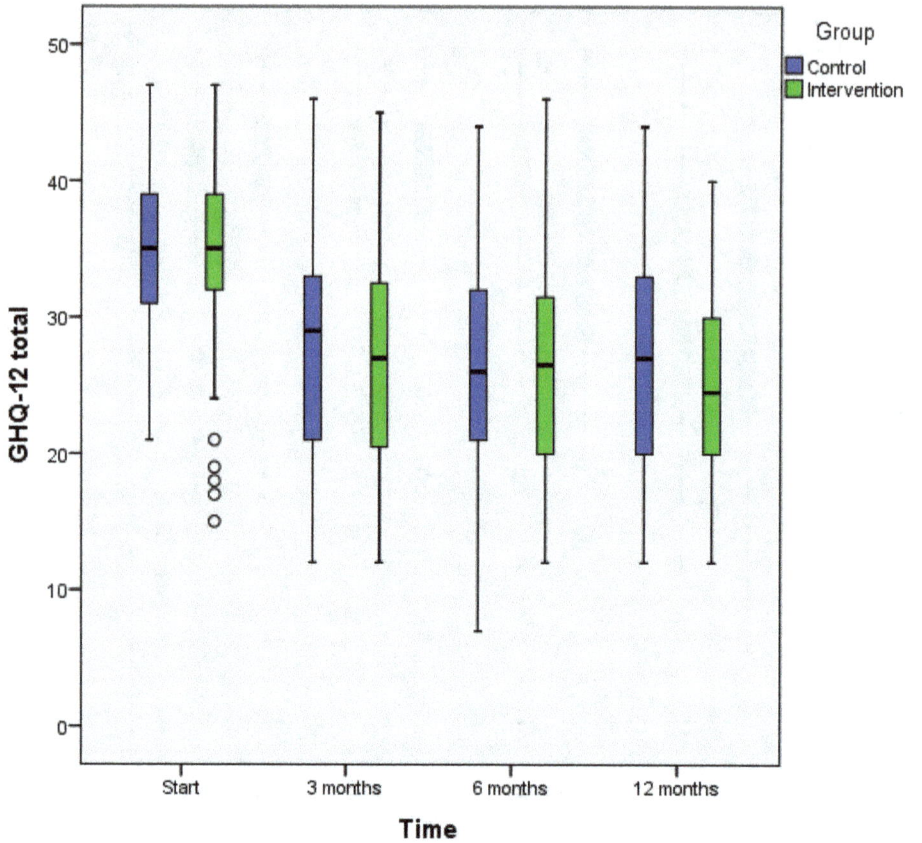

Fig. 4 Overall psychological well-being (GHQ-12 values) in the intervention and TAU groups. Boxplots for baseline, 3-months follow up, 6-months follow up, and 12-months follow up. The outcome variable is presented as box plot with medians, minimum and maximum values and lower and upper quartiles. Y-axis: GHQ-12, X-axis: time 0, 3, 6, 12 months. Outliers (*circle*) are cases with values between 1.5 and 3 times the interquartile range

All patients included had a new episode of mild/moderate depression, but the selection procedure did not differentiate between recurrent or first episode patients. There is some evidence that recurrent depression has slower remission [29], but according to the similar frequency of maintenance antidepressant medication in both intervention and TAU groups at inclusion, we can assume that the rate of recurrent depression disorder was the same in both arms. Further, the high number of outcomes, assessed at baseline and at 3, 6, and 12 months, necessitated multiple statistical comparisons, thus increasing the possibility of type I errors. Although the low p-values indicated that the few significant findings were not likely due to chance, the results need further confirmation in other studies. A limitation is also that we did not use more advanced statistical models to account for the correlation between patients treated by the same GP and to handle all observations of the patient instead of pairwise comparisons (e.g. mixed models).

Table 2 Number and percent of patients who had prescriptions for antidepressants and sedatives and stated medication at baseline and 3-, 6-, and 12-months follow up, respectively, in the intervention and TAU groups

	Baseline		3 months follow-up		6 months follow-up		12 months follow-up	
	n	(%)	*n*	(%)	*n*	(%)	*n*	(%)
Antidepressants								
Intervention (n = 125)	27	(22)	90	(72)	86	(69)**	74	(59)
TAU (n = 133)	43	(32)	96	(72)	78	(59)	77	(58)
Sedatives								
Intervention	26	(21)	64	(51)	53	(42)	52	(42)
TAU[a]	32	(24)	73	(55)	56	(42)	51	(38)

[a]*TAU* treatment as usual

**Significantly higher proportion of patients in intervention group still on antidepressants after 6 months, $p = 0.007$

Table 3 Number and percent of individuals on sick leave, mean days of sick leave, and p-values for difference in mean days of sick leave between participants in intervention and TAU groups, based on information obtained from electronic patient records

	Intervention			TAU			
	n (%)	Mean days of sick leave	SD	*n* (%)	Mean days of sick leave	SD	*P* for difference mean days
0-3 months	31(25)	63.1	29.8	48 (36)	55.8	27.7	0.221
4-12 months	35(28)	100.8	87.3	47(35)	102.7	85	0.922
Total 0-12 months	49(39)	124.8	102.5	64 (48)	123.3	85.0	0.942

Drop outs

Among the study drop outs, 37 individuals belonged to the intervention group and 48 to the TAU group. At the 3 and 6 month follow-up, participation rate was somewhat lower in the control group, but at the 12 month follow up, participation rate was almost the same in intervention and control groups; 70% and 69%, respectively (Fig. 1).

Generalisability

The study population represented patients treated by GPs for mild and moderate depression in primary health care. It included patients from health care centres in urban and rural areas and areas characterised by differing socioeconomic status. Health care is heavily subsidised in Sweden; patients pay a small per-visit fee and their yearly total co-payment is capped at approximately £100. The study results can be generalised to other countries with similar health care systems.

The RCT had a representative selection among the Swedish speaking population. One could argue that the exclusion of non-speaking Swedish patients may have limited the study's generalisability. Unfortunately, it was not possible to translate and validate the instruments or to use an interpreter at every contact with study staff.

In this study, we chose to use MADR-S as the basis for patient education and collaborative care. These two factors can facilitate better depression outcomes [29–31]. Depression is complex, and the outcome of treatment often depends on the GP's ability to connect with the patient during the consultation and her/his ability to choose proper treatment in agreement with the patient. Use of self-rating scales may function as one piece of the depression treatment puzzle, but as in many difficult jigsaw puzzles, more than one piece is needed to complete the picture. Thus, the Swedish National Board of Health and Welfare, i.e. the body that establishes the national guidelines for depression treatment, has expressed interest in whether it is meaningful to routinely use self-rating scales for patients with mild to moderate depression in primary care. We chose to use MADRS-S because it is the most commonly used depression self-rating scale in Sweden. About one third of all GPs state that they sometimes use MADRS-S, although not regularly [13, 32]. MADRS-S is designed to be sensitive to change and is often used in RCT studies that evaluate antidepressant treatment [12].

Table 4 Number of patients' contacts with GPs, nurses, and psychologists between baseline to 3 months, and 4 to12 months for intervention and TAU groups, based on information obtained from electronic patient records

Profession	Type of contact	Intervention 0-3 months m (SD)	TAU 0-3 months m (SD)	*p*
GP	visit	3.44 (1.214)	2.59 (1.354)	0.066
Nurse	visit	0.32 (0.829)	0.32 (0.875)	0.878
Psychologist/Therapist	visit	0.40 (1.320)	0.89 (1.776)	**0. 0001**
Total visits to PHCC	visit	4.16 (2.398)	3.81 (2.692)	**0.006**
		Intervention 4-12 months m (SD)	TAU 4-12 months m (SD)	*p*
GP	visit	2. 54 (2.337)	2.38 (2.595)	0.301
Nurse	visit	0. 68 (1.484)	0.62 (1.551)	0.581
Psychologist/Therapist	visit	0. 90 (2.504)	0.83 (1.908)	0.401
Total visits to PHCC	visit	4. 11 (4.586)	3.83 (4.403)	0.619
		Intervention total 0-12 months m (SD)	TAU total 0-12 months m (SD)	*p*
GP	visit	8.26 (5.842)	7.64 (5.976)	0.304
Nurse	visit	0.99 (1.978)	0.94 (2.088)	0.967
Psychologist/Therapist	visit	1.30 (3.129)	1.73 (3.222)	0.167
Total visits to PHCC	visit	8.26 (5.842)	7.64 (5.976)	0.812

Bold numeral indicates statistically significant *p*-value

The study shows that use of self-rating scales during regular visits facilitates adherence to pharmacological treatment according to guidelines, in that once medication with antidepressants has been initiated, this treatment should be continued for at least 6 months [5]. On the other hand, the study also shows that treatment as usual, as it is practiced in the Swedish primary care of today, in most cases not including the use of self-rating scales, is just as efficient concerning reduction of depressive symptoms, perceived quality of life and general health, as well as sick leave frequency and duration, which is supported by the results from several international studies [33].

Strengths and weaknesses in relation to other studies

To our knowledge there have been few or no studies that have evaluated the effect of recurrent use of self-rating scales regarding depression in relation to the above described outcomes.

Use of antidepressants for the period mandated by current guidelines was associated with neither an improvement nor a worsening of patients' symptoms during the one-year study period. However, using antidepressants for the length of time called for in guidelines has been shown to reduce risk of relapse [34].

Clinical importance of the study

More discussion is needed as to how self-rating scales might be best implemented in primary care, how to manage depressed patients using these instruments, and how to integrate this into the consultation. The feasibility of meaningful and person-centred use of self-rating scales, continuity, and accessibility in the care of mild to moderate depression in the clinical setting is of great interest. Engaging the patient with a cognitive and person-centred approach and with regular consultations and follow-ups is a way to empower the patient, give the patient knowledge and tools to handle depression, follow his or her illness course, and create a basis for regaining of function [2, 6, 30]. Continuity and close regular follow-ups facilitate care that is adjusted to the individual's explicit needs and requirements and is an absolute condition for person-centred care [35]. Requirements for treatment are also reached in cooperation and collaboration with the patient, facilitating understanding and communication [36]. The continuous use of self-rating scales in the treatment of primary care patients with depression might support this process of care.

Conclusions

When GPs used a depression self-rating scale in recurrent consultations, patients more often continued antidepressant medication according to guidelines, compared to TAU patients. However, concerning outcomes in terms of depression symptoms, quality of life, overall psychological well-being, consumption of care, and sick leave the use of self-rating scales did not seem to increase treatment effects compared to the usual treatment provided in primary care. Thus, the use of depression self-rating scales should perhaps not be mandatory in primary health care but rather left to the discretion of the GP and the patient.

Abbreviations

GP: General practitioner; MADRS-S: Montgomery-Asberg Depression Rating Scale (Self-administered); PHCC: Primary health care centre; PRI-SMA: PRImary care Self-assessment Montgomery-Asberg; RCT: Randomised controlled trial

Acknowledgements

We would like to thank all participating PHCCs for their concentrated efforts and active involvement in the study.

Funding

The study was financed by grants from Rehsam RS11-013 (PRI-SMA/MADRS trial) and the Region Västra Götaland of Sweden. The study sponsors had no role in the collection, analysis, interpretation of data, or the writing of the report or the decision to submit the article for publication. All authors were independent from funders.

Authors' contributions

CB was chief investigator and initiated the project, designed the RCT, chaired the trial management group (TMG), drafted and revised the paper and is guarantor. JW participated in the design of the RCT, was member of the TMG, drafted and revised the paper. CW assisted during the whole conduct of the RCT at the PHCC sites and was member of the TMG, monitored data, drafted and revised the paper. E-L P was trial manager, monitored data collection for the whole RCT, was member of the TMG, drafted and revised the paper. HÅ, ML, MA, RE, JT were members of the TMG, contributed to the trial design, drafted and revised the paper. All authors had full access to all of the study data and take responsibility for the integrity and accuracy of the data. All authors have read and approved the final version of this manuscript.

Competing interests

The authors declare that they have no competing interests.

Consent for publication

Not applicable.

Author details

[1]Department of Primary Health Care/Public Health and Community Medicine, Institute of Medicine, Sahlgrenska Academy, University of Gothenburg, Gothenburg, Sweden. [2]Division for Family Medicine, Department of Neurobiology, Care Sciences and Society, Karolinska Institutet, Stockholm, Sweden. [3]Region Västra Götaland, Närhälsan Research and Development Primary Health Care, Gothenburg, Sweden. [4]Department of Health and Rehabilitation, Unit of Physiotherapy, Institute of Neuroscience and Physiology, University of Gothenburg, Gothenburg, Sweden. [5]Department of Public Health and Caring Sciences - Family Medicine and Preventive Medicine, Uppsala University, Uppsala, Sweden. [6]Institute of Neuroscience and Physiology, University of Gothenburg, Gothenburg, Sweden.

References

1. Ferrari AJ, Charlson FJ, Norman RE, Patten SB, Freedman G, Murray CJ, et al. Burden of depressive disorders by country, sex, age, and year: findings from the global burden of disease study 2010. PLoS Med. 2013;10:e1001547.
2. World Health Organization. The global burden of disease: 2004 update. Geneva: WHO; 2008.
3. Swedish National Board of Health and Welfare 2013. National Evaluation – care and treatment in depression, anxiety and schizophrenia (In Swedish). Supplement 3, p 27. Available from: http://www.socialstyrelsen.se/SiteCollectionDocuments/2013-6-7-Bilaga3.pdf. Accessed 7 Jan 2017.
4. Bijl RV, Ravelli A. Psychiatric morbidity, service use, and need for care in the general population: results of The Netherlands Mental Health Survey and Incidence Study. Am J Public Health. 2000;90(4):602–7.
5. National Collaborating Centre for Mental Health (UK). Depression: the Treatment and Management of Depression in Adults (Updated edition). Leicester (UK): British Psychological Society; 2010. (Nice Clinical Guidelines, No. 90). Available from: https://www.ncbi.nlm.nih.gov/books/NBK63748/. Accessed 10 Oct 2016.
6. National Board of Health and Welfare. National guidelines for treatment of depression and anxiety 2010: Support for governance and management. Stockholm (in Swedish); 2010. Available at: http://www.angest-stockholm.se/wp-content/uploads/2013/01/Socialstyrelsens-riktlinjer-depression-och-angestsyndrom.pdf. Accessed 6 Jan 2017.
7. Groot PC. Patients can diagnose too: How continuous self-assessment aids diagnosis of, and recovery from, depression. J Ment Health. 2010;19(4):352–62.
8. Gilbody S, Sheldon T, House A. Screening and case-finding instruments for depression: a meta-analysis. CMAJ. 2008;178(8):997–1003.
9. Montgomery SA, Asberg M. A new depression scale designed to be sensitive to change. Br J Psychiatry. 1979;134:382–9.
10. Svanborg P, Asberg M. A new self-rating scale for depression and anxiety states based on the Comprehensive Psychopathological Rating Scale. Acta Psychiatr Scand. 1994;89(1):21–8.
11. Royal College of General Practitioners Curriculum. 3.10 Care of people with Mental Health Problems. http://www.rcgp.org.uk/clinical-andresearch/toolkits/~/media/B9B066784CED42518D2E5F80E141D504.ashx. Accessed 15 June 2016.
12. Fantino B, Moore N. The self-reported Montgomery-Asberg Depression Rating Scale is a useful evaluative tool in Major Depressive Disorder. BMC Psychiatry. 2009;9:26.
13. Pettersson A, Björkelund C, Petersson EL. To score or not to score: a qualitative study on GPs views on the use of instruments for depression. Fam Pract. 2014;31(2):215–21.
14. Spitzer RL, Williams JB, Kroenke K, Linzer M. deGruy FV3rd, Hahn SR, et al. Utility of a new procedure for diagnosing mental disorders in primary care. The PRIME-MD 1000 study. JAMA. 1994;272(22):1749–56.
15. Malterud K. Key questions–a strategy for modifying clinical communication. Transforming tacit skills into a clinical method. Scand J Prim Health Care. 1994;12(2):121–7.
16. Maguire P, Pitceathly C. Key communication skills and how to acquire them. BMJ. 2002;325(7366):697–700.
17. Beck AT, Steer RA, Carbin MG. Psychometric properties of the Beck Depression Inventory: Twenty-five years of evaluation. Clin Psychol Rev. 1988;8(1):77–100
18. Arnau RC, Meagher MW, Norris MP, Bramson R. Psychometric evaluation of the Beck Depression Inventory-II with primary care medical patients. Health Psychol. 2001;20(2).112–9.
19. The EuroQol Group. EuroQol - a new facility for the measurement of health-related quality of life. Health Policy. 1990;16(3):199–208.
20. Dolan P. Modeling valuations for EuroQol health states. Med Care. 1997; 35(11):1095–108.
21. Hardy GE, Shapiro DA, Haynes CE, Rick JE. Validation of the General Health Questionnaire-12: Using a sample of employees from England's health care services. Psychol Assess. 1999;11(2):159–65.
22. Björkelund C. Structured use of a self rating instrument in the primary care consultation with patients with mild and moderate depression. ClinicalTrials gov Identifier: NCT01402206. https://clinicaltrials.gov/ct2/show/NCT01402206.
23. Schulz KF, Altman DG, Moher D. CONSORT 2010 Statement: updated guidelines for reporting parallel group randomised trials. Trials. 2010;11:32.
24. Khan A, Brown WA. Antidepressants versus placebo in major depression: an overview. World Psychiatry. 2015;14(3):294–300.
25. Zhu Z, Zhang L, Jiang J, Li W, Cao X, Zhou Z, et al. Comparison of psychological placebo and waiting list control conditions in the assessment of cognitive behavioral therapy for the treatment of generalized anxiety disorder: a meta-analysis. Shanghai Arch Psychiatry. 2014;26(6):319–31.
26. Hange D, Björkelund C, Svenningsson I, Kivi M, Eriksson MC, Petersson EL. Experiences of staff members participating in primary care research activities: a qualitative study. Int J Gen Med. 2015;8:143–8.
27. Richter-Sundberg L, Nystrom ME, Krakau I, Sandahl C. Improving treatment of depression in primary health care: a case study of obstacles to perform a clinical trial designed to implement practice guidelines. Prim Health Care Res Dev. 2015;16(2):188–200.
28. Roy-Byrne PP, Sherbourne CD, Craske MG, Stein MB, Katon W, Sullivan G, et al. Moving treatment research from clinical trials to the real world. Psychiatr Serv. 2003;54(3):327–32.
29. Garrison GM, Angstman KB, O'Connor SS, Williams MD, Lineberry TW. Time to Remission for Depression with Collaborative Care Management (CCM) in Primary Care. J Am Board Fam Med. 2016;29(1):10–7.
30. Katon WJ, Lin EH, Von Korff M, Ciechanowski P, Ludman EJ, Young B, et al. Collaborative care for patients with depression and chronic illnesses. N Engl J Med. 2010;363(27):2611–20.
31. Richards DA, Hill JJ, Gask L, Lovell K, Chew-Graham C, Bower P, et al. Clinical effectiveness of collaborative care for depression in UK primary care (CADET): cluster randomised controlled trial. BMJ. 2013;347:f4913.
32. Swedish Council for Health Technology Assessment. Diagnosis and follow up of affective disorders- a systematic review. Report 212/2012 ISBN 978-91-85413-52-2 ISSN 1400–1403 [in Swedish]
33. Blais MA, Malone JC, Stein MB, Slavin-Mulford J, O'Keefe SM, Renna M, et al. Treatment as usual (TAU) for depression: a comparison of psychotherapy, pharmacotherapy, and combined treatment at a large academic medical center. Psychotherapy. 2013;50(1):110–8.
34. Geddes JR, Carney SM, Davies C, Furukawa TA, Kupfer DJ, Frank E, et al. Relapse prevention with antidepressant drug treatment in depressive disorders: a systematic review. Lancet. 2003;361(9358):653–61.
35. Solberg LI, Crain AL, Sperl-Hillen JM, Hroscikoski MC, Engebretson KI, O'Connor PJ. Effect of improved primary care access on quality of depression care. Ann Fam Med. 2006;4(1):69–74.
36. Sighinolfi C, Nespeca C, Menchetti M, Levantesi P, Belvederi Murri M, Berardi D. Collaborative care for depression in European countries: a systematic review and meta-analysis. J Psychosom Res. 2014;77(4):247–63.

7

Partner notification and partner treatment for chlamydia: attitude and practice of general practitioners in the Netherlands

Ingrid V. F. van den Broek[1*], Gé A. Donker[2], Karin Hek[3], Jan E. A. M. van Bergen[4,5], Birgit H. B. van Benthem[4] and Hannelore M. Götz[4,6,7]

Abstract

Background: Chlamydia prevalence remains high despite scaling-up control efforts. Transmission is not effectively interrupted without partner notification (PN) and (timely) partner treatment (PT). In the Netherlands, the follow-up of partners is not standardized and may depend on GPs' time and priorities. We investigated current practice and attitude of GPs towards PN and PT to determine the potential for Patient-Initiated Partner Treatment, which is legally not supported yet.

Methods: Multiple data-sources were combined for a landscape analysis. Quantitative data on (potential) PT were obtained from prescriptions in the national pharmacy register (2004–2014) and electronic patient data from NIVEL-Primary Care Database (PCD) and from STI consultations in a subgroup of sentinel practices therein. Furthermore, we collected information on current practice via two short questionnaires at a national GP conference and obtained insight into GPs' attitudes towards PN/PT in a vignette study among GPs partaking in NIVEL-PCD.

Results: Prescription data showed Azithromycin double dosages in 1–2% of cases in the pharmacy register (37.000 per year); probable chlamydia-specific repeated prescriptions or double dosages of other antibiotics in NIVEL-PCD (115/1078) could not be interpreted as PT for chlamydia with certainty. STI consultation data revealed direct PT in 6/100 cases, via partner prescription or double doses. In the questionnaires the large majority of GPs (>95% of 1411) reported to discuss PN of current and ex-partner(s) with chlamydia patients. Direct PT was indicated as most common method by 4% of 271 GPs overall and by 12% for partners registered in the same practice. Usually, GPs leave further steps to the patients (83%), advising patients to tell partners to get tested (56%) or treated (28%). In the vignette study, 16–20% of 268 GPs indicated willingness to provide direct PT, depending on patient/partner profile, more (24–45%) if patients would have the chance to notify their partner first.

Conclusion: GPs in the Netherlands already treat some partners of chlamydia cases directly, especially partners registered in the same practice. Follow-up of partner notification and treatment in general practice needs more attention. GPs may be open to implement PIPT more often, provided there are clear guidelines to arrange this legally and practically.

Keywords: Partner notification, Partner treatment, Expedited partner therapy, Patient-initiated partner treatment, General practice, Sexually transmitted infections, Chlamydia trachomatis

* Correspondence: Ingrid.van.den.Broek@rivm.nl
[1]Epidemiology and Surveillance Unit, Centre for Infectious Diseases Control, RIVM, Bilthoven, The Netherlands
Full list of author information is available at the end of the article

Background

Chlamydia trachomatis (hereafter "chlamydia") incidence remains high in the Netherlands despite targeted control efforts. The estimated report rate was 310/100,000 in 2015 and 272/100.000 in 2010. [1] STI centres provide low-threshold additional care prioritising high-risk groups. Young people under 25 years of age and other high-risk groups can be tested for chlamydia without cost at STI clinics. The general practitioner (GP) still performs the largest number of STI consultations (estimated at two thirds or more) [1]; a minority uses private (self-)care and some get tested in the hospital (gynaecologist) after referral. The number of chlamydia tests has increased over the years but diagnostic rates have not gone down: an estimated 54,000 infections were detected at GPs and STI clinics in 2015: 35,000 at the GP and 19,000 in STI clinics. [1] New routes of chlamydia control need to be explored and integrated in the STI care system.

Effective partner notification (PN) and partner treatment (PT) are essential to prevent re-infection and further spread. Re-infections for chlamydia are common, occurring in 14–20% of cases [2–5].The importance of PN for chlamydia has been demonstrated in several studies [6] and is addressed in all Dutch STI care manuals and guidelines [7, 8]. Persons notified by a sexual partner are at high risk of infection; in Dutch STI clinics the infection rate was 36% among women and 32% among heterosexual men who visited due to notification for chlamydia. [1]

Dutch guidelines advise PN for chlamydia patients (a) in case of symptomatic infections for partners in the period 6 weeks prior to the onset of symptoms and (b) in case of asymptomatic infections for all partners in the last 6 months. According to GP guidelines, [7, 8] PN should be discussed in order to motivate chlamydia-patients to inform their sex partners, or alternatively, GPs should offer to help with notification or refer to other services. The advice is to tell the partner to see a health professional to get tested or to get treated directly. GPs can offer presumptive treatment for a partner presenting for consultation. Online tools for patients and GPs are available: 'www. Thuisarts.nl' gives instructions on how to perform PN and 'partnerwaarschuwing.nl' [9] can be used to arrange individual PN after diagnosis, but uptake at GPs is still limited [10].

A way to improve partner management is to provide practical tools to simplify procedures for both patients and GPs. A systematic review showed that providing direct treatment for the current sexual partner, so-called Expedited Partner Therapy (EPT), can be an effective strategy. [6] Patients give a prescription or medication to their sexual partners to treat the infection or, alternatively, partners obtain medication from the pharmacy directly. [11] EPT is efficacious in reducing repeated infections in index patients and increasing the number of partners treated. [12–15] The implementation of EPT reduced the chlamydia test positivity in a large scale pilot in Washington State, USA, although this may not have been an exclusive effect of the intervention. [16] The method is used widely in the USA: EPT is permissible in 38 states and potentially allowable in 8 states. [17] Also in the UK, EPT or similarly, Accelerated partner therapy (APT), is seen as a viable option. [18–20]

In the Netherlands, direct PT via the partner, referred to as Patient Initiated Partner Therapy (PIPT), is not officially implemented, because a physician is legally required to have contact with a patient before prescribing medication, to explain the reason for medication and to check medical history and allergies. In 2016, the Project Investigating options for Patient Initiated Contact treatment for Chlamydia in the Netherlands (PICC-UP) started, with the objective to investigate the potential of PIPT as an effective method for improving PT. The project covers other issues of PIPT, including the legal steps needed for implementation. Here we describe an initial landscape analysis on the current level of practice of PN/PT and (potential) direct PT for chlamydia in the general practice, as well as the attitude and opinions of Dutch GPs towards implementation of direct PT, provided it would be possible in future. [21]

Methods

This study was set up to combine multiple sources to explore PN/PT practices among GPs in the Netherlands, both prescription data (paragraph 1) and questionnaire data (paragraph 2) were used.

Quantitative data on current practice

Chlamydia-specific double dosage prescriptions as (potential) indicator for PIPT

1.1 The SFK database (*'Stichting Farmaceutische Kengetallen'*[1]) contains anonymous data on prescriptions covering 95% of public pharmacies (i.e. extramural pharmacies) in the Netherlands. Information is available on the date of issue, delivered amount of tablets, average daily dose recommended to be taken, delivered Defined Daily Dose (DDD); the indication for the prescribed medication is not registered in the SFK. We selected (2004–2015) Azithromycin prescriptions typical and thought to be exclusively used for chlamydia (single dose of 1 g Azithromycin for 1 day or multiple dose thereof), and calculated the proportion of double/ multiple dosage prescriptions that could reflect simultaneous PT for chlamydia. This method had been validated before in a previous (unpublished) report, showing that prescriptions of Azithromycin single dose as specific treatment for chlamydia compare well to estimates of the number of chlamydia infections reported nationally.

1.2 The NIVEL-PCD was used to study episode-based data from the electronic patient registration (2015). This network includes over 400 practices, nationally representative by age and gender and by population density and geographical practice distribution.[2] The database system records data on morbidity, prescriptions and referrals. Analyses were performed with the aim to tabulate single versus double dosages with a diagnosis code for chlamydia infection, as well as repeated prescriptions within a period of 2 weeks after the initial prescription, seen as (potential) cases of PIPT. Chlamydia episodes were identified by ICPC codes (vaginitis (X84), cervicitis (X85) and Pelvic Inflammatory Disease (PID) (X74) in women, and orchitis/epididymitis (Y74) and other genital diseases (Y99) in men) combined with specific chlamydia-prescriptions, based on an earlier developed definition of chlamydia in the absence of a specific ICPC code for chlamydia. [22] Prescription data are ATC-coded. Standard first choice treatment for genital chlamydia is Azithromycin (1 g single dose; ATC-code J01FA10); we also looked at dosages of Doxycycline (2 dd 100 mg 7 days; J01AA02), given for anal infections or epididymitis/orchitis and Amoxicillin (during pregnancies, 3dd 500 mg 7 days; J01CA04). We studied the dosage prescribed, based on frequency (times per day), unit, total number of units prescribed and whether it was a repeat prescription. Episodes with one of the ICPC codes and one of the ATC codes were selected. Episodes with no prescription of antibiotics were assumed not to be chlamydia; those with missing information on dosage were excluded from the analyses.

Consultations

1.3 Sentinel practices ($N = 42$) of NIVEL Primary Care Database (NIVEL-PCD), collect data specific for STI-consultations. GPs are requested to routinely complete a questionnaire for each registered new disease episode in a patients' electronic record with an ICPC-code (International Classification of Primary Care (ICPC-1)) concerning STI/HIV issues. This contains, with anonymous identification numbers, information on testing and diagnosis, patient demographics, reason for consultation and sexual risk behaviour. Since January 2015, questions concerning PN and PT were added; we used 2015 data for the current analyses.

Questionnaire data on current practice of PN/PT and attitude towards PIPT

1.4 For a large pre-conference survey, GPs were asked to fill in an online questionnaire at the time of registration for a national GP conference (November 2015). This survey included a question on partner notification of current and ex-partners for patients diagnosed with STIs.

1.5 At the same national GP conference, a short questionnaire was handed out on site to GP participants. This contained questions on the most common methods for PN and PT in the general practice.

1.6 In the NIVEL-PCD, a vignette study on practice and attitude of GPs towards partner management was performed. An annual online questionnaire is distributed among GPs in this network. We included in this questionnaire (in 2016) two case descriptions or 'vignettes', known as a useful way to measure reported and/or intended physician practices in an outpatient setting. [23, 24] The vignettes described two hypothetical chlamydia positive patients: (i) a 'low risk' case, woman with a steady relationship (25 years, Dutch; partner patient in the same practice), chlamydia probably acquired through an incidental casual partner and (ii) a presumed 'higher risk' case: young man (17 years, migrant background), who had 4 different female partners in the last 4 months, and was still seeing one of these. We asked for the GPs intention for PN and PT and his/her attitude towards PIPT.

Results

Prescription data

1.1 In total, 443,512 chlamydia-specific prescriptions of Azithromycin (1 g 1d) were registered in the SFK between 2004 and 2015 (increasing, average 37,000 per year). Of these, 99.3% had a single dosage prescription and 0.7% a double or (incidental) triple or more, which may have been direct partner treatment. A clear increase in double dose prescriptions was observed from 2013 onwards: it rose from below 0.5% to 1.5% in the period 2013–2015, much more obvious in men than in women (see Fig. 1).

1.2 For the pilot study on potential PT in the NIVEL PCD, data from 311 general practices in 2015 was available. We identified 18,599 episodes with one of the five relevant ICPC codes; for a large part of these no antibiotic was prescribed which were therefore assumed not to be chlamydia infections

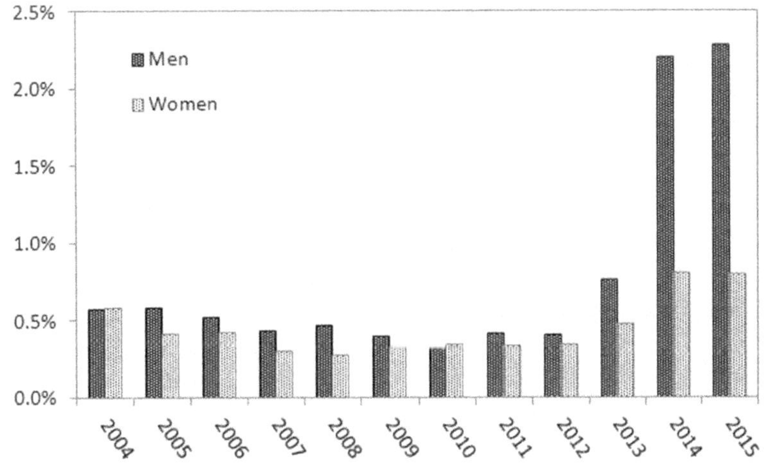

Fig. 1 Proportion of double dosages of Azithromycin (1 g single dose) prescribed in public pharmacies in The Netherlands 2004–2015, in men and women

and excluded. For 902 chlamydia episodes (in 891 patients), a total of 1078 chlamydia-related antibiotic prescriptions were recorded with dosage information. The major part of the prescriptions was Azithromycin, a smaller part Doxycycline and a few Amoxicillin (with specified dosages or a multiple dose thereof, see Table 1). Double dosages were prescribed in 2.1% of Azithromycin-treated chlamydia episodes: in 2.8% of women and 1.3% of men (12/427 women and 5/372 men; difference not significant; 3 cases gender unknown), most commonly in the age group 30–39 years (3.1%; 6/191) versus 2.1% in <20 years (2/97) and 2.1% in 20–29 years old (9/420).

Furthermore, double dosages were found for 31.1% of Doxycycline episodes and in none of the Amoxicillin-treated ones. The double-dosed Doxycycline were prescriptions of 28 dosages instead of 14 dosages, unlikely to be PT, probably prescriptions for 2 weeks instead of 1 week, as indicated for epididymitis caused by chlamydia (but duration was not consistently reported). Double-dosages were indeed more common among men than among women (46.2% of men treated with doxycycline and 11.1% of women). The proportion of chlamydia episodes with repeated prescriptions was 12.6%, of which 7.6% was registered on the same day (66/902). Of the total, 11.9% was treated with the same antibiotic and 0.8% with a different antibiotic. These proportions did not relate to age group or gender.

1.3 In the 42 sentinel practices, 100 chlamydia cases were recorded in 470 STI-consultations (reported in 2015). The most common way for GPs to inform the patient of his/her chlamydia infection was by phone ($n = 65$) or personal consultation ($n = 29$). The remaining cases heard it from another care provider (under whose responsibility they were tested; $n = 5$) or no follow-up was done ($n = 1$), as the GP stated 'the patient had already been treated blind, so no follow-up visit was needed'. PN was discussed with the 94 cases contacted: most GPs ($n = 85$) left it to the patient to take further steps; for two cases PN was done by the GP or assistant, while two cases were referred to PN services (five no answer). For 72 of the 94 cases (77%) GPs indicated they did not treat the partner, while 12 said they advised to tell the partner to come to the practice (13%), either for a test ($n = 6$) or for direct treatment ($n = 5$) or both

Table 1 Type of antibiotics used for chlamydia: per prescription and per episode, in 2015

Antibiotics	Chlamydia prescriptions N %		Chlamydia episodes N %		Episodes with double dose N %		Episodes with repeated Ct-prescriptions[a]	
Azithromycin (1 g 1d)	937	86.9	802	88.9	17	2.1	93	11.6
Doxycycline (2dd 100 mg 7d)	123	11.4	106	11.8	33	31.1	20	18.9
Amoxicillin (3dd 500 mg 7d)	18	1.7	15	1.7	0	0	2	13.3
Total	1078		902		50		115	

[a]episodes had multiple prescriptions of the same or different antibiotics (maximum 4 recorded)

(*n* = 1); four gave no answer. PIPT was applied in six cases (6.4%): the GPs wrote a direct, extra medical prescription for partners of four cases, while they prescribed a double dosage for two cases to treat partners simultaneously (Fig. 2). No clear correlations were found between patient characteristics (gender, sexual preference, age, reason for consultation) and PN/PT.

Current practice of PN/PT and attitude towards PIPT

1.4 The online pre-conference survey was filled-in by 1411 GPs (53% of a total of 2650 conference participating GPs). The majority of GPs discusses PN of the current partner and the ex-partner with the patient. Of all GPs, 80% indicated to discuss PN always and 18% mostly with their STI-patients (Fig. 3). The GPs discussed PN significantly less frequently for ex-partners than for current partners (Chi-square $p < 0.001$).

1.5 The short hand-out questionnaire was completed by 271 participants at the GP conference. The most common method of PN reported was to discuss this and leave it to the patient to take further steps (83%). In most cases, the GP would advise the patient to tell his/her partner to get tested (56%) or get treated (28%). Direct PT was used for some cases: 4% of GPs treat partners directly: 2% through prescription for the partner and 2% through a double dosage to the index. When the partner is also a patient in the same practice, 12% of GPs write a prescription for him/her at the same time as the index (Fig. 4).

1.6 The vignette study in the annual questionnaire to NIVEL PCD was answered by 289 of 438 persons (response 66%), of which we included the GPs (*n* = 268) for our analysis (21 questionnaires were filled in by GP assistants or managers). The large majority of GPs (87%) indicated they would discuss PN with the patient and leave it to the patient to notify the partner(s) (Table 2). PN via the MHS or another (online) service was more commonly suggested for the high risk than for the low risk case (74% vs 37%). PT advice was via the patient, to inform the partner to consult a doctor to either get tested (76%) or to get direct treatment (55%). PIPT was an option for about one in five GPs: 16% would write a prescription for the partner, while 6% would write a double dosage prescription for the patient to treat the partner simultaneously. In the hypothetical situation that a patient could notify the partner first, prescription for the current partner was considered as an option, more commonly for the low risk than the high risk case (45% vs 24%). Notification and treatment of ex-partners or casual partners was largely left to the responsibility of the patient. In additional comments GPs made clear that PN/PT steps depend on patient- and partner profiles and the character of their relationship (e.g. steady, long-term or casual) as well as the connection between GP and patient.

Most of the GPs agreed PIPT can be a means to reduce re-infections from chlamydia (62%). GPs said to be open to the idea of PIPT: a considerable

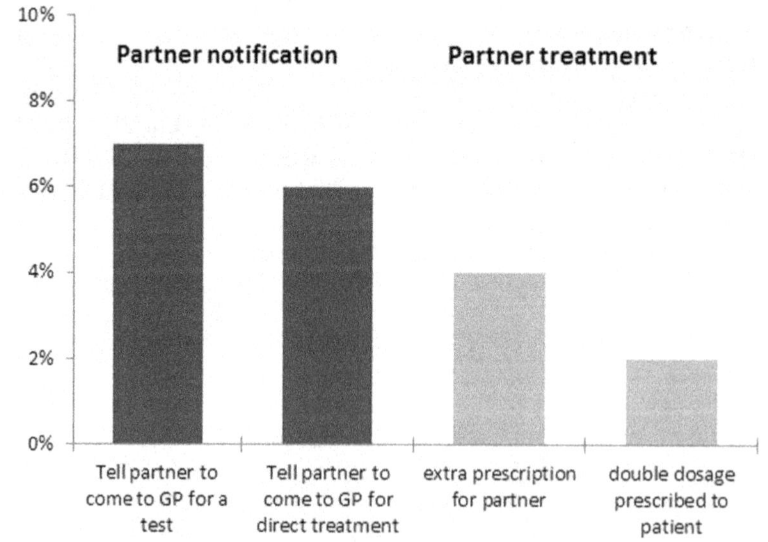

Fig. 2 Proportion of 94 chlamydia-positive cases seen by GP for whom one of the specified partner treatments was applied (Sentinel Practices, NIVEL PCD 2015)

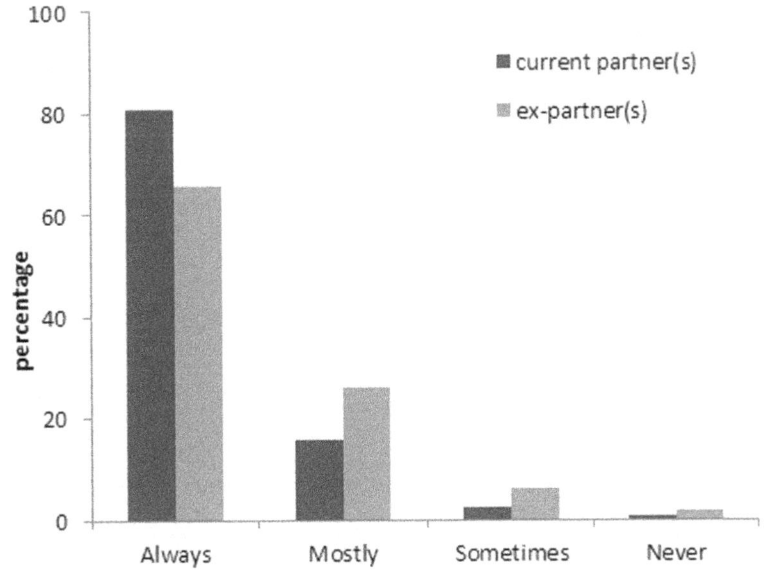

Fig. 3 Proportion of 1411 GPs (answering pre-conference questionnaire, Nov 2015) indicating to discuss partner notification with patients diagnosed with an STI, for current partner(s) and for ex-partners

proportion of GPs indicated it should be an option for some patients (36%), for most patients (21%) or all (10%). Important advantages were mentioned, especially better infection control and better chances to treat the partner, also practical ones in the sense that it would make PT easier and cheaper. On the other hand, a range of disadvantages were also mentioned. The main objections seem to lie in the uncertainty whether the medication will reach the right person and that there is no chance to give advice to the partner or check his/her risk for allergies or contra-indications. Furthermore over-treatment, potentially leading to resistance, issues on patient privacy, and the fact that the partner may have other STIs or have contact with other partners were mentioned.

Discussion

Findings

This first study about PN and PT of chlamydia in the general practice in the Netherlands shows that GPs currently perform an advisory rather than active, facilitating

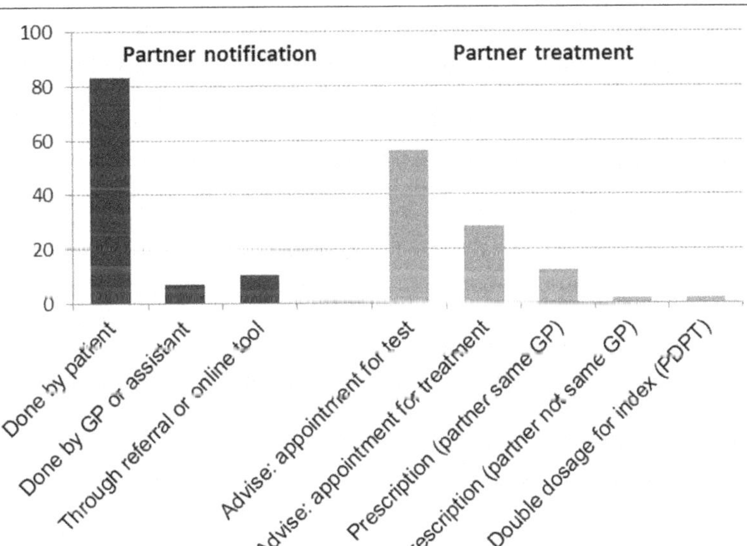

Fig. 4 Proportion of 271 GPs (answering 'multiple choice' questions at conference, Nov 2015) reporting on most common method used for partner notification and partner treatment for patients diagnosed with chlamydia

Table 2 Partner notification and partner treatment practices indicated by 289 GPs for the two 'vignettes' of chlamydia cases presented in the questionnaire (NIVEL PCD 2016)

	Case 1: low risk	Case 2: higher risk	Total
Partner notification (PN)[a]			
Discuss with patient, let patient do PN him/herself	93%[b]	81%[b]	87%
Discuss and offer to do PN by GP or assistant	22%	26%	24%
Refer to MHS or use PN website	37%[b]	74%[b]	55%
Partner treatment (PT)a			
Advise to get the partner to consult the GP for a test	72%[b]	81%[b]	76%
Advise to get the partner to consult a GP for direct treatment	52%	59%	55%
Prescribe antibiotics for the partner	18%	14%	16%
Prescribe a double dosage to patient to treat his/her partner	5.6%	6.9%	6.3%
Prescribe AB to partner after patient has done PN	45%[b]	24%[b]	34%

[a]multiple choice questions, more than 1 answer possible
[b]significant difference between low risk and high risk, at $p < 0.05$. PN = partner notification; PT = Partner Treatment

role in chlamydia PN and PT. In some cases they provide actual PIPT. In general, GPs discuss PN of current and ex-partners with chlamydia patients but leave it to the patient to carry it out. PIPT is applied in an estimated 2–6% of chlamydia cases, based on questionnaires and available electronic consultation- and prescription-data. We found that when the partner is also registered as a patient in the same practice, GPs are more inclined to implement PIPT, i.e. in 12–21% of chlamydia cases. PIPT for unseen/unknown partners is not yet in line with legal regulations.

Follow-up of partner notification and treatment in general practice needs more attention. GPs appeared to be open to the idea of PIPT, although they also expressed concerns, disadvantages and risks. PIPT was an option for about one in five GPs. PN/PT intentions may depend on the STI-risk behaviour of the patient: a high-risk case (with multiple recent partners) would be referred to (online) PN services more often than a low risk case, while a low-risk case with a steady relationship and a partner registered in the same practice was more likely to receive PIPT, especially if the patient would have notified the partner first. PN/PT steps also depend on the connection between GP and patient.

Strengths and limitations

The strength of our study was the use of multiple data-sources (questionnaires, consultation- and pharmacy data) and the access to representative groups of GPs for questionnaire surveys (via the large national GP conference and the NIVEL-PCD network). We have combined data on intentions and opinions with estimates of PN/PT from GP registers and thereby obtained much better insight into practice and attitude towards PN and PIPT.

Some sources provided more in-depth information than others. The questionnaires used for the (pre)conference surveys were short and with the instruction to choose one 'most applicable' answer (multiple choice), more subtle nuances may have been lost. The vignette study on the other hand offered more room for opinions and thoughts, giving insight in opportunities and challenges foreseen for PIPT implementation. Intentions to use PIPT seemed higher than actual practice, maybe due to the discrepancy between intention and implementation but might also indicate that GPs would like to apply PIPT more often but are restricted by guidelines or regulations. Risk profiles of patients (e.g. sexual preference) are not described in regular patient records, so the actual insight into PN/PT practice of GP's in high risk groups was limited.

The information on PIPT from prescription data had major limitations. The national pharmacy data showed a small but increasing proportion of Azithromycin prescribed as double dosage, but without the indication for the medication, we cannot be certain these were for chlamydia. Moreover, the recent update of the GP STI guideline (end of 2013), [7] provides a 3rd choice treatment option of Azithromycin 2 g single dose for gonorrhoea, for patients for whom Ceftriaxone is contra-indicated and the resistance pattern unavailable. We saw a clear rise in double dosages from 2013 onwards as well as an unequal gender distribution of the double dosages, which suggests these prescriptions may be for gonorrhoea rather than for chlamydia, because gonorrhoea is seen more commonly in men than in women [1], due to the sexual network (MSM) and symptomatic nature of infections in men, urging them to visit their GP. Probably, the level before 2013 (0.4–0.5%) shows the actual proportion of double dosages for patient and partner prescription. In the NIVEL-PCD, part of the double/repeated prescriptions of antibiotics seems unlikely to be PIPT. Double dosages of Doxycycline were prescribed in more than 30% of cases, especially in men (46%); we suspect these relate to other diagnoses including (acute) epididymitis or PID, for which a prolonged course is indicated. The repeated prescriptions on 1 day may also have been registration artefacts, due to back reporting from pharmacies after patients receive the medication. Hence, to be able to use prescription data to monitor PIPT, more reliable information on the prescription and its indication is required. The registration in the national pharmacy database would be improved by including the indication of prescriptions. Prescription data from the GP electronic patient registration would be improved by adapting software to extract more exact dosage schemes and clarifying whether or not back-reporting from the pharmacy takes place in the one or more of the current registration software systems in use.

Comparison to other studies and countries

We found that the implementation of PIPT for chlamydia is currently low among GPs in the Netherlands, while GPs showed a higher intention to use PIPT when presented with hypothetical chlamydia cases and after PIPT principles were explained briefly. The low level is not surprising, as in the current legal system in the Netherlands the GP should have contact with the partner, before prescribing antibiotics, to check medical history and allergies and inform about the reason for prescription. [25] In fact, some of the cases of PIPT in the records may have been given without observing the law. In other countries where PIPT is legal, levels of uptake are still relatively low: in the US, in a national survey of more than 3000 physicians who treat patients for STIs, approximately 50% reported ever using PIPT, while only 11%–14% of physicians reported usually or always using PIPT. [26] In New York City, the number of expedited partner therapy prescriptions was found to be low and vary greatly between pharmacies in New York City. [27] In the UK, in a pilot RCT the proportion of partners treated after partner details (medical history and allergies) were communicated via the phone (35%) or at pharmacy (46%) did not exceed that by standard patient referral (45%). [18]

In our vignette study, GPs have shown to be aware of the beneficial effects of PIPT in preventing further transmission and facilitating partner management procedures for chlamydia, as has been assessed in effectiveness studies in other countries (US [13 16], UK [28]) and reviews reporting an overall 20–29% reduction of reinfection. [6, 29, 30] Besides the effect on transmission, PIPT can simplify procedures for the partner, which will make treatment much faster. The few cases that may receive PIPT, according to the present study, appear to be at relatively low risk, with a steady partner who is patient in the same practice. Successful treatment of current partners is most important for preventing reinfection of index cases and reducing further transmission of chlamydia at the population level. On the other hand, also for casual partners, or when it is likely that partners will not seek treatment and are at high risk of infection, PIPT is a good last option or 'better than nothing' [31]. Modelling studies by Althaus [32, 33] showed that PN for partners up to 18 months back would identify 10% infections in notified partners.

The GPs in our study also mentioned important barriers to implement PIPT, which have been reported in the literature as well. [30, 31] GPs stated in the questionnaire that PIPT reduces the opportunity for the partner to see a professional and get further STI counselling and advice. [34] Current legislation requires direct contact with partners. It remains unclear if contact by telephone is sufficient to meet the legal requirements for the prescription of a drug. It is defendable that under certain conditions contact by telephone with a partner will suffice, but the applicable law nor the existing case law gives a decisive answer to that question. Contacting partners via internet would however certainly require a change in legal requirements. Current GP guidelines on partner notification should be extended with a specification of how and when PIPT can be applied (for partners in the same practice and/or when timely treatment is impossible without PIPT). A further concern is that the patient may not reach his/her partner(s) so partner uptake is not guaranteed. [19, 35] The partner may have other STIs or have sexual contact with other partners, which would not be traced with PIPT. [36] Potential over-treatment by PIPT is a real concern, as only 35% of those notified for chlamydia are found infected. [1] Following antibiotic stewardship, careful use of antibiotics is advocated and embedded in the Dutch habit of relatively low use of antibiotics in patient care in general (the lowest in Europe [37]). Resistance of chlamydia to Azithromycin is not an urgent threat, [38] but for gonorrhoea, a common co-infection with chlamydia which could go unnoticed with PIPT, it is on the rise. [39] Furthermore, in case of an anal (co)infection, chlamydia should be treated with Doxycycline and not just Azithromycin. [7, 8]

Conclusions/recommendations

GPs in the Netherlands are open to implement PIPT for some chlamydia cases but not for all, provided there are clear guidelines, including clarity about legal options, and indications how PIPT can be applied and which patients and partners would be eligible for PIPT. We advise recommendations for partner treatment in GP guidelines to be extended with a specification of when and how PIPT can be applied.

Endnotes

[1]See: https://www.sfk.nl/english (accessed may 2017)

[2]See: www.nivel.nl/NZR/zorgregistraties-eerstelijn (accessed may 2017)

Abbreviations

APT: Accelerated Partner Therapy; ATC: Anatomical Therapeutic Chemical classification system; EPT: Expedited Partner Therapy; GP: General Practitioner; ICPC: International Coding Primary Care; MHS : Municipal Health Services; PIPT: Patient Initiated Partner Therapy; PN: Partner Notification; PT: Partner Treatment; STI: Sexually Transmitted Infection

Acknowledgements

We want to acknowledge all GPs for their participation in questionnaires. We are grateful to the GPs in the NIVEL-PCD network for their cooperation in supplying anonymised patient data and especially the GPs of the sentinel practices (*Peilstations*) for the extra questionnaires on STI consultations. Furthermore, the authors appreciate the input from the other PICCUP project members: F van Aar, G Haringhuizen (RIVM), A Watzeels, A Nanhoe (GGD Rotterdam Rijnmond), C Phillips-Santman (Leiden UMC) and G Kok (Maastricht University).

Funding

The project received funding from ZonMW (The Netherlands Organisation for Health Research and Development), research grant number 5220020.

Authors' contributions

IvdB coordinated the data collection and analyses of the various datasources and wrote the draft versions of the manuscript. GD was involved in the parts of study on NIVEL-PCD (questionnaire and data), KH analysed the prescription data from NIVEL-PCD and drafted the related part of the manuscript. All authors, including JEvB, BHvB and HMG, were involved in the overall design of the study, follow-up of progress and commenting on earlier versions of the manuscript. All authors read and approved the final manuscript.

Ethics approval and consent to participate

For patient-derived data from the NIVEL-PCD and the national pharmacy data (SFK), ethics approval via an METC was not needed, as explained in the 'Privacy statement NIVEL PCD': Dutch law allows the use of electronic health records for research purposes under certain conditions. According to this legislation, neither obtaining informed consent from patients nor approval of a medical ethics committee is obligatory for this type of observational studies containing no directly identifiable data (Dutch Civil Law, Article 7:458; http://www.dutchcivillaw.com/civilcodebook077.htm). This study has been approved by the applicable governance bodies of NIVEL Primary Care Database under nr. NZR00316.012).

For the national pharmacy database, SFK, privacy regulations guarantee the privacy of the participating pharmacists. With regard to the prescribing doctor and the patient, the SFK only uses anonymously gathered data. Respondent GPs (questionnaires) gave informed consent for use of anonymised data for publication.

Consent for publication

Not applicable.

Competing interests

The authors declare that they have no competing interests.

Author details

[1]Epidemiology and Surveillance Unit, Centre for Infectious Diseases Control, RIVM, Bilthoven, The Netherlands. [2]NIVEL Primary Care Database, Sentinel Practices, Utrecht, The Netherlands. [3]NIVEL Primary Care database, Utrecht, The Netherlands. [4]Epidemiology and Surveillance Unit, Centre for Infectious Diseases Control, RIVM, Bilthoven, The Netherlands. [5]Department of General Practice, Academic Medical Center, Amsterdam; STI AIDS Netherlands, Amsterdam, The Netherlands. [6]Department of Infectious Disease Control, Municipal Public Health Service Rotterdam-Rijnmond, Rotterdam, The Netherlands. [7]Department of Public Health, Erasmus MC—University Medical Center Rotterdam, Rotterdam, The Netherlands.

References

1. van den Broek I, van Aar F, van Oeffelen A, et al.: Sexually transmitted infections in the Netherlands in 2015. In: *RIVM report*. vol. 2016–0027. Bilthoven, The Netherlands: RIVM; 2016.
2. Götz H, Wolfers M, Luijendijk A, van den Broek I. Retesting for genital Chlamydia trachomatis among visitors of a sexually transmitted infections clinic: randomized intervention trial of home- versus clinic-based recall. BMC Infect Dis. 2013;13:239.
3. Hosenfeld C, Workowski K, Bouman S, Zaidi A, Dyson J, Mosure D, Bolan G, Bauer H. Repeat infection with Chlamydia and gonorrhea among females: a systematic review of the literature. Sex Transm Dis. 2009;36(8):478–89.
4. Kampman C, Koedijk F, Driessen-Hulshof H, Hautvast J, van den Broek I. Retesting young STI clinic visitors with urogenital Chlamydia trachomatis infection in the Netherlands; response to a text message reminder and reinfection rates: a prospective study with historical controls. Sex Transm Infect. 2016;92(2):124–9.
5. Geisler W, Lensing S, Press C, Hook E. Spontaneous resolution of genital Chlamydia trachomatis infection in women and protection from reinfection. J Infect Dis. 2013;207(12):1850–6.
6. Ferreira A, Young T, Mathews C, Zunza M, Low N. Strategies for partner notification for sexually transmitted infections, including HIV. Cochrane Database Syst Rev. 2013;3(10):CD002843.
7. Van Bergen J, Dekker J, Boeke A, Kronenberg E, Van der Spruit R, Burgers J, Bouma M, Verlee E. Dutch GP guideline on STI consultations [guidelines in Dutch: NHG-Standaard het soa-consult (Eerste herziening)]. Huisarts en Wetenschap. 2013;56:450–63.
8. de Vries H, van Doornum G, Bax C, al. e: Multidisciplinary guidelines sexually transmitted diseases secondary care [guidelines in Dutch: Multidisciplinaire Richtlijn Seksueel Overdraagbare Aandoeningen voor de 2e Lijn]. In. Nederlandse Vereniging voor Dermatologie en Venereologie; 2012. www.huidarts.info.
9. Gotz HM, van Rooijen MS, Vriens P, Op de Coul E, Hamers M, Heijman T, van den Heuvel F, Koekenbier R, van Leeuwen AP, Voeten HA. Initial evaluation of use of an online partner notification tool for STI, called 'suggest a test': a cross sectional pilot study. Sex Transm Infect. 2014;90(3):195–200.
10. Voeten HACM: Anoniem sekspartners waarschuwen? Het kan via www.partnerwaarschuwing.nl. Medisch Farmaceutische Mededelingen, praktijkgerichte nascholing over farmacotherapie, 27 oktober 2016 (https://www.pil-nascholing.nl/tijdschrift/editie/artikel/t/anoniem-sekspartners-waarschuwen).
11. Centers for Disease Control and Prevention: Expedited partner therapy in the management of sexually transmitted diseases.. In. Edited by US DEpartment of Health and Human Services. Atlanta, GA,; 2006.
12. Oliver A, Rogers M, Schillinger J: The Impact of Prescriptions on Sex Partner Treatment Using Expedited Partner Therapy for Chlamydia trachomatis Infection, New York City, 2014–2015. Sex Transm Dis. 2016;43(11):673-78.
13. Schillinger J, Kissinger P, Calvet H, Whittington W, Ransom R, Sternberg M, Berman S, Kent C, Martin D, Oh M, et al. Patient-delivered partner treatment with azithromycin to prevent repeated Chlamydia trachomatis infection among women: a randomized, controlled trial. Sex Transm Dis. 2003;30(1):49–56.
14. Golden M, Whittington W, Handsfield H, Hughes J, Stamm W, Hogben M, Clark A, Malinski C, Helmers J, Thomas K, et al. Effect of expedited treatment of sex partners on recurrent or persistent gonorrhea or chlamydial infection. N Engl J Med. 2005;352(7):676–85.
15. Kissinger P, Mohammed H, Richardson-Alston G, Leichliter J, Taylo S, Martin D, Farley T: Patient-delivered partner treatment for male urethritis: a randomized, controlled trial. *Clin Infect Dis* 2005, **41**(5):623-629.
16. Golden M, Kerani R, Stenger M, Hughes J, Aubin M, Malinski C, Holmes K. Uptake and population-level impact of expedited partner therapy (EPT) on Chlamydia trachomatis and Neisseria gonorrhoeae: the Washington state community-level randomized trial of EPT. PLoS Med. 2015;12(1):e1001777.
17. Legal Status of EPT - Summary Totals (July 1, 2016). See: website Centers for Disease Control and Prevention, section Sexually Transmitted Diseases: https://www.cdc.gov/std/ept/legal/totals.htm.

18. Estcourt C, Sutcliffe L, Copas A, Mercer C, Roberts T, Jackson L, Symonds M, Tickle L, Muniina P, Rait G, et al. Developing and testing accelerated partner therapy for partner notification for people with genital Chlamydia trachomatis diagnosed in primary care: a pilot randomised controlled trial. Sex Transm Infect. 2015;91(8):548–54.
19. Cameron S, Glasier A, Muir A, Scott G, Johnstone A, Quarrell H, Oroz C, McIntyre M, Miranda D, Todd G. Expedited partner therapy for Chlamydia trachomatis at the community pharmacy. BJOG. 2010;117(9): 1074–9.
20. Dombrowski J, Golden M. Accelerated partner therapy: a promising new partner treatment option. Sex Transm Infect. 2012;88(1):2–3.
21. Van den Broek IV, Donker GA, Hek K, Van Benthem BHB, van Bergen JEAM, Götz HM P3.224 Partner notification and partner treatment for chlamydia: atttitude and practice of general practitioners in the Netherlands. Sexually Transmitted Infections. 2017,93(Suppl 2):A177. doi:10.1136/sextrans-2017-053264.459.
22. van den Broek I, Verheij R, van Dijk C, Koedijk F, van der Sande M, van Bergen J. Trends in sexually transmitted infections in the Netherlands, combining surveillance data from general practices and sexually transmitted infection centres. BMC Fam Pract. 2010;11:39.
23. Peabod J, Luck J. P G, Jain S, Hansen J, spell M: measuring the quality of physician practice by using clinical vignettes: a prospective validation study. Ann Intern Med. 2004;141(10):771–80.
24. Peabody J, Luck J, Glassman P, Dresselhaus T, Lee M. Comparison of vignettes, standardized patients, and chart abstraction: a prospective validation study of 3 methods for measuring quality. JAMA. 2000; 283(13):1715–22.
25. Geneesmiddelenwet. Hoofdstuk 6: Terhandstelling van geneesmiddelen en het voorschrijven daarvan (Artikelen 61–68), See: http://wetten.overheid.nl/BWBR0021505/2016-08-01#Hoofdstuk6 (accessed May 2017).
26. Hogben M, McCree DH, Golden MR. Patient-delivered partner therapy for sexually transmitted diseases as practiced by U.S. physicians. Sex Transm Dis. 2005;32(2):101–5.
27. Okah E, Arya V, Rogers M, Kim M, Schillinger JA. Sentinel surveillance for expedited partner therapy prescriptions using pharmacy data, in 2 new York City neighborhoods, 2015. Sex Transm Dis. 2017;44(2):104–8.
28. Cameron S, Glasier A, Scott G, Young H, Melvin L, Johnstone A, Elton R. Novel interventions to reduce re-infection in women with chlamydia: a randomized controlled trial. Hum Reprod. 2009;24(4): 888–95.
29. Hogben M, Collins D, Hoots B, O'Connor K: Partner Services in Sexually Transmitted Disease Prevention Programs: a review. Sex Transm Dis 2016, 43(2 Suppl 1):S53-S62.
30. Gannon-Loew K, Holland-Hall C, Bonny A: A Review of Expedited Partner Therapy for the Management of Sexually Transmitted Infections in Adolescents. *J Pediatr Adolesc Gynecol* 2017, Feb 3. pii: S1083–3188(16)30276–5. doi: https://doi.org/10.1016/j.jpag.2017.01.012. [Epub ahead of print].
31. Pavlin N, Parker R, Piggin A, Hopkins C, Temple-Smith M, Fairley C, Tomnay J, Bowden F, Russell D, Hocking J, et al. Better than nothing? Patient-delivered partner therapy and partner notification for chlamydia: the views of Australian general practitioners. BMC Infect Dis. 2010;10:274. https://doi.org/10.1186/1471-2334-1110-1274.
32. Althaus C, Turner K, Mercer C, Auguste P, Roberts T, Bell G, Herzog S, Cassell J, Edmunds W, White P, et al. Effectiveness and cost-effectiveness of traditional and new partner notification technologies for curable sexually transmitted infections: observational study, systematic reviews and mathematical modelling. Health Technol Assess. 2014;18(3):1–100.
33. Althaus CL, Heijne JC, Herzog SA, Roellin A, Low N. Individual and population level effects of partner notification for Chlamydia trachomatis. PLoS One. 2012;7(12):e51438.
34. Rosenfeld E, Marx J, Terry M, Stall R, Flatt J, Borrero S, Miller E. Perspectives on expedited partner therapy for chlamydia: a survey of health care providers. Int J STD AIDS. 2016;27(13):1180–6.
35. Goldsworthy R, Fortenberry D. Patterns and determinants of patient-delivered therapy uptake among healthcare consumers. Sex Transm Dis. 2009;36(1):25–32.
36. Forbes G, Clutterbuck D. How many cases of chlamydial infection would we miss by not testing partners for infection? Int J STD AIDS. 2009;20(4):267–8.
37. OECD Health Statistics: Health at a Glance: Europe 2016: State of Health in the EU Cycle. Overall volume of antibiotics prescribed, 2014 (or nearest year). In. DOI:https://doi.org/10.1787/health_glance_eur-2016-graph115-en: OECD; 2016.
38. Kong F, Hocking J: Treatment challenges for urogenital and anorectal Chlamydia trachomatis. BMC Infect Dis 2015, **15**(293):doi: https://doi.org/10.1186/s12879-12015-11030-12879.
39. Wind CM, van der Loeff MF S, van Dam AP, de Vries HJ, van der Helm JJ. Trends in antimicrobial susceptibility for azithromycin and ceftriaxone in Neisseria gonorrhoeae isolates in Amsterdam, the Netherlands, between 2012 and 2015. Euro surveillance. 2017;22:1.

8

Impact of a continuing medical education meeting on the use and timing of urgent cancer referrals among general practitioners

Berit Skjødeberg Toftegaard[1,2,3*], Flemming Bro[1,3], Alina Zalounina Falborg[1,2,3] and Peter Vedsted[1,2,4]

Abstract

Background: Detection of cancer in general practice is challenging because symptoms are diverse. Even so-called alarm symptoms have low positive predictive values of cancer. Nevertheless, appropriate referral is crucial. As 85% of cancer patients initiate their cancer diagnostic pathway in general practice, a Continuing Medical Education meeting (CME-M) in early cancer diagnosis was launched in Denmark in 2012. We aimed to investigate the effect of the CME-M on the primary care interval, patient contacts with general practice and use of urgent cancer referrals.

Methods: A before-after study was conducted in the Central Denmark Region included 396 general practices, which were assigned to one of eight geographical clusters. Practices were invited to participate in the CME-M with three-week intervals between clusters. Based on register data, we calculated urgent referral rates and patient contacts with general practice before referral. Information about primary care intervals was collected by requesting general practitioners to complete a one-page form for each urgent referral during an 8-month period around the time of the CME-Ms. CME-M practices were compared with non-participating reference practices by analysing before-after differences.

Results: Forty percent of all practices participated in the CME-M. There was a statistically significant reduction in the number of total contacts with general practice from urgently referred patients in the month preceding the referral and an increase in the proportion of patients who waited 14 days or more in general practice from the reported date of symptom presentation to the referral date from before to after the CME-M in the CME-M group compared to the reference group.

Conclusions: We found a reduced number of total patient contacts with general practice within the month preceding an urgent referral and an increase in the reported primary care intervals of urgently referred patients in the CME-M group. The trend towards higher urgent referral rates and longer primary care intervals may suggest raised awareness of unspecific cancer symptoms, which could cause the GP to register an earlier date of first symptom presentation. The standardised CME-M may contribute to optimising the timing and the use of urgent cancer referral.

Keywords: Denmark, General practice, Continuing medical education meeting, Diagnosis, Early detection of cancer, Behavioural change, Referral rate, Primary care interval, Use of health care

* Correspondence: berit.toftegaard@feap.dk
[1]Research Unit for General Practice, Department of Public Health, Aarhus University, Bartholins Allé 2, Aarhus DK-8000, Denmark
[2]Research Centre for Cancer Diagnosis in Primary Care (CaP), Department of Public Health, Aarhus University, Bartholins Allé 2, Aarhus DK-8000, Denmark
Full list of author information is available at the end of the article

Background

Danish cancer patients have lower survival and more advanced disease stages at treatment initiation than many other European countries [1, 2]. The ability among general practitioners (GPs) to interpret and respond to symptoms plays a pivotal role in cancer detection as 85% of all cancer patients initiate their diagnostic pathway in general practice [3, 4]. Increasing evidence suggests that prompt referral from general practice matters [5–7], and a UK study found that a high propensity to use urgent referrals was associated with better survival of cancer patients [8].

Cancer detection in general practice is, however, a challenging task. The symptoms of cancer are diverse, they develop over time, and they tend to mimic symptoms of trivial and common conditions [9]. Some symptoms are unspecific, e.g. fatigue and weight loss. Others are considered to be alarm symptoms [10] although they have a low positive predictive value of cancer of only 2-10%, depending on age, gender and cancer type [11–13]. Danish cancer patients have increased visits in general practice already six months before the diagnosis [14], and one in four waits for more than 20 days in general practice until referral [4, 15]. Consequently, there may be room for improvements.

To support the GPs' decision strategies for referral, a specific Continuing Medical Education meeting (CME-M) was developed and implemented as part of the Danish National Cancer Plan III in 2012 [16]. The developed CME-M consisted of central elements for cancer detection in primary care [17]. So far, the initial evaluation has shown that the CME-M has affected the knowledge among GPs on cancer diagnosis and their attitude towards own role in cancer detection. The CME-M also lowered the GPs' assessed risk of cancer in urgently referred patients [18]. Yet, we need to explore whether the change in GPs' knowledge and attitude was translated into a behavioural change.

The aim of this study was to investigate the effect of the CME-M on the use of urgent cancer referrals by investigating urgent referral rates and the timing of urgent referrals in terms of length of primary care interval and number of patient contacts with general practice before referral.

Methods

The setting of the study was the Central Denmark Region with approx. 1.3 million inhabitants and 8,000 new cancer patients annually [19]. The Danish healthcare system is tax-funded with free access for citizens to medical advice and treatment in general practice and hospitals. More than 98% of the Danish citizens are listed with a specific general practice, which they must consult for medical advice. GPs serve as gatekeepers to specialised care, such as diagnostic investigations and hospital care [20]. In order to ensure consistency in the GPs' selection of patients for urgent cancer referrals, national referral guidelines were made for each cancer fast-track pathway [21, 22]. As an example, the referral guideline for colorectal cancer state that cancer should be considered if a patient above 40 years of age presents at least one of the following symptoms: visible rectal bleeding, discharge of mucus or changes in bowel habits or stools for a four-week period, iron-deficiency anaemia and unspecific symptoms as pain or weight loss [21]. All Danish citizens have a civil personal registration (CPR) number, which enables linkage of information at the individual level between national registries and allows identification of the practice at which each citizen is listed [23].

Design

We conducted a before-after study with a stepwise enrolment of GPs in the CME-Ms [17]. All practices in the Central Denmark Region were allocated to one of eight clusters by exploiting the already existing municipal units. The Regional Cancer Quality Unit assigned the random order in which all GPs (practices) in the cluster were offered the CME-M at 3-week intervals within the period 1 September 2012 to 1 May 2013 (Fig. 1). GPs were registered if they participated in the CME-M [17].

Intervention: continuing medical education meeting

The content of the CME-M was developed through a comprehensive process, which has been described previously in detail [17]. The CME-M provided the GPs with new knowledge on symptoms of cancer and presented risk assessment tools (RATs) for lung, colorectal, ovarian and prostate cancer [13, 24]. Use of investigations and reasons for missed opportunity [25, 26] were discussed in terms of risk of false reassurance [27, 28]. Mechanisms affecting referral thresholds were debated based on patient cases [29].

Outcomes

Use of urgent referrals was operationalised as: 1) *urgent referral rate per GP* (i.e. number of urgently referred patients during six months per GP in the practice) and 2) *urgent referral rate per 1000 patients in the practice* (i.e. number of urgently referred patients during six months per 1000 listed patients aged > 40 years in the practice). Timing of urgent referrals was operationalised as: 1) *prior contacts* (i.e. number of daytime contacts with general practice from urgently referred patients before referral) and 2) *primary care interval* (i.e. number of days from first presentation in general practice until urgent referral to secondary care) [30].

Practice population

The practices were identified in the Danish provider number registry. The number of included practices

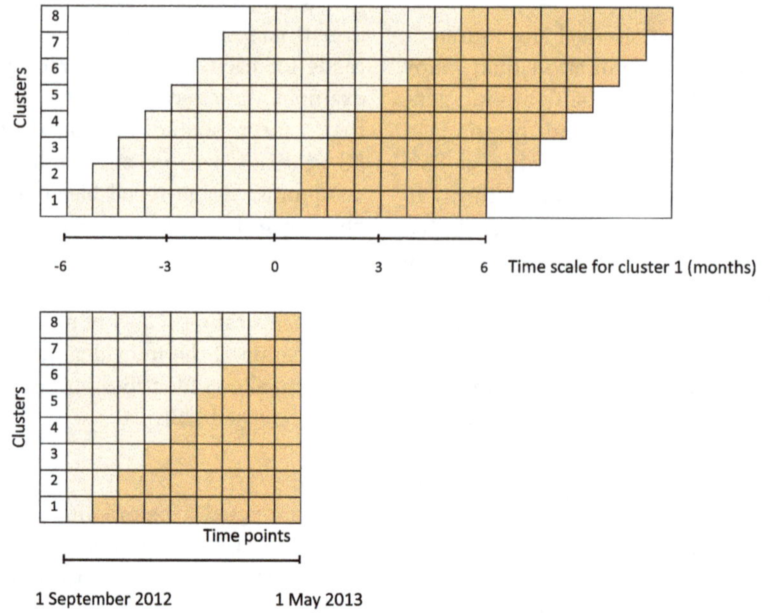

Fig. 1 Time periods used for classifying patient populations. The cluster-specific time period used for identifying urgently referred patients in the primary care referral database (*light boxes* = time before CME-M; *dark boxes* = time after CME-M). The method at the top was applied for evaluating CME-M effect on referral rates and patient contacts with general practice. The method at the bottom was used for evaluating CME-M effect on primary care intervals

depended on the outcome to be measured. For *urgent referral rates,* practices were included if registered from six months before to six months after their CME-M date. For prior *contacts,* practices were included if registered from 18 months before to six months after their CME-M date. For *primary care interval,* practices were included if registered in the period from 1 September 2012 to 1 May 2013 provided that they had completed one-page forms (Additional file 1).

Patient populations

The urgently referred patients were identified by applying an algorithm, which was developed for the purpose, to the primary care referral database [31]. The algorithm had a sensitivity of 93.6%, a specificity of 97.3%, a positive predictive value of 83.6% and a negative predictive value of 99.0% for identifying urgently referred patients aged ≥ 40 years without prior cancer among all referred patients aged ≥ 40 years [31].

For *urgent referral rates,* patients were included if: 1) identified by the algorithm, 2) referred from an included practice from six months before until six months after the CME-M date of the practice, 3) age ≥ 40 years and 4) no prior cancer.

For *prior contacts,* patients were included on the same criteria as above. Furthermore, they were also required to have been listed with the same practice for one year prior to the referral date.

For *primary care interval,* patients were included if: 1) identified by the algorithm, 2) referred from an included practice from 1 September 2012 to 1 May 2013, 3) age ≥ 40 years, 4) no prior cancer and 5) receipt of one-page form stating the date of first symptom presentation and the date of referral.

Patients already diagnosed with cancer were excluded based on data in the Danish Cancer Registry [32] registered in accordance with the International Classification of Diseases, 10th revision: C0-C9, except for non-melanoma skin cancer (C44) [33].

Variables

Patient contacts with general practice were obtained from the Danish National Health Service Register [34]. The registration is based on fee-for-service remuneration of the providing GP, and the records in this registry are generally considered highly complete [35]. We used two variables: 1) face-to-face (F2F) contacts and 2) total contacts, which included F2F, phone and e-mail contacts.

Date of first presentation of symptom in general practice and date of referral were collected by requesting GPs to complete a one-page form including the patient's CPR number each time a patient was referred for suspected cancer during an 8-month period around the CME-Ms (1 September 2012 to 1 May 2013) (Fig. 1) [17]. Furthermore, in the hospital patient administrative system, patients registered as investigated as part of an urgent referral were identified every other week. If the one-page form was missing, the relevant GP was requested to complete a form and to specify the patient's route to investigation. This was done to increase the completeness of data for urgently referred patients.

The development, pilot-testing, coding and data transfer of the forms have been reported elsewhere [17].

Age and gender distribution of the patient population for each practice was obtained from the patient list system on 1 January 2013.

The Danish Deprivation Index (DADI), which is used to adjust for differences in socioeconomic factors, was calculated based on data from the Integrated Database for Labour Market Research [36]. The DADI has a value between 10 and 100; the higher the number, the more deprived population. The variables used were: (i) proportion of adults aged 20–59 years with no employment, (ii) proportion of adults aged 25–59 years with no professional education, (iii) proportion of adults aged 25–59 years with low income, (iv) proportion of adults aged 18–59 years receiving public welfare benefits (transfer payments or social security benefits), (v) proportion of children from parents with no education and no professional skills, (vi) proportion of immigrants, (vii) proportion of adults aged 30+ years living alone and (viii) proportion of adults aged 70+ years with low income (= the lowest national quartile).

A modified Charlson Comorbidity Index score [37] was obtained for each referred patient by using data from the Danish National Patient Register with the referral date as the index date [38]. We divided the comorbidity scores into "none" (no recorded disease), "moderate" (score of 1 or 2) and "high" (score of 3 or more) [15].

The suspected cancer type stated at the one-page form was divided into two groups of cancer detection difficulty based on the available evidence [39]. Cancers considered *easier to detect* included suspected cancer in kidney, bladder, breast, head and neck, female genitalia, nevus (melanoma), penis, testis and gastrointestinal system, whereas cancers considered *harder to detect* included suspected cancer in pancreas, liver and gall bladder, brain, lymph node and bone marrow, lung, prostate, connective tissue including fat, muscle and bones, and suspicion based on unspecific serious symptoms.

Statistical analyses

Practices were divided into two groups: practices with at least one CME-M-participating GP ("CME-M practices") and practices without any CME-M-participating GPs ("reference practices").

The time point for a CME-M session for each cluster was defined as the point that separated the time of observation in "before CME-M" and "after CME-M" (Fig. 1). The data collected before and after the CME-M provided paired responses for each outcome. The practice and patient populations were described by their characteristics.

Urgent referral rates were indirectly age-sex standardised as we used the full patient population in the Central Denmark Region as standard population divided into ten-year age groups (40–49, 50–59, etc.).

The CME-M effect on *urgent referral rates* was analysed using mixed-effects negative binomial regression [40] with a random effect associated with the intercept for each practice to make comparisons before and after CME-M within and between groups. The model allowed dealing with repeated observations on practice level. The time of observation (before and after CME-M) was treated as a fixed-effect variable. In the analysis of *urgent referral rates per GP*, the number of GPs per practice was treated as an exposure variable. The effects within groups were reported as incidence rate ratios (IRRs). Comparison of effects between groups was reported as a ratio of the IRRs. The analyses were adjusted for cluster, type of practice (single-handed/partnership) and DADI index. A single-handed practice was defined as a practice with only one GP. A stratified analysis was performed on practice type.

Prior contacts were measured in different time intervals: 0–1 month, 0–3 months and 4–6 months preceding referral. The number of contacts during the 7–12 months preceding referral was calculated to estimate an average habitual contact rate per month for each patient.

The CME-M effect on *prior contacts* was analysed using mixed-effects negative binomial regression with a random effect associated with the intercept for each practice and time of observation as a fixed-effect variable to make comparisons before and after CME-M within and between groups while adjusting for patient clustering in the practices. The results were reported as IRRs or a ratio of the IRRs. Due to convergence problems for F2F within the last month preceding the referral, the analysis was based on ordinary negative binomial regression applying cluster robust variance at practice level.

For the 10% of patients with most frequent contact, the number of F2F contacts and total contacts were dichotomised based on the 90th percentile (number of contacts within 0–1 month was 4 for F2F and 5 for total contacts). A mixed-effects logistic regression [41] allowed for random effects at practice level, and the observation time (before and after) was treated as a fixed-effect variable. The effects were reported as odds ratios (ORs) for having most contacts within groups and ratio of the ORs between groups.

The analyses were adjusted for cluster, practice type, patient gender, age, habitual monthly contact rate and comorbidity. Furthermore, a stratified analysis on practice type was performed.

The *primary care intervals* were calculated as medians, 75th and 90th percentiles. We dichotomised the intervals based on the 75th and 90th percentiles from before the CME-M. Comparisons within and between groups were estimated with mixed-effects logistic regression with a random effect associated with the intercept for each practice adjusting for patient clustering in the practices. The results were reported as ORs or a ratio of the ORs. The analyses were adjusted for cluster, practice type, patient gender, age, co-morbidity and cancer detection difficulty. Furthermore, stratified analyses were performed on cancer detection difficulty and type of practice.

The statistical software Stata 13.0 (StataCorp LP, TX, USA) was used for the analyses [42].

Results

Study population

A total of 148 of the 396 general practices (37.4%) participated in the CME-M (Table 1). Compared to the reference practices, the CME-M practices were more often partnership practices, the GPs were slightly younger and more often female, the practice population size per GP was lower, the practice population consisted of fewer male and slightly less deprived patients (Tables 1 and 2).

The patients used for calculation of the *primary care interval* were included by 139 CME-M practices and 199 reference practices (Table 3).

Impact of CME-M on urgent referral rates

The CME-M was associated with a two-fold relative rise in *urgent referral rates per GP* when comparing CME-M practices with reference practices. Within the CME-M group, this increase was statistically significant (IRR: 1.05 (95% CI: 1.01;1.08) (Table 4). Each CME-M practice referred one patient more per 1000 patients in their underlying practice population during the 6-month period after the CME-M compared to before; this increase was three times higher than the increase in

Table 1 Characteristics of practices, GPs and patients used for CME-M impact on urgent referral rates

	Reference group		CME-M group	
Study base, Practices, *N*	248		148	
Proportion of solo practices (95% CI)	0.60 (0.54;0.66)		0.30 (0.23;0.38)	
GPs per practice, mean (range)	1.72 (1–5)		2.60 (1–10)	
GPs, *N*	*425*		*385*	
Proportion of males (95% CI)	0.59 (0.54;0.64)		0.48 (0.43;0.53)	
Mean age (95% CI)	52.6 (51.7;53.4)		51.6 (50.8;52.4)	
Underlying practice populations, *N*	661,805		570,926	
Mean list size, patients ≥ 40 yrs. per practice	1353		1920	
Mean list size, patients ≥ 40 yrs. per GP in practice	787		738	
Proportion of male patients aged ≥ 40 yrs. (95% CI)	0.50 (0.49;0.50)		0.48 (0.47;0.49)	
Age groups (yrs.), proportion of all patients ((%)(95% CI))				
0–39	48.6 (47.4; 49.9)		49.9 (48.4; 51.3)	
40–49	14.1 (13.8;14.4)		14.0 (13.7;14.4)	
50–59	13.4 (13.0;13.7)		12.7 (12.2;13.1)	
60–69	12.5 (12.0;12.9)		12.1 (11.6;12.6)	
70–79	7.3 (6.9;7.6)		7.2 (6.8;7.6)	
80–90	3.5 (3.3; 3.7)		3.4 (3.2; 3.6)	
Above 90	0.76 (0.7; 0.8)		0.73 (0.7; 0.8)	
Mean DADI index (95% CI)	26.9 (25.9;27.8)		25.5 (24.4;26.5)	
Referred patients (age ≥ 40 yrs.)	*Before CME-M, N = 8,388*	*After CME-M, N = 8,534*	*Before CME-M, N = 7,579*	*After CME-M, N = 7,942*
Proportion of males (95% CI)	0.47 (0.45;0.48)	0.45 (0.44;0.46)	0.44 (0.43;0.46)	0.44 (0.43;0.45)
Mean age (95% CI)	63.0 (62.7;63.3)	63.1 (62.9;63.4)	62.6 (62.3;62.9)	62.8 (62.5;63.1)
Comorbidity[a] (%)				
None	75.5	74.8	76.2	75.2
Medium	20.9	21.3	19.9	21.0
High	3.6	3.9	3.9	3.8

Abbreviations: CME-M continuing medical education meeting, *GP* general practitioner, *CI* confidence interval; yrs., years, *DADI* Danish Deprivation Index
[a]Comorbidity scores were divided into "none" (no recorded disease)," moderate" (score of 1 or 2) and "high" (score of 3 or more)

Table 2 Characteristics of practices, GPs and patients used for CME-M impact on patients' prior contacts

	Reference group		CME-M group	
Practices, *N*	240		144	
Proportion of solo practices (95% CI)	0.60 (0.54;0.66)		0.29 (0.22;0.37)	
GPs per practice, mean (range)	1.73 (1–5)		2.63 (1–10)	
GPs, *N*	415		377	
Proportion of males (95% CI)	0.60 (0.55;0.64)		0.48 (0.43;0.53)	
Mean age (95% CI)	52.9 (52.0;53.7)		51.7 (50.9;52.5)	
Referred patients (age ≥ 40 yrs.), *N*	*Before CME-M, N = 7,659*	*After CME-M, N = 7,731*	*Before CME-M, N = 7,121*	*After CME-M, N = 7,417*
Proportion of males (95% CI)	0.46 (0.45;0.47)	0.46 (0.45;0.47)	0.44 (0.43;0.46)	0.44 (0.43;0.45)
Mean age (95% CI)	63.1 (62.8;63.4)	63.2 (62.9;63.5)	62.7 (62.4;63.0)	62.9 (62.6;63.2)
Comorbidity (%)[a]				
None	75.9	75.3	76.4	75.7
Medium	20.7	21.1	19.8	20.8
High	3.4	3.6	3.8	3.6
Mean habitual F2F monthly contact rate[b] (95% CI)	0.60 (0.58;0.61)	0.57 (0.56;0.59)	0.61 (0.59;0.62)	0.60 (0.58;0.61)
Mean habitual total monthly contact rate[b] (95% CI)	1.05 (1.03;1.08)	1.02 (1.00;1.05)	1.07 (1.05;1.10)	1.04 (1.01;1.06)

Abbreviations: CME-M continuing medical education meeting, *GP* general practitioner, *CI* confidence interval; yrs., years, *DADI* Danish Deprivation Index, *F2F* face-to-face
[a]Comorbidity scores were divided into "none" (no recorded disease), " moderate" (score of 1 or 2) and "high" (score of 3 or more)
[b]Mean habitual monthly contact rate: average contacts per month based on number of contacts 7–12 months preceding referral for each patient

reference practices (Table 4). When we stratified on practice type, the partnership practices who participated in the CME-M increased their *urgent referral rate per GP* (IRR: 1.06 (95% CI: 1.02;1.10) and their *urgent referral rate per 1000 patients* (IRR: 1.06 (95% CI: 1.01;1.12) from before to after the CME-M.

Compared with the reference practices, none of these findings were statistically significant (Table 4). Note that the stratified analyses on practice type showed a higher use of *urgent* referrals among CME-M-participating single-handed practices compared to non-participating single-handed practices (Table 4).

Impact of CME-M on prior contacts
There was a statistically significant reduction in the number of total contacts within the last month before referral in the CME-M group compared to the reference group (IRR-ratio: 0.97 (95% CI: 0.94;0.99)) (Table 5). Note the tendency that the proportion of patients contacting the most in terms of total contacts decreased from before to after in the CME-M group (OR-ratio: 0.90 (95% CI: 0.86;1.02)) (Table 5).

Impact of CME-M on primary care intervals
The proportion of patients who waited 14 days or more in the CME-M practices statistically significantly increased from before to after the CME-M compared to the reference practices (OR-ratio: 1.47 (95% CI: 1.06;2.03)) (Table 6). This was also seen as a tendency for other estimates although these figures were not statistically significant. When we stratified on cancer detection difficulty, no statistically significant differences were found in the primary care intervals (Table 6).

Sensitivity analyses
When we excluded patients urgently referred within one or two months after the CME-M date, the CME-M effect on *urgent referral rates* and *prior contacts* did not differ considerably from the main results (Additional file 2).

Discussion
Main findings
Forty percent of general practices participated in the cancer diagnostic CME-M. Increased use of urgent referrals was found in the CME-M group from before to after the CME-M. However, this increase was only small in absolute numbers and was not statistically significantly different from the figures for the reference group. Compared with the reference group, the CME-M seemed to reduce the number of total contacts with general practice in the CME-M group during the last month before the urgent referral. Furthermore, the proportion of patients with more than five contacts in total during the last month decreased in the CME-M group; together this indicates a lower referral threshold.

The CME-M was associated with an increase in the reported primary care intervals.

Strength and limitations
The before-after design allowed us to perform a robust evaluation with corrections for baseline measures of a natural experiment. We controlled for calendar time by

Table 3 Characteristics of practices, GPs and patients used for CME-M impact on patients' primary care interval

	Reference group		CME-M group	
Practices, *N* (proportion of study base %)	199 (82.9%)		139 (93.9%)	
Proportion of solo practices (95% CI)	0.53 (0.46;0.60)		0.26 (0.19;0.35)	
GPs per practice, mean (range)	1.85 (1–5)		2.66 (1–10)	
GPs, *N*	369		370	
Proportion of males (95% CI)	0.57 (0.52;0.62)		0.47 (0.42;0.53)	
Mean age (95% CI)	52.1 (51.2;53.0)		51.4 (50.6;52.2)	
Total referred patients during 8 months (age ≥ 40 yrs.)	*Before CME-M, N = 5,749*	*After CME-M, N = 4,607*	*Before CME-M, N = 4,935*	*After CME-M, N = 5,303*
Proportion of males (95% CI)	0.46 (0.45;0.47)	0.45 (0.44;0.47)	0.44 (0.43;0.46)	0.44 (0.43;0.46)
Mean age (95% CI)	62.8 (62.5;63.1)	63.0 (62.6;63.4)	62.5 (62.1;62.8)	62.8 (62.5;63.2)
Comorbidity (%)				
None	75.3	74.7	75.8	74.8
Medium	20.7	21.3	19.9	21.2
High	4.0	4.0	4.3	3.9
Referred patients with known primary care intervals (age ≥ 40 yrs.) (Response (%))	*Before CME-M, N = 1,227 (21.3%)*	*After CME-M, N = 753 (16.3%)*	*Before CME-M, N = 990 (20.0%)*	*After CME-M, N = 1,102 (20.8%)*
Proportion of males (95% CI)	0.52 (0.49;0.55)	0.54 (0.50;0.57)	0.48 (0.45;0.51)	0.47 (0.44;0.50)
Mean age (95% CI)	64.9 (64.2;65.6)	64.5 (63.6;65.3)	64.5 (63.8;65.3)	64.8 (64.1;65.5)
Comorbidity[a] (%)				
None	76.7	75.4	76.1	75.6
Medium	19.7	20.2	20.1	21.0
High	3.6	4.4	3.8	3.4
Cancer detection difficulty[b] (%)				
Easier to detect	72.2	68.4	69.2	70.2
Harder to detect	23.1	25.4	26.4	24.9
Missing information	4.6	6.2	4.4	4.9

Abbreviations: CME-M continuing medical education meeting, *GP* general practitioner, *CI* confidence interval; yrs., years

[a]Comorbidity scores were divided into "none" (no recorded disease), " moderate" (score of 1 or 2) and "high" (score of 3 or more)

[b]The suspected cancer was divided based on cancer detection difficulty: 1) easier to detect included kidney, bladder, breast, head and neck, female genitalia, nevus (melanoma), penis, testis and gastrointestinal and 2) harder to detect included unspecific symptoms, pancreas, liver and gall bladder, brain, lymph node and bone marrow, lung, prostate and connective tissue, including fat, muscle and bones

comparing CME-M group and reference group and by including the stepwise enrolment of GPs in the CME-M into the modelling of data, which diminished the influence of increasing cancer-related knowledge over time.

Another strength was the well-defined and well-described study population and the valid identification of the individuals listed with the studied practices. Additionally, we were able to link selected information on all included individuals to relevant register data at the individual level.

The main limitation of this study was the natural selection to participate in the CME-M. Participating practices and GPs differed from non-participating practices and GPs, particularly single-handed practices differed on the use of urgent referrals (Table 4). This indicates that CME-M participating practices cannot be directly compared to non-participating practices. The CME-M practices had a higher use of urgent referrals among 1000 patients at baseline; this indicates that their potential for improvement was lower than for the entire study base, which may have underestimated the effect of the CME-M. However, the true direction of such bias is difficult to establish.

The use of the referral algorithm allowed us to base the identification of urgently referred patients on register data [31]. We have no reason to believe that patients from CME-M practices had different chances of being identified by the algorithm than patients from reference practices. On the contrary, the patient population used for the evaluation of the CME-M effect on the primary care interval required that the referring GP completed the one-page form about the urgently referred patient. The CME-M practices were more likely to complete one-page forms (Table 2), whereas the reference practices lost

Table 4 The CME-M impact on urgent referral rates

	Reference group					CME-M group					Comparison between groups		
	Before CME-M	After CME-M	Before vs. after			Before CME-M	After CME-M	Before vs. after					
			Δ0	IRR0[b] (95% CI)	P			Δ1	IRR1[b] (95% CI)	P	Δ1/Δ0	IRR1/IRR0[b] (95% CI)	P
All data, N practices (GPs)	248 (425)		-			148 (385)		-	-		-		-
Referral rate[a] per GP, mean	20.4	20.8	0.4	1.02[c] (0.98;1.05)	0.316	20.6	21.4	0.8	**1.05[c] (1.01;1.08)**	**0.009**	2.0	1.03[c] (0.98;1.08)	0.214
Referral rate[a] per 1000 patients, mean	25.0	25.3	0.3	1.01[c] (0.98;1.05)	0.435	27.1	28.1	1.0	1.04[c] (0.99;1.08)	0.111	3.3	1.02[c] (0.97;1.08)	0.454
Single-handed practices, N practices (GPs)	149 (149)		-			45 (45)		-	-		-		-
Referral rate[a] per GP, mean	21.3	21.7	0.4	1.02 (0.96;1.08)	0.481	24.0	23.9	−0.1	0.99 (0.89;1.09)	0.796	−0.25	0.97 (0.86;1.08)	0.566
Referral rate[a] per 1000 patients, mean	24.2	24.3	0.1	1.01 (0.95;1.07)	0.763	26.9	26.2	−0.7	0.98 (0.88;1.08)	0.626	−7.0	0.97 (0.86;1.09)	0.567
Partnership practices, N practices (GPs)	99 (276)		-			103 (340)		-	-		-		-
Referral rate[a] per GP, mean	18.9	19.3	0.4	1.02 (0.97;1.05)	0.540	19.0	20.2	1.2	**1.06 (1.02;1.10)**	**0.002**	3.0	1.04 (0.99;1.10)	0.105
Referral rate[a] per 1000 patients, mean	26.3	26.9	0.6	1.02 (0.97;1.08)	0.457	27.2	28.9	1.7	**1.06 (1.01;1.12)**	**0.019**	2.8	1.04 (0.97;1.12)	0.280

Indirectly age-sex standardised referral rates for 6 months before and after CME-M, respectively, are shown for 1000 patients (age ≥ 40 yrs.) per practice and per GP in the practice. Practices are divided into CME-M group and reference group. The referral rates are further stratified on practice type. The effect within a group is shown as an incidence rate ratio (IRR0: Reference group; IRR1: CME-M group). Comparisons between groups are shown as the ratio of the incidence rate ratios

Abbreviations: CME-M continuing medical education meeting, *GP* general practitioner, *IRR* incidence rate ratio, *CI* confidence interval

[a]Indirectly age-sex standardised

[b]Adjusted for cluster and Danish Deprivation index

[c]In addition, adjusted for practice type

Bold = significance level of $p \leq 0.05$

Table 5 The CME-M impact on patients' prior contacts with general practice

	Reference group $N = 240$ practices				CME-M group $N = 144$ practices					
N patients	Before CME-M 7,659	After CME-M 7,731	Before vs. after		Before CME-M 7,121	After CME-M 7,417	Before vs. after		Comparison between groups	
Prior contacts			IRR0[a] (95% CI)	P			IRR1[a] (95% CI)	P	IRR1/IRR0[a] (95% CI)	P
F2F contacts (mean)										
0–1 month	1.91	1.89	1.00 (0.98;1.02)	0.662	1.92	1.90	0.99 (0.97;1.01)	0.190	0.99 (0.96;1.02)	0.525
0–3 months	3.24	3.20	1.00 (0.98;1.02)	0.868	3.23	3.22	1.00 (0.98;1.02)	0.950	1.00 (0.97;1.03)	0.872
4–6 months	1.82	1.81	1.01 (0.98;1.05)	0.536	1.84	1.83	0.99 (0.96;1.03)	0.870	0.99 (0.94;1.04)	0.583
Total contacts (mean)										
0–1 month	2.84	2.87	1.01 (0.99;1.03)	0.189	2.95	2.87	**0.98 (0.94;0.99)**	**0.044**	**0.97 (0.94;0.99)**	**0.019**
0–3 months	5.17	5.21	1.01 (0.99;1.03)	0.233	5.31	5.19	0.99 (0.97;1.02)	0.369	0.98 (0.95;1.01)	0.137
4–6 months	3.22	3.24	1.00[b] (0.97;1.04)	0.980	3.27	3.21	0.97[b] (0.94; 1.01)	0.138	0.97[b] (0.93;1.02)	0.296
Most contacting patients in the month preceding referral			OR0[a] (95% CI)	P			OR1[a] (95% CI)	P	OR1/OR0[a] (95% CI)	P
F2F contacts ≥ 4[c] (%)	10.4	10.4	1.02 (0.92;1.14)	0.726	10.8	10.8	0.99 (0.89;1.11)	0.911	0.97 (0.84;1.14)	0.745
Total contacts ≥ 5[c] (%)	16.9	17.2	1.04 (0.95;1.13)	0.426	18.5	17.5	0.94 (0.86;1.02)	0.148	0.90 (0.86;1.02)	0.112

Prior contacts are shown as face-to-face and total contacts for three time periods: 0–1, 0–3 and 4–6 months and as the proportions of patients who had most contacts within the last month before referral. Practices are divided into CME-M group and reference group. The effect within a group is shown as an incidence rate ratio (IRR0: Reference group; IRR1: CME-M group), and comparisons between groups are shown as a ratio of incidence rate ratios. The effect on the proportion of the most attending patients within a group is shown as an odds ratio (OR0: Reference group; OR1: CME-M group), and comparisons between groups are shown as a ratio of odds ratios

Abbreviations: CME-M continuing medical education meeting, *F2F* face-to-face, *IRR* incidence rate ratio, *OR* odds ratio, *CI* confidence interval

Face-to-face (F2F) contacts include contacts with GP and patient in same room. Total contacts include face-to-face contacts, e-mails and phone contacts

[a]Adjusted for cluster, practice type, patient's age, gender and habitual contact rate, Charlson Comorbidity Index

[b]Adjusted for cluster, patient age and gender, Charlson Comorbidity Index

[c]90th centile based on all data for F2F contacts and for total contacts

Bold = significance level of $p \leq 0.05$

Table 6 The CME-M impact on patients' primary care interval (PCI)

	Reference group $N = 199$ practices				CME-M group $N = 139$ practices				Comparison between groups	
	Before CME-M	After CME-M	Before vs. after		Before CME-M	After CME-M	Before vs. after			
			OR0[a] (95% CI)	P			OR1[a] (95% CI)	P	OR1/OR0[a] (95% CI)	P
All data, N patients	*1,227*	*753*	-		*990*	*1,102*	-		-	
PCI, median days (percentiles: 75th, 90th)	1 (13. 43)	1 (12, 46)	-		1 (14, 42)	1 (17, 53)	-		-	
PCI ≥ baseline 75th percentile[c] %	25.8	24.4	0.81[2] (0.63;1.04)	0.099	25.1	27.9	1.19[b] (0.95;1.49)	0.135[b]	**1.47[b] (1.06;2.03)**	**0.021**
PCI ≥ baseline 90th percentile[c] %	10.1	10.6	1.12[b] (0.79;1.57)	0.532	10.4	12.5	1.27[b] (0.92;1.74)	0.146	1.13[b] (0.72;1.78)	0.583
Easier to detect, N patients	*887*	*515*	-		*685*	*774*	-		-	
PCI, median days (percentiles 75th, 90th)	0 (8, 34)	0 (7, 35)	-		0 (7, 35)	0 (9, 41)	-		-	
PCI ≥ baseline 75th percentile[c] %	26.2	23.9	0.87 (0.66;1.15)	0.345	27.2	29.7	1.18 (0.92;1.52)	0.187	1.35 (0.94;1.94)	0.101
PCI ≥ baseline 90th percentile[c] %	10.5	10.1	0.97 (0.66;1.44)	0.888	10.2	11.9	1.24 (0.87;1.77)	0.241	1.27 (0.76;2.12)	0.353
Hard to detect, N patients	*284*	*191*	-		*261*	*274*	-		-	
PCI, median days (percentiles: 75th, 90th)	7 (26.5, 71)	5 (28, 79)	-		7 (27, 58)	8 (30, 80)	-		-	
PCI ≥ baseline 75th percentile[c] %	25.0	25.7	1.12 (0.69;1.79)	0.653	25.7	30.3	1.35 (0.87;2.08)	0.180	1.21 (0.66;2.21)	0.543
PCI ≥ baseline 90th percentile[c] %	10.2	11.5	1.20 (0.62;2.34)	0.584	10.3	13.1	1.34 (0.73;2.46)	0.348	1.11 (0.48;2.59)	0.805

Primary care intervals were measured as median, 75th and 90th percentile and the proportion of patients who had the longest primary care interval before and after the CME-M. The analyses are also stratified on cancer detection difficulty. Practices are divided into CME-M group and reference group. An effect within a group is shown as an odds ratio (OR0: Reference group; OR1: CME-M group). Comparisons between groups are shown as a ratio of odds ratios

The suspected cancer types were divided into two groups based on cancer detection difficulty: 1) easier to detect included suspected cancer in kidney, bladder, breast, head and neck, female genitalia, nevus (melanoma), penis, testis and gastrointestinal and 2) harder to detect included suspected cancer in pancreas, liver and gall bladder, brain, lymph node and bone marrow, lung, prostate, connective tissue including fat, muscle and bones, and non-specific serious symptoms

Abbreviations: PCI primary care interval, *CME-M* continuing medical education meeting, *OR* Odds ratio, *CI* confidence interval

[a]Adjusted for cluster, practice type, patient gender, age and comorbidity

[b]In addition, adjusted for cancer detection difficulty

[c]75th and 90th percentiles of baseline measurements (before the CME-M) were used for each group as basis

Bold = significance level of $p \leq 0.05$

compliance over time. We do not know whether this was a differentiated non-response (e.g. in cases with long primary care intervals), but it could be the case as also indicated by the paradoxical result. However, the proportion of patients in the "harder to detect" group of referrals actually increased in the reference group after the CME-M [39].

To investigate the reasons for the observed increase in the primary care interval combined with an indication of lowered referral threshold, we performed sensitivity analyses. These did not point towards a delayed effect of the CME-M or a "cleaning up process" of patients who had recently been seen in general practice because of unspecific symptoms. The most likely explanation of our finding is a change in the awareness of unspecific symptoms among GPs in CME-M practices, which could have led the GPs to report an earlier date of first symptom presentation. Thus, the GPs may have gained a more realistic idea about the usual time intervals in general practice for patients suspected of cancer.

Comparison with other studies and clinical implications

To our knowledge, this study is among the first to evaluate a CME-M on GPs' use and timing of urgent cancer referrals. In accordance with our findings, an English before-after study found that the use of RATs for lung and colorectal cancer in general practice was associated with an increased number of urgent referrals during a 6-month period [43]. The reason for this could be that the GPs' awareness of potential cancer symptoms and attitude towards urgent cancer referral changed through the CME-M. Similar results have also been found in qualitative studies about the use of RATs [44, 45] and in our previous analysis of the impact of the CME-M on GP knowledge, attitude and intentions [18].

Our intervention was developed on the basis of theoretical frameworks and reviews of empirical results to ensure optimal likelihood of positive effect [44–47]. The CME-M consisted of a variety of elements [18], and we could not validly identify the most effective parts of the CME-M; this calls for further research in changing the GPs' behaviour [46].

In our study, the non-participating practices were more often single-handed, the GPs were more often males, and their practice population was larger, more deprived and with more male patients than in participating practices. Similar findings were also reported in a comprehensive quality development project on chronic diseases conducted in the Central Denmark Region in 2010 [47]. These findings may result from differences in the GPs' possibility to participate (e.g. time constraints) [48]. However, it may also be explained by the theories of varying readiness for change of behaviour [49]; some GPs belong to a group known to be susceptible for new knowledge (innovators, early adopters and early majority), whereas other GPs are known to be sceptical (late majority and laggards). One way to change the pattern of non-participation could perhaps be to develop specific CME initiatives to better fit the GPs' preferences for education and individual learning style [50].

Conclusion

We found a statistically significant reduction in the number of total contacts with general practice within the month preceding an urgent referral and an increase in the reported primary care intervals from before to after in the CME-M group compared to the reference group. A CME-M may contribute to changing the threshold for referring the patients and the GPs' understanding of the primary care interval.

Additional files

Additional file 1: One page forms used for collection of patient information.

Additional file 2: Tables on sensitivity analyses. Additional file 2 includes Additional Tables I-V. Additional **Table I**: The CME-M impact on patients' prior contacts with general practice stratified on practice type. Additional **Table II**: The CME-M impact on patients' primary care interval stratified on both practice type and cancer detection difficulty. Additional **Table III**: The CME-M impact on patients' prior contacts with general practice with exclusion of patients referred within 30 days following the CME-M-date. Additional **Table IV**: The CME-M impact on patients' primary care interval with exclusion of patients referred within 30 days following the CME-M-date. Additional **Table V**: The CME-M impact on patients' primary care interval with exclusion of patients referred within 61 days following the CME-M-date.

Abbreviations

CME-M: Continuing medical education meeting; CPR: Civil personal registration; DADI: Danish deprivation index; F2F: Face to face; GP: General practitioner; IRR: Incidence rate ratio; OR: Odds ratio; RATs: Risk assessment tools

Acknowledgements

We thank Rikke Pilegaard and Jens Rubak, hospital-GP liaison advisors, Marianne Lentz, CME supervisor, and Gry Stie, academic coordinator at the Regional Cancer Quality Unit, for their contributions to the operationalisation of the CME-M programme. We thank Anne Gammelgaard, specialised consultant at Quality and Informatics, Central Denmark Region, and the four radiology departments in Aarhus, Holstebro, Randers and Viborg for the data on patients referred to a fast-track cancer pathway. We thank Kaare Rud Flarup, data manager at the Research Unit for General Practice at Aarhus University, for creating the database. We thank the general practitioners from the Central Denmark Region who generously contributed with their time and experience to this study.

Funding

The project was supported by the Foundation for Primary Health Care Research (Praksisforskningsfonden) of the Central Denmark Region, the Committee for Quality Improvement and Continuing Medical Education (KEU) of the Central Denmark Region, the Committee of Multi-practice Studies in General Practice (MPU) of the Danish College of General Practitioners (DSAM), the Danish Cancer Society and the Novo Nordisk Foundation. The sponsoring organisations were not involved in any part of the study.

Authors' contributions
BST, PV and FB planned the design of the study. BST conducted the data collection. AZF and BST performed the statistical analyses. BST wrote the first draft of the article. PV, FB and AZF critically reviewed the article and provided comments to improve the manuscript. All authors have read and commented on the final manuscript.

Competing interests
PV was a lecturer at seven CME-Ms; FB was a lecturer at one CME-M. The authors declare to have no competing interest.

Consent for publication
Not applicable.

Author details
[1]Research Unit for General Practice, Department of Public Health, Aarhus University, Bartholins Allé 2, Aarhus DK-8000, Denmark. [2]Research Centre for Cancer Diagnosis in Primary Care (CaP), Department of Public Health, Aarhus University, Bartholins Allé 2, Aarhus DK-8000, Denmark. [3]Section for General Medical Practice, Department of Public Health, Aarhus University, Bartholins Allé 2, Aarhus DK-8000, Denmark. [4]Department of Clinical Medicine, University Clinic for Innovative Health Care Delivery, Silkeborg Hospital, Aarhus University, Aarhus DK-8000, Denmark.

References
1. Coleman MP, Forman D, Bryant H, Butler J, Rachet B, Maringe C, et al. Cancer survival in Australia, Canada, Denmark, Norway, Sweden, and the UK, 1995–2007 (the International cancer benchmarking partnership): an analysis of population-based cancer registry data. Lancet. 2011;377(9760):127–38.
2. Ferlay J, Steliarova-Foucher E, Lortet-Tieulent J, Rosso S, Coebergh JW, Comber H, et al. Cancer incidence and mortality patterns in Europe: estimates for 40 countries in 2012. Eur J Cancer. 2013;49(6):1374–403.
3. Allgar VL, Neal RD. Delays in the diagnosis of six cancers: analysis of data from the national survey of NHS patients: cancer. Br J Cancer. 2005;92(11):1959–70.
4. Hansen RP, Vedsted P, Sokolowski I, Sondergaard J, Olesen F. Time intervals from first symptom to treatment of cancer: a cohort study of 2,212 newly diagnosed cancer patients. BMC Health Serv Res. 2011;11(1):284.
5. Richards MA, Smith P, Ramirez AJ, Fentiman IS, Rubens RD. The influence on survival of delay in the presentation and treatment of symptomatic breast cancer. Br J Cancer. 1999;79(5):858–64.
6. Neal RD, Tharmanathan P, France B, Din NU, Cotton S, Fallon-Ferguson J, et al. Is increased time to diagnosis and treatment in symptomatic cancer associated with poorer outcomes? Systematic review. Br J Cancer. 2015;112(Suppl):S92–S107.
7. Torring ML, Frydenberg M, Hansen RP, Olesen F, Vedsted P. Evidence of increasing mortality with longer diagnostic intervals for five common cancers: A cohort study in primary care. Eur J Cancer. 2013;49(9):2187–98.
8. Moller H, Gildea C, Meechan D, Rubin G, Round T, Vedsted P. Use of the English urgent referral pathway for suspected cancer and mortality in patients with cancer: cohort study. BMJ. 2015;351:h5102.
9. Hamilton W. Cancer diagnosis in primary care. Br J Gen Pract. 2010;60(571): 121–8.
10. Nielsen TN, Hansen RP, Vedsted P. Symptom presentation in cancer patients in general practice. Ugeskr Laeger. 2010;172(41):2827–31.
11. Shapley M, Mansell G, Jordan JL, Jordan KP. Positive predictive values of >5% in primary care for cancer: systematic review. Br J Gen Pract. 2010;60(578):e366–77.
12. Jones R, Latinovic R, Charlton J, Gulliford MC. Alarm symptoms in early diagnosis of cancer in primary care: cohort study using general practice research database. BMJ. 2007;334(7602):1040.
13. Hamilton W. The CAPER studies: five case–control studies aimed at identifying and quantifying the risk of cancer in symptomatic primary care patients. Br J Cancer. 2009;101 Suppl 2:S80-6.
14. Christensen KG, Fenger-Gron M, Flarup KR, Vedsted P. Use of general practice, diagnostic investigations and hospital services before and after cancer diagnosis - a population-based nationwide registry study of 127,000 incident adult cancer patients. BMC Health Serv Res. 2012;12:224–6963. 12-224.
15. Jensen H, Torring ML, Olesen F, Overgaard J, Fenger-Gron M, Vedsted P. Diagnostic intervals before and after implementation of cancer patient pathways - a GP survey and registry based comparison of three cohorts of cancer patients. BMC Cancer. 2015;15:308–015. 1317-7.
16. Sundhedsstyrelsen. Kræftplan III Styrket indsats på kræftområdet - et sundhedsfagligt oplæg. København; 2010. Available from: http://www.sst.dk/~/media/702E936E9979422D9591BA0DBDCEDA8F.ashx. Accessed 2 Nov 2016.
17. Toftegaard B, Bro F, Vedsted P. A geographical cluster randomised stepped wedge study of continuing medical education and cancer diagnosis in general practice. Implement Sci. 2014;9(1):159.
18. Toftegaard BS, Bro F, Falborg AZ, Vedsted P. Impact of continuing medical education in cancer diagnosis on GP knowledge, attitude and readiness to investigate - a before-after study. BMC Fam Pract. 2016 Jul 26;17:10.1186/s12875,016-0496-x.
19. National Board of Health Data [in Danish: Sundhedsdatastyrelsen] The Cancer Registry 2013. Available from: http://sundhedsdatastyrelsen.dk/da/tal-og-analyser/analyser-og-rapporter/sygdomme/cancerregisteret. Accessed 6 Jun 2016.
20. Pedersen KM, Andersen JS, Sondergaard J. General practice and primary health care in Denmark. J Am Board Fam Med. 2012;25(Suppl 1):S34–8.
21. Cancer fast-track pathways [in Danish: Pakkeforløb på Kræftområdet]. Available from: https://sundhedsstyrelsen.dk/da/sygdom-og-behandling/kraeft/pakkeforloeb. Accessed 2 Nov 2016.
22. Probst HB, Hussain ZB, Andersen O. Cancer patient pathways in Denmark as a joint effort between bureaucrats, health professionals and politicians-a national Danish project. Health Policy. 2012;105(1):65–70.
23. Pedersen CB. The Danish civil registration system. Scand J Public Health. 2011;39(7):22–5.
24. Hamilton W, Peters TJ, Bankhead C, Sharp D. Risk of ovarian cancer in women with symptoms in primary care: population based case–control study. BMJ. 2009;339(0959–535):b2998.
25. Jensen H, Nissen A, Vedsted P. Quality deviations in cancer diagnosis: prevalence and time to diagnosis in general practice. Br J Gen Pract. 2014; 64(619):e92–8.
26. Lyratzopoulos G, Vedsted P, Singh H. Understanding missed opportunities for more timely diagnosis of cancer in symptomatic patients after presentation. Br J Cancer. 2015;112 Suppl 1:S84–91.
27. Quekel LG, Kessels AG, Goei R, van Engelshoven JM. Miss rate of lung cancer on the chest radiograph in clinical practice. Chest. 1999;115(3):720–4.
28. Stapley S, Sharp D, Hamilton W. Negative chest X-rays in primary care patients with lung cancer. Br J Gen Pract. 2006;56(529):570–3.
29. Rubin G, Berendsen A, Crawford SM, Dommett R, Earle C, Emery J, et al. The expanding role of primary care in cancer control. Lancet Oncol. 2015;16(12):1231–72.
30. Weller D, Vedsted P, Rubin G, Walter FM, Emery J, Scott S, et al. The Aarhus statement: improving design and reporting of studies on early cancer diagnosis. Br J Cancer. 2012;106(7):126210–1267.
31. Toftegaard BS, Guldbrandt LM, Flarup KR, Beyer H, Bro F, Vedsted P. Development of an algorithm to identify urgent referrals for suspected cancer from the Danish primary care referral database. Clin Epidemiol. 2016;8:751–9.
32. Gjerstorff ML. The Danish cancer registry. Scand J Public Health. 2011;39(7):42–5.
33. WHO. International Classification of Diseases (ICD). Available from: http://apps.who.int/classifications/icd10/browse/2016/en. Accessed 2 Nov 2016.
34. Olivarius NF, Hollnagel H, Krasnik A, Pedersen PA, Thorsen H. The Danish national health register. A tool for primary health care research. Dan Med Bull. 1997;44(4):449–53.
35. Storm HH, Michelsen EV, Clemmensen IH, Pihl J. The Danish cancer registry-history, content, quality and use. Dan Med Bull. 1997;44:535–9.
36. Timmermans B. The Danish integrated database for labor market research: towards demystification for the English speaking audience. Aalborg: Aalborg University; 2010.
37. Quan H, Li B, Couris CM, Fushimi K, Graham P, Hider P, et al. Updating and validating the charlson comorbidity index and score for risk adjustment in hospital discharge abstracts using data from 6 countries. Am J Epidemiol. 2011;173(6):676–82.

38. Lidegaard O, Hammerum MS. The national patient registry as a tool for continuous production and quality control. Ugeskr Laeger. 2002;164(38):4420–3.
39. Lyratzopoulos G, Saunders CL, Abel GA, McPhail S, Neal RD, Wardle J, et al. The relative length of the patient and the primary care interval in patients with 28 common and rarer cancers. Br J Cancer. 2015;112 Suppl 1:S35–40.
40. Cameron A, Trivedi P. Regression analysis of count data. Econometric Society Monograph. 53rd ed. Cambridge: Cambridge University Press; 2013.
41. Fitzmaurice G, Laird N, Ware J. Applied Longitudinal Analysis. 2nd ed. New York: Wiley; 2004.
42. StataCorp. 2013. Stata: Release 13. Statistical Software. College Station, TX: StataCorp LP. Available from: http://www.stata.com/manuals13/u.pdf. Accessed 2 Nov 2016.
43. Hamilton W, Green T, Martins T, Elliott K, Rubin G, Macleod U. Evaluation of risk assessment tools for suspected cancer in general practice: a cohort study. Br J Gen Pract. 2013;63(606):e30–6.
44. Green T, Martins T, Hamilton W, Rubin G, Elliott K, Macleod U. Exploring GPs' experiences of using diagnostic tools for cancer: a qualitative study in primary care. Fam Pract. 2015;32(1):101–5.
45. Dikomitis L, Green T, Macleod U. Embedding electronic decision-support tools for suspected cancer in primary care: a qualitative study of GPs' experiences. Prim Health Care Res Dev. 2015;16(6):548–55.
46. Moore GF, Audrey S, Barker M, Bond L, Bonell C, Hardeman W, et al. Process evaluation of complex interventions: medical research council guidance. BMJ. 2015;350:h1258.
47. Ribe AR, Fenger-Gron M, Vedsted P, Bro F, Kaersvang L, Vestergaard M. Several factors influenced general practitioner participation in the implementation of a disease management programme. Dan Med J. 2014;61(9):A4901.
48. Ross S, Grant A, Counsell C, Gillespie W, Russell I, Prescott R. Barriers to participation in randomised controlled trials: a systematic review. J Clin Epidemiol. 1999;52(12):1143–56.
49. Rogers EM. Diffusions of innovations. New York: Simon & Schuster Ltd; 2013.
50. Robinson G. Do general practitioners' risk-taking propensities and learning styles influence their continuing medical education preferences? Med Teach. 2002;24(1):71–8.

Blood transfusion in elderly patients with chronic anemia: a qualitative analysis of the general practitioners' attitudes

Sylvain Le Calvé[1*], Dominique Somme[2,3,4], Joaquim Prud'homm[2,4] and Aline Corvol[2,4]

Abstract

Background: Blood transfusion in chronic anemia is not covered by guidelines specific to older adults. When they consider that this treatment is necessary in elderly patients, French general practitioners (GPs) contact a hospital specialist to plan a transfusion.

Methods: Twenty French GPs were questioned individually regarding their approach to blood transfusion using semi-structured interviews. Each interview was recorded, typed up verbatim and then coded using an inductive procedure by theme, in a cross-over design (two researchers) in two phases: analysis and summary, followed by grouping of the recorded comments.

Results: The criteria for transfusion were hemoglobin level < 8 g/dL and cardiac comorbidities. Some geriatric issues, such as cognitive disorder or dependence, were considered, either as aspects of frailty favoring transfusion or as markers of reduced life expectancy that limit care. Falls and fear of an unpleasant death from anemia prompted GPs to order blood transfusion. The patient's family provided guidance, but the patient was not routinely consulted. The specialists were rarely asked to participate in decision making. GPs' perceptions were ambivalent: they considered transfusion to be extraordinary and magical, but also pointless since its effects are transient.

Conclusion: The decision to give a transfusion to an elderly patient with chronic anemia is deemed complex, but GPs seem to take it alone, sometimes guided by the patient's family. The drawing up of an advance care plan could help involve the patient in decision making.

Keywords: Anemia, Transfusion, Elderly, GP, Decision, Referral

Background

Anemia and transfusion for older patients

Chronic anemia in elderly patients is frequent (affecting >20% of the over-85 s) [1–3] and associated with increased morbidity-mortality [4]. In France, General practitioners (GPs) collaborate with specialists in the follow-up of patients living at home with chronic diseases by prescripting most usual laboratory tests. In the case of chronic anemia, GPs receive results of blood cell counts and can be confronted with a lowering of hemoglobin. So they are called upon to decide whether or not to order a transfusion, which in France can only be given in hospital, mostly in internal or hematology departments. This referral process is peculiar, as GPs don't expect from the specialist they call (hematologist, internist, or geriatrician) a medical advice; they want him to approve and enact their choice. On his side, the specialist can accept or refuse the transfusion, but will usually organize it after a simple phone call, often in a day hospital, before he can meet the patient.

There are no blood transfusion guidelines specific to chronic anemia in elderly patients [5], and the World Health Organization considers that the definition of anemia is independent of age [6]. However, there is a proven statistical link between anemia and increased cognitive disorders, risk of fall, and hospitalization. Anemia is also associated with reduced muscle

* Correspondence: s.le-calve@ch-stmalo.fr
[1]Unité de Soins de Longue Durée, Centre Hospitalier de Saint Malo, La Briantais, 78, boulevard du rosais, 35400 Saint-Malo, France

strength, decreased bone density, and with reduced quality of life [7].

Several reports indicate that one-third of anemia cases are explained by chronic illness (anemia of chronic disease, including inflammatory diseases and myelodysplasia) and/or by renal insufficiency, one-third by nutritional deficiency (essentially in iron), and one-third are unexplained [4, 5, 7]. As anemia is caused by an underlying illness in two-thirds of cases, the guidelines recommend treatment of the cause. However, symptomatic treatment by blood transfusion may prove necessary if there is no effective etiological treatment or if the anemia is of unknown etiology. Several studies have reported that half of patients receiving blood transfusions are elderly [8–10]. French studies show that blood transfusions have better outcomes in the elderly [11–13], in whom low rates of adverse reactions have been reported [14–16]. Analyses of Medicare databases show increased occurrence of febrile non-hemolytic transfusion reaction and transfusion-related acute lung injury and decreased occurrence of transfusion-associated circulatory overload in the over-80s, compared with patients aged 65–79 [17–19].

Current guidelines

The official French guidelines on tranfusion [20, 21] are the subject of professional agreement, albeit without a high level of scientific proof. They do not differentiate between the elderly and the general population or between acute and chronic anemia. The guidelines do, however, specify that people aged 80 or over tolerate anemia less well than children and younger adults, that the clinical signs of anemia depend mainly on speed of onset, and that it is the context that matters and not the hemoglobin level [21].

In the United States, the American Association of Blood Banks guidelines [22] concern a hemodynamically stable population, with no mention of any age criterion, and recommend a restrictive transfusion strategy based on a hemoglobin threshold ≤7 g/dL, or ≤8 g/dL in patients with a history of cardiovascular disease. The authors specify, however, that the strength of these guidelines is limited by the small number of clinical trials in some populations and that clinical trials in the elderly are needed [22]. Comparisons of so-called restrictive and liberal strategies have failed to define precise hemoglobin targets in the elderly with chronic anemia [5, 23–25].

The decision to ask for a blood transfusion to an elderly patient with chronic anemia is complex because various factors have to be taken into account and because GPs are uncertain what benefits to expect for a given patient. The decision is based on the patient's condition and preferences, and on scientific data and the clinical conditions. These factors are included in the decision-making process through clinical expertise, which is central to decision making and which reflects the skill-set and judgment that the clinician has acquired through experience and clinical practice [26]. Clinical expertise incorporates the data of evidence-based medicine and the patient's preferences and values, so as to assess the problem and work towards a decision [27]. The lack of precise guidelines derived from evidence-based medicine means that a GP's judgment becomes central.

Objectives

The aim of this survey was to identify GPs' attitudes regarding blood transfusion in cases of chronic anemia in older adults, so as to understand how they decide whether or not to contact a transfusion center.

Methods

The decision to order a transfusion is essentially subjective, so it seemed appropriate to use a qualitative approach, with semi-structured recorded interviews. We gathered a purposive sample of GPs, with heterogeneous age, gender, place of work (rural ou urban) and seniority. A single physician interviewed GPs likely to care for elderly outpatients in the Calvados Department (Normandy) in northwestern France.

Data collection

Twenty GPs seemed to be a number of participants high enough so the probability of reaching data saturation, ie, that no new property, dimension, or relation will emerge during the analysis, was high. Twenty-nine GPs chosen at professional meetings were telephoned to explain the study aims and procedure and to ask them to participate. Twenty agreed and were recontacted to organize a meeting at their office. Had this saturation not been reached, a new sample would have been recruited [28]. An interview guide (Additional file 1) designed for a 30-min individual interview served as a basis. This semi-structured approach was based on the following themes relevant to older adults (>80 years): definition, consequences and prevalence of chronic anemia, indications, non-indications, and consequences of transfusion. These non-remunerated interviews guaranteed confidentiality and anonymity and were conducted between January and July 2013. They were recorded and typed up verbatim.

Data analysis

Each interview was coded inductively, based on content, using observed data leading to a hypothesis or model. No a priori hypothesis was applied. Emergent themes, related to the GPs' attitudes, were sought. Two researchers who are GPs experienced in geriatrics and worked independently to code all interviews by themes and categories, before cross-referencing the results. This coding was done in two stages: first, analysis and summary of statements, interview by interview, and second, organization of statements by target theme. Validation of the survey results confirmed that the statements were reproduced faithfully.

Results

Characteristics of the population and interviews

The 20 GPs (13 men, 7 women) interviewed were aged 30 to 65, and worked in rural [9], semi-rural [6], or urban [5] settings. They had more than 15 years (12 GPs), 5 to 15 years [5], or less than 5 years [3] of experience of general medicine. Thirteen of the interviewed GPs worked within 30 km of several transfusion centers. The interviews lasted 16 to 43 min.

The Table 1 summarizes main spontaneous replies to our questions, with the number of occurrence. Two questions do not appear in that table as the replies were too heterogeneous.

Table 1 Main replies to the interview guide

Theme of questions	Main replies	Number of occurrence out of 20
Applied transfusion treshold	< 8 g/dL Hb	16
	< 9 g/dL Hb	1
	< 7 g/dL Hb	3
Definition and attitude toward anemia	Same definition and attitude	6
	Different definition and attitude	12
	No answer	2
Apprehended geriatric complications	General complications	20
	Speficic geriatric complications	14
	Falls	10
Influence of cognitive impairments	No influence	6
	Influence	14
Influence of autonomy loss	Fear of autonomy loss or autonomy loss as a treshold	6
	Positif effect of transfusion over anemia	5
Family opinion over transfusion decision-making process	Family opinion in a palliative care context	5
	Family opinion about withholding tranfusion	4
	Family opinion in a cognitive impairment context	6
Image of transfusion	Positive image for GPs	19
	Family satisfaction	4
Improved items thanks to transfusion	General status	15
	Psychomotor status	12
Feared complications of transfusion	Circulatory overload	13
	No fear	5

Patient-related decision criteria

Most GPs applied an absolute hemoglobin level of 8 g/dL as a transfusion threshold. None of the GPs referred to any specific guidelines. Cardiac comorbidities were considered to increase this threshold. The cause of anemia did not appear as a determining factor in the decision-making process of transfusion. The poor clinical safety of anemia was considered as the most important factor, without consideration of the threshold.

"If the patient's clinical condition is poor, I don't bother with figures [...] I always think first of the patient. Because statistics are all very well, but they also make us do stupid things. There's common sense and there's experience." (GP man 18).

These elements can be found in French or American recommendations [20–22], in fact used without being cited.

Age seems to have paradoxical effect on GPs attitudes: they tolerate a lower hemoglobin concentration before starting lab tests for older patients, but propose transfusion earlier. In other terms, the presence of a moderate anemia will be trivialized, but in case of worsening they will react faster.

Falls strongly motivated GPs to order a transfusion. The GPs apprehended other geriatric complications like loss of autonomy, worsening of cognitive disorders, and orthostatic hypotension. More than the slow and insidious complications of chronic anemia, the events of rapid occurrence trigger the process of requesting a transfusion.

The presence of cognitive impairments makes the situation more complex. GPs freely mentioned cognitive disorders and their influence on decision making. However, the GPs' comments revealed contradictions regarding how cognitive disorders affect their attitudes. Fear of worsening cognitive disorders linked to anemia leads to earlier transfusion, but cognitive disorders also complicate assessment of the safety of chronic anemia, and the risk of behavioral problems during transfusion tends to reduce requests.

"It's true that if a patient with dementia starts pulling all the tubes out..."(GP man 13).

Overall, GPs' attitudes varied greatly, ranging from those for whom transfusion is conditional upon preservation of higher functions to those who assert that cognitive disorders do not influence their decision, not to mention those who above all are baffled.

Institutionalization of the patient was spontaneously associated with severe cognitive disorders and dependence, with a twofold effect: it complicates assessment of the impact of anemia and potentially worsens its effects, through loss of residual autonomy.

When cognitive disorders are severe, or loss of autonomy major, or sometimes just because of a very old age, transfusion may appear futile.

"If the patient is in a wheelchair all day, we're not really going to see any difference, are we?" (GP man 14).

The GPs held differing opinions regarding palliative care for an incurable disease. Some favored transfusion at the end of life, while others were in theory opposed, perhaps because they lacked experience. A perceived unpleasantness of death caused by anemia (drawn out, physical and mental discomfort) increased the likelihood that a transfusion would be ordered.

"I won't let somebody die of anemia. It would be like letting someone die of hunger." (GP man 18).

All GPs were of the opinion that there is no indication for blood transfusion when death is imminent, citing cost and availability. So palliative care situations, as cognitive impairment, very old age or loss of autonomy, can lead to opposite decisions: early transfusions because of patients' frailty, or transfusion avoidance because this treatment is seen as invasive and useless.

Attitudes to transfusion

Physicians unanimously see transfusion as "magical", with "spectacular" effects.

"We prolong life." (GP woman 7).

"It's crazy, almost like vitamins, like doping [...]Suddenly they wake up!" (GP man 13).

This excellent image of transfusion seems to be shared with the patients and their families, who retain the immediate effects of this quite simple therapeutic act. One GP recalled a patient with end-stage kidney disease who refused dialysis but agreed to transfusion.

"He didn't want to be dialyzed: he already had been once or twice [...], but he did want transfusions, because he experienced an immediate effect" (GP man 13).

The satisfaction of patients, and consequently of their families, is for the physician a token of recognition.

Furthermore, most GPs interviewed considered the risk-benefit ratio as always being favorable, and pointed to psychomotor improvement, as well as improved general condition or mood, and a favorable impact on daily activities. Cognitive improvement in particular was highlighted. No concern was expressed regarding the risk of infection or of incompatibility. The only risks mentioned were volume overload and sometimes delirium.

"If it bothers a patient to undergo transfusion, if he comes back afterwards highly agitated and with behavioral problems..."(GP man 14).

Compared with the extraordinary efficacy of transfusion, these risks seem insignificant.

Despite these very positive descriptions of transfusion, GPs frequently expressed unease when taking the decision to recommend a transfusion, as they did not feel sufficiently competent or experienced.

"I don't feel comfortable with it [...]I haven't had enough training, or perhaps I haven't been interested enough, or maybe I haven't had to face the problem often enough." (GP man 16).

The impression of lack of competence is easily understandable since there are no precise recommendations in this type of situation. Moreover, the low frequency of confrontation with this situation does not allow learning by experience. But beyond lack of knowledge and experience, the unease expressed may be linked to ambivalence regarding transfusion, which is seen as extraordinarily effective in the short term, but completely useless in the long term.

"We make do by filling a vase with a hole in it." (GP man 1).

So the patient and/or the patient's family bestow recognition on the GP, who feels at a loss in the more or less long term. The power of medicine therefore seems illusory if the question of disease progression has not been addressed with the patient.

A lone decision

GPs faced with decisions regarding transfusions feel that they are responsible for a weighty decision, as they attribute to transfusion the power to prolong or even to restore life. But despite the complexity of the decision, few practitioners reported seeking support of specialists or decision sharing with patients and family. The relation with the specialist who performs the transfusion was mentioned by only two of the 20 GPs interviewed. One GP anticipated a refusal by the specialist, with no possibility of dialogue, above a hemoglobin threshold of 8 g/dL. The other was the only one thinking in terms of a collaborative approach, useful in decision making.

"I'd propose it jointly with the specialist. We could agree on it together." (GP man 16).

It is surprising, in a complex situation where the physician feels uncomfortable and uncertain, that the specialist physician is not contacted either for decision support or for shared responsibility, but rather to confirm the orientation proposed by the general practitioner and to perform the act as a service provider.

Patient's family circle finally appears as more influent than specialist in decision making. First of all, because the very presence of the family made an order for transfusion more likely. And second, because the GPs involved the family in decision making, notably in complex situations such as transfusion at the end of life and in the case of cognitive disorders.

"And then afterwards, regarding the family... To know whether or not they wish to prolong their loved one's life." (GP woman 11).

Only one of the GPs interviewed generally preferred not to include the family in decision making.

Interestingly, the patient's opinion was not explicitly referred to as guiding decision making, and did not seem to be systematically sought, even if some patients expressed weariness after repeated transfusions.

"There are a lot of patients over 80 who don't want to be bothered anymore, who don't want a transfusion." (GP woman 12).

Discussion

Summary of results

Our results, summarized in Fig. 1, show that GPs are ambivalent regarding blood transfusion, which is seen as life-giving, but also as useless because of the transience of its effects. This creates a sense of unease, which is worsened by GPs' isolation. One GP apart, they did not refer to the hospital specialist as someone likely to help them in their decision making: they considered that it is up to them to assess the expected benefit for the patient. GPs interviewed were aware of specifically geriatric problems, but were unsure how to include them in a line of reasoning.

The notion of quality of life does not appear explicitly in the decision making process, and patients' opinions have little place. GPs give thought to the patient's comfort and to whether the family, which here takes on the mantle of authority, wishes to prolong the patient's life, but not to what value the patient may attach to his or her current life. More generally, the attitude of French GPs appears paternalistic and lacks consideration for the decisional independence of patients debilitated by age and illness.

Comparison with previous literature

Decision making under uncertainty

Decision making regarding blood transfusion in elderly patients with chronic anemia is clouded by uncertainty, because in a high proportion of patients the etiology of chronic anemia is unknown 4,5,7, and because we lack guidelines specific to such patients [20–22]. Conventionally, in complex situations two ways can be used independently or simultaneously to make a decision [29, 30]: the analytical method, based on scientific data, and the intuitive method, which is based on experience and reasoning by analogy. GPs faced with decisions regarding transfusions in the elderly may experience unease because they cannot base decisions on compelling data or on substantial clinical experience.

A geriatric assessment is clearly valuable when making complex decisions regarding elderly patients, in particular dialysis or the choice of cancer treatment [31–33]. However, our study has showed that GPs currently don't know how to integrate geriatric factors in transfusion decision making. Furthermore, the question of transfusion in chronic anemia is different from dialysis for exemple because it is not a single important decision involving the long-term therapeutic strategy, but rather

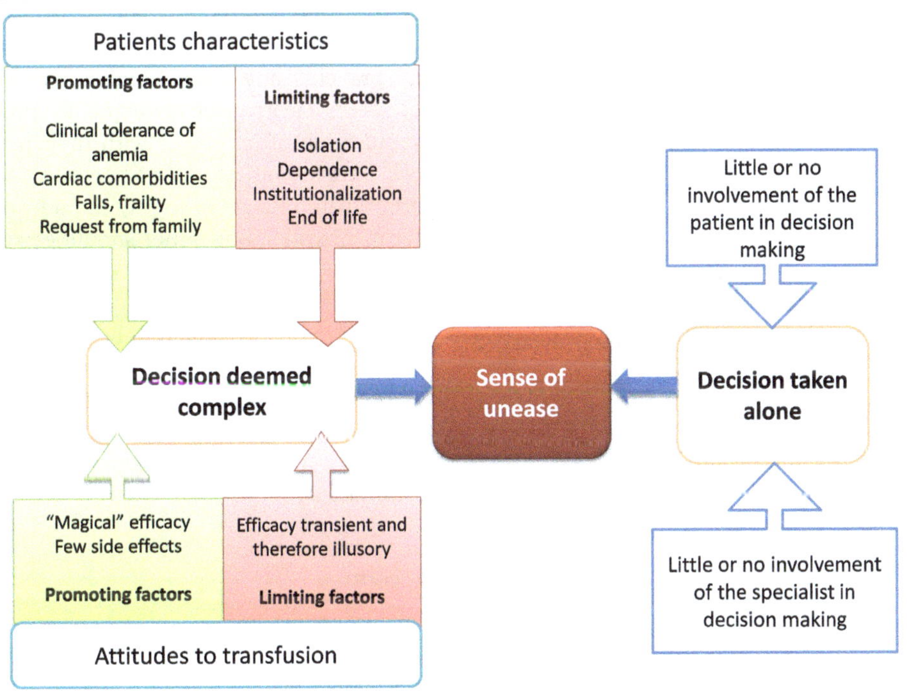

Fig. 1 Transfusion

lots of "small" decisions, with an approach that in all cases will have to be adapted in light of the patient's progress. A geriatric assessment could be useful in the process of discussing an advanced care plan, but is usually not feasible at the time of the decision.

Shared decision making

The GPs did not feel that their isolation could be lessened by taking the decision together with the patient. It is striking how infrequently the patient's opinion is taken into account, which raises the question of ageist stereotypes among GPs.

Shared decision making would yet seem realistic and relevant in the context of repeated transfusions: the patient knows the procedure and its associated discomfort, and experiences, or not, its positive effects. Discussion with the patient appears relatively simple, since immediate discomfort must be balanced against the immediate benefit experienced by the patient. The fact that few GPs referred to shared decision making is surprising considering the literature: the absence of strong preference of the medical practitioner considering treatment options and end of life care have been identified as facilitators for shared decision making [34]. If GPs adopted a clearly paternalistic approach, viewing patients as passive and vulnerable, it may be the consequences of GPs' stereotype and lack of training: the concept of patient-centered care [35] is poorly developed in France [36], and older patients are sometimes deemed incapable of deciding. As in other clinical situations [37, 38], GPs do act according to ageist stereotypes [39]. However, patients factors limiting decision sharing, such as not being empowered or having cognitive limitations [34, 40], have to be considered as well.

Conversely, the families seem to be actively involved in decision-making. It is possible that the participation of the family is sought to share the responsibility for the decision and/or to avoid a conflict in case of disagreement. However, this opposition between patients and family in shared decision should be taken with caution: a study on admission of elderly patients in intensive care units demonstrated that physicians who frequently asked patients about their preferences may be more inclined to asked relative for an opinion [41].

GP-specialist relationship

GPs who order a blood transfusion are requesting a procedure that they will neither perform nor are trained to perform. Yet, they don't seek for specialists' advice. We can suppose that they regard themselves as the best able to make the decision, acting as "specialist" of patient centered comprehensive care [42]. They consider that transfusion decisions don't rely on a technical knowledge owned by the specialist, but on their comprehensive approach. Motivation of GPs for collaboration with specialist is known to be largely knowledge driven [43]. It could explain that they don't seek for collaboration, if they can't acquire new knowledge this way.

We found in the interviews no elements arguing for a lack of approachability of transfusion specialists. In the absence of economic or organizational constraints, transfusion specialists generally seemed to agree to all requests for transfusion (one exception was related to a hemoglobin level > 8 g), particularly as in the French health care system a blood transfusion is a profitable procedure that takes up little of the specialist's time.

The interviews did not explicitly address the question of whether the specialist or the GP should explain to the patient the palliative nature of transfusions and involve him in drawing up an advance care plan [44].

Strengths and limitations

To our knowledge ours is the only survey to have analyzed decisions taken by GPs regarding blood transfusion in elderly patients with chronic anemia. The heterogeneity of the sample of GPs (sex, age, experience, conditions of medical practice) resulted in great variation in their attitudes. A cross-analysis has limited interpretation bias in data slicing and data aggregation. Further studies in different organizational and cultural contexts would be necessary to better describe and understands GPs attitudes.

Conclusion

Failure to draw up an advance care plan puts the GP in the awkward situation of deciding on an ad hoc basis and prevents any dispassionate discussion with the patient. GPs clearly feel inadequately prepared to address the question of prognosis with their patients and to discuss a treatment plan. The specialist, whether internist, geriatrician, or hematologist, should not act as a simple service provider, but rather should explain the prognosis. A closer collaboration between specialists and GPs would enable the drawing up of an advance care plan, discussed with the patient, and possibly with the family. The GP could refer to such a plan, anticipating the symptoms that should prompt transfusion, when taking decisions in light of disease progression. Such an advance care plan seems essential to facilitate GP-patient communication.

Abbreviation

GP: General Practitioner

Acknowledgements

We thank Dr. Benjamin Mordellet for his help in data analysis, and the interviewed GPs.

Funding
No.

Authors' contributions
SLC wrote the interview guide, conduct the interviews, analysed the data, wrote the first draft of the article, revised the manuscript and gave his final approval to the submission. JP made substantial contribution to the interpretation of the data, revised the manuscript and gave his final approval to the submission. DS designed the study, participated to the interpretation of the data, revised the manuscript and gave his final approval to the submission. AC made substantial contribution to the interpretation of the data, revised in-depth the manuscript, made the submission, and replied the reviewers. All authors read and approved the final manuscript.

Consent for publication
Not Applicable.

Competing interests
The authors declare that they have no competing interests.

Author details
[1]Unité de Soins de Longue Durée, Centre Hospitalier de Saint Malo, La Briantais, 78, boulevard du rosais, 35400 Saint-Malo, France. [2]CHU de Rennes, Service de gériatrie, Rennes, France. [3]Université Rennes 1, Faculté de Médecine, Rennes, France. [4]Centre de recherche sur l'action politique en Europe, UMR 6051, Rennes, France.

References
1. Patel KV. Epidemiology of anemia in older adults. Semin Hematol. 2008;45:210–7.
2. Artz AS. Anemia and the frail elderly. Semin Hematol. 2008;45:261–6.
3. Beghe C, Wilson A, Ershler WB. Prevalence and outcomes of anemia in geriatrics: a systematic review of the literature. Am J Med. 2004;116 Suppl 7A:3S–10S.
4. Berliner N. Anemia in the elderly. Trans Am Clin Climatol Assoc. 2013;124:230–7.
5. Beyer I, Compte N, Busuioc A, Cappelle S, Lanoy C, Cytryn E. Anemia and transfusions in geriatric patients: a time for evaluation. Hematology. 2010;15:116–21.
6. WHO. Nutritional anaemias. Tech Rep Ser. 1968;405:1–37.
7. Eisenstaedt R, Penninx BW, Woodman RC. Anemia in the elderly: current understanding and emerging concepts. Blood Rev. 2006;20:213–26.
8. Vamvakas EC, Taswell HF. Epidemiology of blood transfusion. Transfusion. 1994;34:464–70.
9. Mathoulin-Pelissier S, Salmi LR, Verret C, Demoures B. Blood transfusion in a random sample of hospitals in France. Transfusion. 2000;40:1140–6.
10. Wells AW, Mounter PJ, Chapman CE, Stainsby D, Wallis JP. Where does blood go? Prospective observational study of red cell transfusion in north England Bmj. 2002;325:803.
11. Gaxatte C, Olejnik C, Renom P, Boulanger E, Puisieux F. Pratique transfusionnelle chez les sujets âgés Rev Med Interne. 2009;30(Suppl 4):S384.
12. Claeys D, Bazin A, Guesdon N, Descatoire P, Leenaert F. Pratique transfusionnelle en court séjour gériatrique cah. année gerontol. 2011;3(Suppl 1):223.
13. Le Guen A, Cattenoz C, Lotton S, Brillant F, Troadec C, Gouezec H. Étude des pratiques transfusionnelles en court séjour gériatrique. Revue Geriatr. 2013;38:501–11.
14. Lubart E, Segal R, Tryhub N, Sigler E, Leibovitz A. Blood transfusion reactions in elderly patients hospitalized in a multilevel geriatric hospital. J Aging Res. 2014;2014:178298.
15. Arewa OP, Akinola NO, Salawu L. Blood transfusion reactions; evaluation of 462 transfusions at a tertiary hospital in Nigeria. Afr J Med Med Sci. 2009;38:143–8.
16. Py JY, Leo-Kodeli S, Fauveau L, Duedari N, Roubinet F. Hypotension and adverse transfusion reactions: from the associated clinical signs to the hypotensive transfusion reaction. Transfus Clin Biol. 2009;16:12–20.
17. Menis M, Anderson SA, Forshee RA, McKean S, Johnson C, Warnock R, Gondalia R, Mintz PD, Holness L, Worrall CM, Kelman JA, Izurieta HS. Transfusion-related acute lung injury and potential risk factors among the inpatient US elderly as recorded in Medicare claims data, during 2007 through 2011. Transfusion. 2014;54:2182–93.
18. Menis M, Forshee RA, Anderson SA, McKean S, Gondalia R, Warnock R, Johnson C, Mintz PD, Worrall CM, Kelman JA, Izurieta HS. Febrile non-haemolytic transfusion reaction occurrence and potential risk factors among the U.S. elderly transfused in the inpatient setting, as recorded in Medicare databases during 2011-2012. Vox Sang. 2015;108:251–61.
19. Menis M, Anderson SA, Forshee RA, McKean S, Johnson C, Holness L, Warnock R, Gondalia R, Worrall CM, Kelman JA, Ball R, Izurieta HS. Transfusion-associated circulatory overload (TACO) and potential risk factors among the inpatient US elderly as recorded in Medicare administrative databases during 2011. Vox Sang. 2014;106:144–52.
20. AFSSAPS. Transfusion de globules rouges homologues: produits, indications, alternatives. Recommandations. 2002.
21. HAS. Transfusion de globules rouges homologues: produits, indications, alternatives. Recommandations. 2014.
22. Carson JL, Grossman BJ, Kleinman S, Tinmouth AT, Marques MB, Fung MK, Holcomb JB, Illoh O, Kaplan LJ, Katz LM, Rao SV, Roback JD, Shander A, Tobian AA, Weinstein R, Swinton McLaughlin LG, Djulbegovic B. Red blood cell transfusion: a clinical practice guideline from the AABB*. Ann Intern Med. 2012;157:49–58.
23. Hebert PC, Wells G, Blajchman MA, Marshall J, Martin C, Pagliarello G, Tweeddale M, Schweitzer I, Yetisir E. A multicenter, randomized, controlled clinical trial of transfusion requirements in critical care. Transfusion requirements in critical care investigators, Canadian critical care trials group. N Engl J Med. 1999;340:409–17.
24. Marik PE, Corwin HL. Efficacy of red blood cell transfusion in the critically ill: a systematic review of the literature. Crit Care Med. 2008;36:2667–74.
25. Rao SV, Jollis JG, Harrington RA, Granger CB, Newby LK, Armstrong PW, Moliterno DJ, Lindblad L, Pieper K, Topol EJ, Stamler JS, Califf RM. Relationship of blood transfusion and clinical outcomes in patients with acute coronary syndromes. JAMA. 2004;292:1555–62.
26. Sackett DL, Rosenberg WM, Gray JA, Haynes RB, Richardson WS. Evidence based medicine: what it is and what it isn't. BMJ. 1996;312:71–2.
27. Haynes RB, Devereaux PJ, Guyatt GH. Clinical expertise in the era of evidence-based medicine and patient choice. Vox Sang. 2002;83 Suppl 1:383–6.
28. Mays N, Pope C. Qualitative research in health care. Assessing quality in qualitative research. BMJ. 2000 Jan 1;320(7226):50–2.
29. Lighthall GK, Vazquez-Guillamet C. Understanding decision making in critical care. Clin Med Res. 2015;13:156–68.
30. van de Luijtgaarden MW, Noordzij M, van Biesen W, Couchoud C, Cancarini G, Bos WJ, Dekker FW, Gorriz JL, Iatrou C, Wanner C, Finne P, Stojceva-Taneva O, Cala S, Stel VS, Tomson C, Jager KJ. Conservative care in Europe–nephrologists' experience with the decision not to start renal replacement therapy. Nephrol Dial Transplant. 2013;28:2604–12.
31. Foote C, Morton RL, Jardine M, Gallagher M, Brown M, Howard K, Cass A. COnsiderations of nephrologists when SuggestIng dialysis in elderly patients with renal failure (CONSIDER): a discrete choice experiment. Nephrol Dial Transplant. 2014;29:2302–9.
32. Murray AM. Cognitive impairment in the aging dialysis and chronic kidney disease populations: an occult burden. Adv Chronic Kidney Dis. 2008;15:123–32.
33. van der Poel MW, Mulder WJ, Ossenkoppele GJ, Maartense E, Wijermans P, Hoogendoorn M, Schouten HC. Comorbidity and treatment decision-making in elderly non-Hodgkin's lymphoma patients: a survey among haematologists. Neth J Med. 2014;72:165–9.
34. Pollard S, Bansback N, Bryan S. 57. Physician attitudes toward shared decision making: a systematic review. Patient Educ Couns. 2015;98(9):1046–57.
35. Care P-C. A definition and essential elements. J Am Geriatr Soc. 2016;64:15–8.
36. Schoen C, Osborn R, Squires D, Doty M, Pierson R, Applebaum S. New 2011 survey of patients with complex care needs in eleven countries finds that care is often poorly coordinated. Health Aff (Millwood). 2011;30:2437–48.
37. Townsley CA, Selby R, Siu LL. Systematic review of barriers to the recruitment of older patients with cancer onto clinical trials. J Clin Oncol. 2005;23:3112–24.
38. Madan AK, Aliabadi-Wahle S, Beech DJ. Ageism in medical students' treatment recommendations: the example of breast-conserving procedures. Acad Med. 2001;76:282–4.
39. Butler RN. Age-ism: another form of bigotry. Gerontologist. 1969;9:243–6.

40. Edwards M, Davies M, Edwards A. What are the external influences on information exchange and shared decision-making in healthcare consultations: a meta-synthesis of the literature. Patient Educ Couns. 2009;75(1):37–52.
41. Le Guen J, Boumendil A, Guidet B, Corvol A, Saint-Jean O, Somme D. Are elderly patients' opinions sought before admission to an intensive care unit? Results of the ICE-CUB study. Age Ageing. 2016;45(2):303–9.
42. Piterman L, Koritsas S. Part I. General practitioner-specialist relationship. Intern Med J 2005;35(7):430–434.
43. Berendsen AJ, Benneker WH, Meyboom-de Jong B, Klazinga NS, Schuling J. Motives and preferences of general practitioners for new collaboration models with medical specialists: a qualitative study. BMC Health Serv Res. 2007;7:4.
44. Piterman L, Koritsas S. Part II. General practitioner-specialist referral process. Intern Med J 2005;35(8):491–496.

10

General practitioners' awareness of depressive symptomatology is not associated with quality of life in heart failure patients – cross-sectional results of the observational RECODE-HF Study

Marion Eisele[1*], Sigrid Boczor[1], Anja Rakebrandt[1], Eva Blozik[1], Jens-Martin Träder[2], Stefan Störk[3], Christoph Herrmann-Lingen[4] and Martin Scherer[1] for the RECODE-HF Study Group

Abstract

Background: Depression is a common comorbidity in patients with chronic heart failure (HF) and linked to a wider range of symptoms which, in turn, are linked to a decreased health-related quality of life (HRQOL). Treatment of depression might improve HRQOL but detecting depression is difficult due to the symptom overlap between HF and depression. Therefore, clinical guidelines recommend to routinely screen for depression in HF patients. No studies have so far investigated the treatment after getting aware of a depressive symptomatology and its correlation with HRQOL in primary care HF patients. Therefore, we examined the factors linked to depression treatment and those linked to HRQOL in HF patients. We hypothesized that GPs' awareness of depressive symptomatology was associated with depression treatment and HRQOL in HF patients.

Methods: For this observational study, HF patients were recruited in primary care practices and filled out a questionnaire including PHQ-9 and HADS. A total of 574 patients screened positive for depressive symptomatology. Their GPs were interviewed by phone regarding the patients' comorbidities and potential depression treatment. Descriptive and regression analysis were performed.

Results: GPs reported various types of depression treatments (including dialogue/counselling by the GP him/herself in 31.8% of the patients). The reported rates differed considerably between GP-reported initiated treatment and patient-reported utilised treatment regarding psychotherapy (16.4% vs. 9.5%) and pharmacotherapy (61.2% vs. 30.3%). The GPs' awareness of depressive symptomatology was significantly associated with the likelihood of receiving pharmacotherapy (OR 2.8; $p < 0.001$) but not psychotherapy. The patient's HRQOL was not significantly associated with the GPs' awareness of depression.

(Continued on next page)

* Correspondence: m.eisele@uke.uni-hamburg.de
[1]Department of Primary Medical Care, Center for Psychosocial Medicine, University Medical Center Hamburg-Eppendorf, Martinistraße 52, 20246 Hamburg, Germany
Full list of author information is available at the end of the article

(Continued from previous page)

Conclusion: GPs should be aware of the gap between GP-initiated and patient-utilised depression treatments in patients with chronic HF, which might lead to an undersupply of depression treatment. It remains to be investigated why GPs' awareness of depressive symptomatology is not linked to patients' HRQOL. We hypothesize that GPs are aware of cases with reduced HRQOL (which improves under depression treatment) and unaware of cases whose depression do not significantly impair HRQOL, resulting in comparable levels of HRQOL in both groups. This hypothesis needs to be further investigated.

Keywords: Depression, Heart failure, Recognition of depression, Quality of life, Depression treatment, Observational study, Primary care, Healthcare research, Depressive symptomatology

Background

About 61.7 billion people worldwide suffer from chronic heart failure (HF) [1], a disease with high rates of mortality and hospital admissions [2, 3]. Depression rates have been found to be higher in HF patients than in patients without HF [4–6] and have been independently predictive of poor clinical outcomes [7]. Furthermore, depression in HF patients has been linked to a wider range of symptoms, which in turn have been linked to a decreased quality of life [8]. Therefore, treatment of depression may significantly improve patients' quality of life, one of the treatment goals specified in the clinical guidelines for the diagnosis and treatment of heart failure [9, 10].

At the same time, detecting depression is particularly difficult due to the symptom overlap between HF and depression. Earlier studies found recognition rates of depression between 57.5% [11] and 63.2% [12] in hospitalised HF patients. The authors investigated to what extent general practitioners (GPs) were aware of their HF patients' depressive symptomatology and found a rate of 35.0%–50.7% (depending on the definition of awareness) [13]. Deficient awareness of depressive symptomatology in HF patients might result in undersupply of depression treatment and reduced quality of life in HF patients. Crystal et al. found that patients with heart disease received significantly less depression treatment in terms of psycho- or pharmacotherapy [14] than patients without heart disease.

Therefore, national and international clinical guidelines recommend to routinely screen patients with HF for depression [10, 15–18]. For a number of years, studies have been investigating if the treatment of depression may also have an effect on HF prognosis, but so far there has not been a definite answer to this question. Interventional trials have found that the pharmacological treatment of depression in HF patients does not reduce the severity of depression nor does it have a positive effect on HF outcomes [19–21]. Conversely, cognitive behavioural therapy has been found to improve depression as well as quality of life [22]. However, so far, no studies have investigated the therapeutic procedures after getting aware of a depressive symptomatology and its potential link to patients' health related quality of life (HRQOL) in primary care HF patients.

Therefore, the study objectives were: (1) To describe how GPs treat depressive symptomatology in HF patients. (2) To describe the congruence between GP-initiated and patient-utilised depression treatment. (3) To examine the factors associated with depression treatment in HF patients. (4) To examine the factors associated with HRQOL of HF patients with depressive symptomatology. We hypothesized that the GPs' awareness of depressive symptomatology is significantly associated with a higher utilisation of pharmacotherapy and psychotherapy. We further hypothesized that the GPs' awareness of depressive symptomatology was significantly associated with a higher HRQOL.

Methods

In this observational study, primary care surgeries and their HF patients were recruited in Germany between 2/2012 and 6/2014. Baseline data were collected between 8/2012 and 11/2014. A detailed description of all study procedures has been described elsewhere [13, 23]. To summarise: All GPs in four German cities and surrounding areas received a written invitation to participate in the study and were contacted by phone, if they had not responded to the invitation letter. Primary care HF patients were recruited by their GP. Those patients who agreed to participate returned the informed consent letters to the study centre and in return received a baseline questionnaire by mail. Inclusion criteria were an age of 18 years or older, a diagnosis of chronic HF documented within the last 5 years, and at least one GP contact within the last 6 months. Exclusion criteria were dementia, death since the last GP visit and HF patients who were not regular patients of the participating GP practice.

Patient questionnaires contained questions regarding patients' psychosocial comorbidity (using the Hospital Anxiety and Depression Scale (HADS) including the anxiety (HADS-A) and depression (HADS-D) subscales [24, 25], Patient Health Questionnaire 9-item depression subscale (PHQ-9) [26–28], as well as selected items from the PROMIS depression and anxiety scales [29, 30]), HRQOL (using the EQ-5D visual analogue scale (EQ-5D VAS) [31]), use of psychotherapy (any psychotherapy, not restricted to those approved by health insurance companies), and current medications taken to treat depression, anxiety, agitation, sleep disturbance or "burnout". Drug names were verified whether they classified as prescription drugs and were then converted to ATC codes. If an ATC code included antidepressant ingredients and the drug was a prescription drug, the drug was coded as "prescription antidepressant".

The questionnaires were analysed by a validated algorithm [13], established to identify depression in patients with HF. All patients with valid criteria 2 of the hierarchical algorithm (PHQ > 8 and HADS-D > 8) were selected. Due to the positive predictive value of 68.8% for a depression diagnosis [13], this included patients with depression and patients with depressive symptoms, later referred to as P(+) patients (patients with depressive symptomatology). A telephone interview was conducted with each GP of the P(+) patients identified by the algorithm regarding the patients' somatic and psychological comorbidities. At the beginning of the interview, the GP was asked to access the patient records in the computer, in order to be able to use all data available (patient record as well as recollections). All questions were answered for each patient separately. If the GP answered "Yes" to the question: "Does the patient currently display depressive symptomatology?", he/she was asked to differentiate whether he/she thought the symptoms indicated a clinical depression or sub-threshold symptoms and what types of measures he had taken to treat said symptoms ("Which treatment did you initiate?"). Of all comorbidities stated by the GP, the numbers of all comorbidities indexed in the MultiCare comorbidity list of chronic conditions [32] were summed up for the comorbidity score.

Patient groups for analyses

Depending on the information given in the GP interview, patients were grouped for analysis (see Fig. 1). P(+) patients, whose GP stated that they currently displayed depressive symptoms or depressive disorder were assigned as P(+/+). P(+) patients, whose GP stated that they currently did not display depressive symptoms or depressive disorder, were assigned as P(+/−).

Statistical analyses

The baseline data were analysed using SPSS Version 20 and 22. Descriptive analyses were performed to address study objectives (1) and (2). To compare the subgroups of P(+/+) and P(+/−) patients, t-tests and chi-squared tests were conducted to test for significant differences where appropriate. Logistic regression models were conducted to examine the factors associated with depression treatment in patients with HF (study objective 3). Besides age, gender, and education, NYHA Class and depression scale PHQ-9 were included as potential confounders to check for disease severity of the study population. Three univariate ANCOVAs were carried out to examine the factors associated with HRQOL of HF patients with depression (study objective 4). Three models with different independent factors were examined: the GP's awareness of depressive symptomatology (model 1), the depression treatment (model 2), and the GP's awareness of depressive symptomatology, depression treatment,and the interaction between both (model 3). All three models were controlled for the patient's age, gender and education. Furthermore - due to their link to HRQOL in HF patients - NYHA Class and severity of depression (PHQ-9 Score) [33] as well as the number of comorbidities [34] were included as potential confounders. The three models were tested for a GP cluster effect. The nominal level of significance was set at $p = 0.05$. No data imputation strategies were applied.

Ethics approval

The study was conducted in compliance with the Declaration of Helsinki. The study protocol was approved by the local ethics committees (Medical Association of Hamburg, Approval No. PV3889; Ethics Committee of the Medical Faculty of the University of Würzburg, Approval No. 125/12, Ethics Committee of the University of Göttingen Medical Center, Approval No. 19/8/11).

Results

Sampling frame

Of 13,830 HF patients invited by their GPs to join the study, 4909 patients consented to participate in the study and returned a completed baseline questionnaire. Of all 4909 incoming questionnaires, 690 (14.1%) screened positive for depressive symptomatology P(+). Of those, 574 patients from 224 GPs were eligible for further analysis (see Fig. 1). On average, each GP referred 2.6 (SD 1.8; range 1–12) patients.

The GPs of 201 of the 574 patients (35.0%) were aware of their patients' depressive symptomatology P(+/+). Patient and GP characteristics are displayed in Tables 1 and 2.

How do general practitioners treat depressive symptomatology in heart failure patients?

Pharmacological and psychological treatment (patient information) stratified by GPs' awareness of depressive symptomatology Regarding all P(+) patients, 6.4% indicated that they utilised psychotherapy, 18.6% reported taking prescription antidepressants and a total

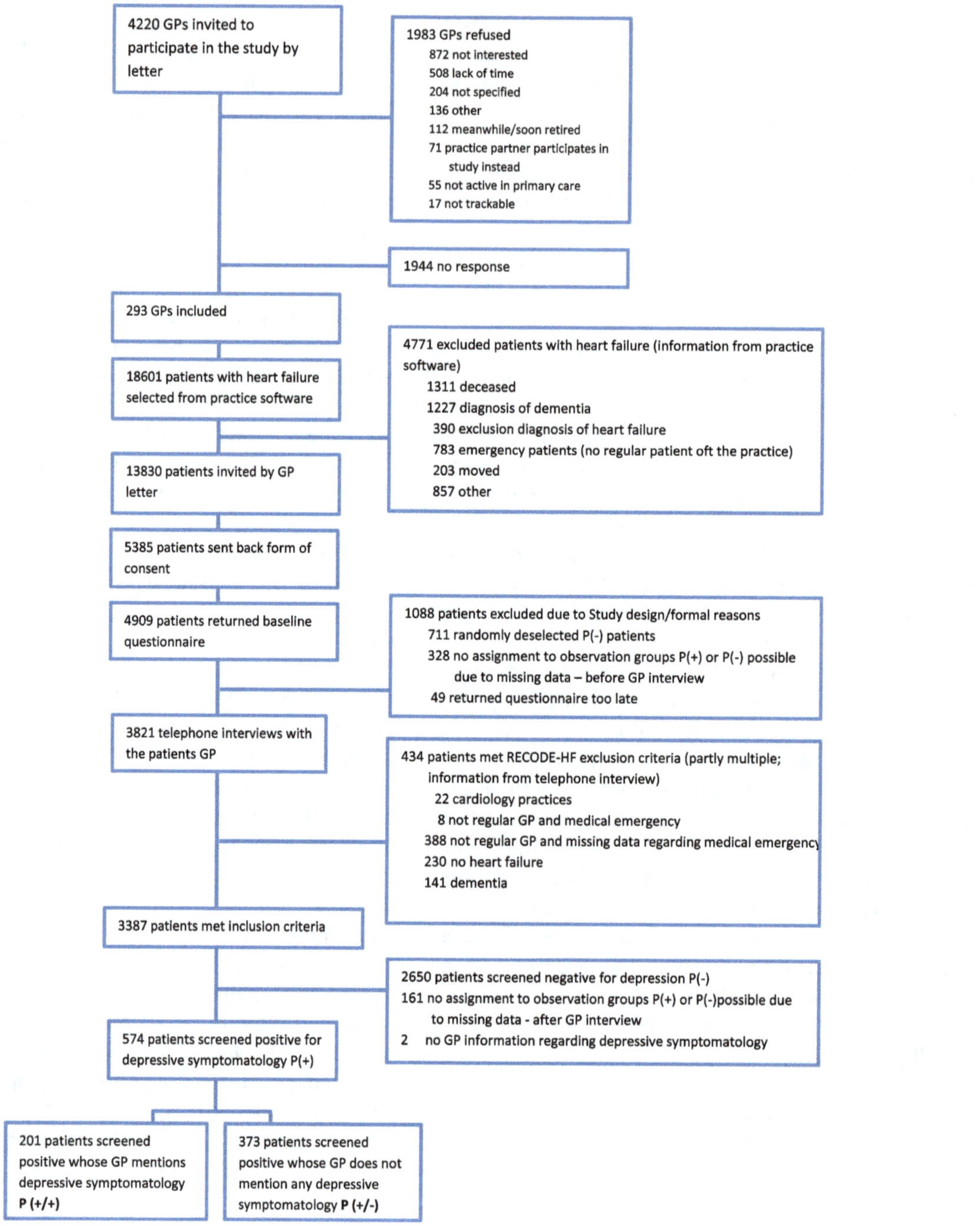

Fig. 1 Sampling frame

of 22.3% utilised psychotherapy, pharmacotherapy or both. All rates were significantly higher in P(+/+) patients than in P(+/−) patients (see Table 3).

Measures taken if GP was aware of depressive symptomatology (GP information) The measures taken if GPs were aware of their patients' depressive symptomatology are displayed in Table 4 for all P(+/+) patients and divided depending on whether GPs stated depressive symptoms or depressive disorder in their patients. No information is displayed for P(+/−) patients, because GPs were not asked about measures taken if no depressive symptoms or depressive disorder were indicated by GPs. GPs prescribed pharmacotherapy to 75.8% of their patients, whom they judged as having a depressive disorder and referred 42.4% to a

Table 1 Patient characteristics

Characteristics	Patients screened positive for depressive symptomatology			Total valid n	Test of significant differences
	GP aware of depressive symptomatology	GP unaware of d epressive symptomatology	Total		
	P (+/+) ($n = 201$)	P (+/−) ($n = 373$)	P (+) ($n = 574$)		
Age, mean (SD)	71.9 (11.7)	73.3 (11.4)	72.8 (11.5)	540	$p = 0.168$
Male gender, N (%)	88 (43.8%)	190 (50.9%)	278 (48.4%)	562	$p = 0.066$
Education level (CASMIN 3)				562	$p = 0.020$
Low	131 (65.2%)	280 (75.1%)	411 (71.6%)		
Middle	51 (25.4%)	67 (18.0%)	118 (20.6%)		
High	16 (8.0%)	17 (4.6%)	33 (5.7%)		
NYHA classification, *N* (%)				566	$p = 0.218$
Class I	30 (14.9%)	60 (16.1%)	90 (15.7%)		
Class II	80 (39.8%)	180 (48.3%)	260 (45.3%)		
Class III	74 (36.8%)	110 (29.5%)	184 (32.1%)		
Class IV	12 (6.0%)	20 (5.4%)	32 (5.6%)		
Comorbidity score, mean (SD)	4.9 (2.5)	5.1 (2.6)	5.0 (2.5)	563	$p = 0.494$
PHQ-9 Score, mean (SD)	14.3 (4.4)	13.0 (3.5)	13.4 (3.9)	574	$p < 0.001$
Health-related quality of life (EQ-5D VAS), mean (SD)	38.2 (19.2)	41.7 (17.6)	40.5 (18.3)	558	$p = 0.029$

specialist. Only 5.3% of the patients judged by their GPs as having a depressive disorder did not receive treatment. If GPs stated that the patients currently displayed depressive symptoms, they still initiated pharmacotherapy in 33.3% of the cases and referred 10.1% to specialists. GPs most often (in 43.5% of the cases) offered this group of patients consultation/counselling carried out by themselves (see Table 4).

Regarding the 123 *P* (+/+) patients whose GPs stated that they had initiated pharmacotherapy, 72 patients (58.5%) did not state that they took any prescription antidepressants. Of those 72 patients, 36.1% received counselling/consultations from their GPs, 23.6% were referred to specialists by their GPs, 2.8% received hospital admission referrals and 4.2% different types of treatment.

Table 2 GP characteristics

GP characteristics		Total valid *n*
Years of GP practice, mean (SD)	15.4 (9.5)	224
Male, *N* (%)	167 (74.6)	217
Type of practice, *N* (%)		223
Single practice	108 (48.4)	
Shared practice	102(45.7)	
Group practice	13 (5.8)	
Any psychological specialisation, *N* (%)	43 (19.2)	224
Medical specialist training in psychiatry, neurology or psychosomatics	4 (1.8)	224
Additional training in psychotherapy	41 (18.3)	224

In total, 40 of the 72 patients (55.6%) received other types of treatment.

Factors associated with depression treatment in heart failure patients

The association between awareness of depressive symptomatology and depression treatment was investigated using two logistic regression models investigating the endpoints: self-reported utilisation of psychotherapy (see Table 5) and of self-reported utilisation of prescription antidepressants (see Table 6). While GPs' awareness of depressive symptomatology was not significantly associated with the probability of self-reported utilization of psychotherapy, older age lowered the chance to utilise psychotherapy. GP's awareness of depressive symptomatology as well as higher PHQ-9 score were both associated with self-reported utilisation of prescription antidepressants.

Factors associated with the health-related quality of life of heart failure patients with depressive symptomatology

Table 7 displays the association between patients' HRQOL and GPs' awareness of depressive symptomatology (model 1), depression treatment (model 2) and awareness of depressive symptomatology, depression treatment as well as the interaction between both (model 3). GPs' awareness of depressive symptomatology was not significantly associated with HRQOL. As there was no significant GP cluster effect, the GP cluster was excluded from the models.

Table 3 Patients' indications regarding utilisation of prescription antidepressants and psychotherapy

	P (+/+) N (%)	P (+/–) N (%)	Total P (+) N (%)	Test of significant differences
Psychotherapy	19 (9.5%)	18 (4.8%)	37 (6.4%)	$p = 0.021$
Taking any prescription antidepressant	61 (30.3%)	46 (12.3%)	107 (18.6%)	$p < 0.001$
Antidepressants and/or psychotherapy	71 (35.3%)	57 (15.3%)	128 (22.3%)	$p < 0.001$
N	201 (100%)	373 (100%)	574 (100%)	

Comparison of patients whose GPs were aware (P(+/+)) of their patients' depressive symptomatology and those whose GPs were unaware (P(+/–)). Compared were cases with utilisation versus all others (no utilisation and cases with no available information, respectively). Absolute and relative frequencies were given

Table 4 GPs indications regarding measures taken by GPs if aware of depressive symptomatology (P(+/+); $N = 201$)

	GP measures if aware of depressive symptomatology P(+/+)		
Measures	GP judgement: depressive symptoms	GP judgement: depressive disorder	Total
Pharmacotherapy	23 (33.3%)	100 (75.8%)	123 (61.2%)
Consultation/Counselling by GP	30 (43.5%)	34 (25.8%)	64 (31.8%)
Referral to specialists	7 (10.1%)	56 (42.4%)	63 (31.3%)
Psychotherapist	5 (7.2%)	28 (21.2%)	33 (16.4%)
Neurologist	1 (1.4%)	18 (13.6%)	19 (9.5%)
Psychiatrist	1 (1.4%)	18 (13.6%)	19 (9.5%)
Other specialist	0 (0%)	1 (0.8%)	1 (0.5%)
Inpatient treatment	0 (0%)	6 (4.5%)	6 (3.0%)
Counselling by others than GP (eg, counselling centre)	0 (0%)	1 (0.8%)	1 (0.5%)
Other	5 (7.2%)	6 (4.5%)	11 (5.5%)
Pain therapy	2 (2.9%)	1 (0.8%)	3 (1.5%)
Physiotherapy/ Rehabilitation	1 (1.4%)	2 (1.5%)	3 (1.5%)
Psychosomatic care	1 (1.4%)	1 (0.8%)	2 (1.0%)
Patient rejects treatment	0 (0%)	2 (1.5%)	2 (1.0%)
Active watchful waiting	2 (2.9%)	0 (0%)	2 (1.0%)
No treatment initiated	14 (20.3%)	7 (5.3%)	21 (10.4%)
N	69 (100%)	132 (100%)	201 (100%)

Absolute and relative frequencies were given

Table 8 displays HRQOL for all P(+) patients depending on GP's awareness of depressive symptomatology and depression treatment.

Discussion

Main results

This observational study revealed that the GPs' awareness of depressive symptomatology was significantly associated with patients' self-reported utilisation of prescription antidepressants and not to patients' self-reported utilisation of psychotherapy. Even though GPs stated that they had referred 16.4% of P(+/+) patients to psychotherapists, only 9.5% of those patients reported utilising psychotherapy. The respective numbers of pharmacotherapy are 61.2% GP-initiated versus 30.3% patient-utilised pharmacotherapy. Patients' HRQOL was not significantly associated with their GPs' awareness of depressive symptomatology.

Strengths and limitations

This has been the first study investigating the treatment of depressive symptomatology and its link to GPs' awareness in a large study of 574 primary care HF patients with comorbid depressive symptomatology. The fact that an algorithm was applied to identify patients with depressive symptomatology, controlling the overlapping symptoms of depression and HF, made this study unique. We believe that fewer false positive cases of HF patients with depressive symptomatology have been included in this study than in other studies using instruments with cut-off values for patients without HF.

This study also has certain limitations. Due to the study procedure, a potential selection bias of patients less impaired by HF and/or depression may have occurred, because severely depressed patients may not have been willing to participate in the study. Therefore, the characteristics of the patients included in the analyses are presented in detail (including the mean PHQ-9 value) in Table 1. Furthermore, due to the study design, patients with depressive symptomatology were identified and included in the study. Next, GPs were asked if they believed these patients to actually display a current depressive symptomatology. Patients with depression who were successfully treated (e.g. with pharmacotherapy), were not identified through the algorithm due to decreased depressive symptomatology. Therefore, we cannot rule out that patients responding less favourably to depression treatment are overrepresented in the study. This may lead to a higher rate of patients who do not adhere to the recommended treatment. Additionally, the number of depression treatment is likely to be underestimated in the present study due to the

Table 5 Association between GPs' awareness of depressive symptomatology and self-reported utilization of psychotherapy in all P(+) patients (logistic regression)

Variable	*P*-Value	Odds Ratio [95% CI]
GPs' awareness of depressive symptomatology (reference: unawareness)	0.081	2.011 [0.919; 4.401]
Education level (reference: Primary education)	0.506	
Secondary education	0.243	1.628 [0.718; 3.688]
Tertiary education	0.821	1.206 [0.238; 6.127]
Age	<0.001	0.926 [0.894; 0.958]
Gender (reference: male)	0.722	1.153 [0.527; 2.522]
NYHA Class (reference: NYHA Class 1)	0.621	
NYHA Class 2	0.273	0.593 [0.233; 1.510]
NYHA Class 3	0.289	0.556 [0.188; 1.645]
NYHA Class 4	0.376	0.366 [0.040; 3.376]
PHQ-9 Score	0.876	1.007 [0.923; 1.099]
Constant	0.059	14.342

$N = 413$; Nagelkerkes $R^2 = 0.197$

selection of patients with acute depressive symptomatology. Those patients undergoing successful treatment and currently free from symptoms may be underrepresented. Also, our results are based on patients with depressive symptomatology and we have not been able to differentiate between patients with depression diagnosis and patients with a subthreshold symptomatology. If only patients with a diagnosis of depression had been included, the results might have been different. However, even though results of our study are not representative for patients diagnosed with depression, there is evidence that patients with subthreshold depressive symptomatology or symptomatology, which is not considered clinically relevant, also experience a reduced quality of life [35] and even higher morbidity and mortality rates after myocardial infarction [36] .

Table 6 Association between GPs' awareness of depressive symptomatology and self-reported utilization of prescription antidepressants in all P(+) patients (logistic regression)

Variable	*P*-Value	Odds Ratio [95% CI]
GPs' awareness of depressive symptomatology (reference: unawareness)	<0.001	2.845 [1.758; 4.604]
Education level (reference: Primary education)	0.670	
Secondary education	0.372	0.765 [0.425;1.377]
Tertiary education	0.868	0.919 [0.338; 2.499]
Age	0.306	0.989 [0.968; 1.010]
Gender (reference: male)	0.136	1.451 [0.889; 2.367]
NYHA Class (reference: NYHA Class 1)	0.421	
NYHA Class 2	0.545	0.821 [0.433; 1.557]
NYHA Class 3	0.217	0.642 [0.318; 1.297]
NYHA Class 4	0.160	0.408 [0.117; 1.424]
PHQ-9 Score	0.001	1.108 [1.045; 1.174]
Constant	0.012	0.089

$N = 525$; Nagelkerkes $R^2 = 0.141$

How do general practitioners treat depressive symptomatology in heart failure patients?

Treatment depending on the GP's rating of symptom severity The initiated treatment of patients whose GP was aware of their depressive symptomatology (P(+/+)), differed depending on the GP's rating whether a patient displayed "depressive symptoms" or "depressive disorder". Consistent with national and international guidelines [37–39], GPs initiated more pharmacotherapy (75.8% vs. 33.3%) and referrals to psychotherapists (21.2% vs. 7.2%) when he/she believed that the patient was suffering from "depressive disorder", than in patients believed to be just displaying "depressive symptoms". Only in 5.3% of patients believed to suffer from "depressive disorder" did GPs not initiate treatment. The respective percentage was higher in patients rated as just displaying "depressive symptoms" (20.3%). This is consistent with the "active monitoring" approach in mild or sub-threshold depression. Even though several GPs referred to this strategy as "treatment", we assumed that most GPs did not refer to this strategy as treatment in our open question "Which treatment did you initiate?". Dialogue or counselling was the most frequent GP-initiated treatment in patients rated as displaying "depressive symptoms" (43.5%). This step-by-step approach corresponds to primary care proceedings and does not indicate any treatment gaps in *P*(+/+) patients.

Incongruences in GP-initiated versus patient-utilised treatment Regarding pharmacotherapy, the reported GP-initiated treatment and the patient-reported treatment utilisation differed considerably in all patients whose GPs were aware of their depressive symptomatology (P(+/+)), (61.2% GP prescription vs. 30.3% patient utilisation) and psychotherapy (16.4% GP referrals to psychotherapists vs. 9.5% patient utilisation of psychotherapy). These differences were in line with prior research focusing on barriers to depression treatment in primary care: The study by Nutting et al. concluded that guideline-appropriate treatment barriers were most frequently caused by patient-centred factors (such as a resistance to the diagnosis, treatment resistance or non-compliance) [40]. In regards to psychotherapy, the authors of the present study assume that a lack of availability may be an additional key factor. Due to social

Table 7 Association between GPs' awareness of depressive symptomatology, depression treatment and HRQOL

Variable	Model 1 F	Model 1 *P*-Value	Model 2 F	Model 2 *P*-Value	Model 3 F	Model 3 *P*-Value
Corrected model	8.968	<0.001	9.107	<0.001	7.602	<0.001
Constant	96.808	<0.001	98.089	<0.001	97.612	<0.001
GPs' awareness of depressive symptomatology	0.122	0.727			0.436	0.510
Utilisation of prescription antidepressants or psychotherapy			1.303	0.254	1.519	0.218
GPs' awareness of depressive symptomatology* Utilisation of prescription antidepressants or psychotherapy					0.087	0.768
Age	4.021	0.045	3.394	0.066	3.512	0.062
Sex (female)	1.440	0.231	1.747	0.187	1.597	0.207
Education	3.052	0.048	3.057	0.048	3.077	0.047
NYHA Class	10.399	<0.001	10.327	<0.001	9.942	<0.001
Comorbidity score	0.447	0.504	0.285	0.594	0.273	0.601
PHQ-9 Score	33.030	<0.001	35.974	<0.001	34.418	<0.001
	$N = 503$; $R^2 = 0.154$		$N = 503$; $R^2 = 0.156$		$N = 503$; $R^2 = 0.157$	

Univariate ANCOVA with endpoint HRQOL (EQ-5D VAS) in patients screened positive for depressive symptomatology P(+). Regarding utilisation of prescription antidepressants or psychotherapy, cases with utilisation were compared with all other cases (no utilisation and cases with no available information, respectively)

desirability and a likely polypharmacy based on the age of the patients, patients might have significantly underreported their utilisation of pharmaco- and psychotherapy while GPs might have reported more measures than they had actually initiated. However, it should be considered that a remaining gap may still be likely between the initiation and utilisation of pharmacotherapy, when treating depression in HF patients. Besides the abovementioned patient barriers found by Nutting et al., interaction effects of antidepressants and HF pharmacotherapy as well as cardiac sideeffects of antidepressants as described in detail by Rustad et al. [41] might decrease patient adherence and lead to the findings in the present study.

Another aspect is the question whether the gap between GP-initiated and patient-utilised pharmacotherapy is filled therapeutically by alternative treatment options, such as counselling by the GP or referrals to other specialists. In our data, 55.6% of patients who did not report the utilising pharmacotherapy although their GP had initiated pharmacotherapy, stated that their GP had also initiated an additional type of treatment. Therefore, even those patients who had not utilised the prescribed pharmacotherapy, might have received (appropriate) treatment. This is what Weel et al. refer to as "treating the patient as a whole" in primary care [42], which cannot be conclusively ascertained by prescription and referral rates.

Lastly, the symptoms of HF in our cohort may have been the GP's highest priority to treat, as these symptoms have been shown to significantly reduce patients' HRQOL [5, 43, 44]. In patients with advanced HF, the disease impairs the mental health scales of quality of life as much as major depression [5]. If patients are depressed because of their poor health status, the treatment of the original disease may be considered to be more important than the depression itself because the depression may improve as soon as the health status improves. To improve HRQOL in HF patients, treating HF symptoms may be as effective as the depression treatment.

Table 8 HRQOL depending on depression treatment and GPs' awareness of all P(+) patients

Utilisation of prescription antidepressants or psychotherapy	GP aware of depressive symptomatology	*N*	mean	SD
No utilization or not specified	No	304	41.7	17.5
	Yes	127	37.5	18.6
Yes	No	56	41.5	18.4
	Yes	71	39.3	20.3

Factors associated with depression treatment in heart failure patients

We hypothesised that GP awareness of depressive symptomatology was significantly associated with a higher utilisation of pharmacotherapy and psychotherapy. We found that HF patients whose GPs were aware of their depressive symptomatology (P(+/+) patients) had a significantly better chance to utilise pharmacotherapy (OR 2.8) than HF patients whose GPs were unaware of their depressive symptomatology (P(+/−) patients). However, we need to interpret these finding with some caution. As GPs had access to their patients' reports, GPs could have used the treatment as a marker for the statement of a patient having shown depressive symptomatology. The link between GPs' awareness of depressive symptomatology and psychotherapy was significant in bivariate analysis but lost significance when controlled for confounding factors. Instead, solely older age was significantly associated with a lesser chance (OR 0.9) of receiving psychotherapy. The significant association with age was consistent with prior research [14, 45, 46] and explained why there were only few cases of this elderly cohort receiving psychotherapy.

These (non-)associations between depression treatment utilisation and GP's awareness of depressive symptomatology reflect the fact that pharmacotherapy can be prescribed by GPs themselves. Psychotherapy does not necessarily require the GP's awareness of depressive symptomatology, nor does the GP's referral to a psychotherapist suffice for a patient to receive psychotherapy. Due to the restricted number of therapy places, the barriers to psychotherapy are higher than to pharmacotherapy. Therefore, a GP's influence on whether or not a patient receives psychotherapy (even though the GP may be aware of the depressive symptomatology and may recommend it) is limited.

Factors associated with health-related quality of life of heart failure patients with depressive symptomatology

HRQOL of all HF patients with depressive symptomatology (P(+) patients) at a mean age of 72.8 years scored 40.5 of 100 points on the EQ-5D VAS Scale. Compared to a 10-year older primary care cohort (65.4 points) [47] and a multimorbid primary care cohort at a similar age (62.4 points) [48], this was a comparably low HRQOL. Studies investigating HF patients found mean EQ-5D VAS scores between 54 and 62.6 points [49–51]). Therefore, besides HF, comorbid depression seems to considerably reduce HRQOL in our study. This impact of depression had been proven in earlier studies [52] and has also been confirmed by our multivariable analysis.

We hypothesised that GPs' awareness of depressive symptomatology was significantly associated with higher HRQOL. Even though, the bivariate analysis showed that HRQOL significantly differed between patients whose GPs were aware of their patients' depressive symptomatology (38.2 of 100 points) and patients whose GPs were unaware (41.7 points), the effect was small and opposed to the objective hypothesised. When controlled for confounders, neither the GP's awareness of depressive symptomatology, nor the depression treatment, nor the interaction of both was significantly linked to HRQOL. Besides the severity of depression, patients' NYHA Class was strongly associated with their HRQOL. This correlation to disease severity had also been shown in other studies [5, 50–52]. The lack of association of both, awareness of depressive symptomatology and depression treatment with HRQOL means that the depression treatment after getting aware of the depressive symptomatology did not suffice to improve HRQOL. Or the reasons might be more complex. The authors hypothesise that the severity of HF symptoms overruled the importance of a GP's awareness of depressive symptomatology in regards to HRQOL in HF patients. Moreover, the GP's awareness of depressive symptomatology might not have been associated with HRQOL because of the following reasons: Patients, whose depressive symptomatology the GP was aware of, might have been more affected by depression despite adequate treatment. At the same time, patients whose GP was unaware of their depressive symptomatology might have been less impaired although they had not received treatment. As a result, both groups did not significantly differ in terms of HRQOL. In other words: The GP was aware of the patients who were impaired by depressive symptoms and overlooked those who were less impaired. This hypothesis was supported by the fact that patients whose GP was unaware of their depressive symptomatology did in fact report a slightly higher HRQOL than patients whose GP was aware of their depressive symptomatology. This was true for both groups of patients (those with depression treatment and those without) as displayed in Table 8.

Overall, the authors did not find that GPs' awareness of depressive symptomatology was significantly associated with patients' HRQOL in contrast to the NYHA Class. Therefore, treating HF symptoms might be more important in improving the HRQOL in HF patients than systematically screening for depression in primary care. In earlier research, certain studies showed similar results and confirmed a positive link between depression treatment and depressive symptomatology [53]. They, however, failed to show a link between depression treatment and cardiac outcome in patients with cardiovascular diseases [53, 54]. Still, the need for depression awareness and treatment remains indisputable to reduce symptoms of depression in HF patients, independent of the possibility of improving HRQOL. We just need to differentiate both outcome criteria.

Implications for research

There are several aspects which need to be considered in future research. Firstly, investigating the treatment of depression in primary care HF patients is more complex than it seems. Treatment options chosen by the GP (eg, dialogue with the patient) are not always hard outcome criteria for research but might be crucial in everyday practice. Outcome criteria need therefore be chosen carefully and qualitative studies may be helpful in regards to depression treatment in HF patients. Secondly, we need to keep in mind that studies focusing on patient utilisation behaviour do not necessarily reflect GPs' efforts to provide treatment. Therefore, future research needs to differentiate between GP efforts to initiate treatment and patients' acceptance and realisation of therapy options, especially in studies based on the claims data of health insurances. Factors leading to patients deciding not to use the recommended therapy options need to be investigated before deciding on the appropriateness of depression treatment in HF patients. Thirdly, the true dimension of a possible treatment gap needs to be further investigated, especially in those patients whose GPs are unaware of their patients' depressive symptomatology. In the present study, the authors have found no significant link between GPs' awareness of a depressive symptomatology and the patients' quality of life. Therefore, one hypothesis may be that GPs are aware of relevant cases of depression in need of treatment and are unaware of less impaired patients without the need for treatment. However, a possible treatment gap should be investigated in longitudinal studies keeping the context of this hypothesis in mind.

Fourthly and last, the condition of HF may have such an impact on patients' HRQOL that depression treatment (which is not significantly linked to HRQOL in the present study) may improve the symptoms of depression but not necessarily HRQOL as long as HF continues to significantly impair patients' HRQOL. If this is the case, the recommendation to screen HF patients for depression and consequently treat depression will not improve patients' HRQOL. Instead, measures beyond standard therapy of HF and depression may be necessary to further improve patients' HRQOL. Especially questions as to why depression treatment does not improve HRQOL in patients with HF and what types of measures beyond standard therapy are necessary to do so should be further investigated. These aspects need to be considered when planning intervention studies in patients with HF and depression.

Implications for practice

GPs should be aware of the gap between GP-initiated and patient-utilised depression treatments in patients with chronic HF, which may lead to a undersupply of depression treatment, even though the GP has initiated treatment. Due to possible interaction effects between antidepressants and HF, close monitoring at the onset of taking antidepressants may improve patient adherence. Furthermore, GPs should critically consider the potentially general reluctance of referring older patients to psychotherapy. Additionally, there are probably patients who display depressive symptomatology and do not receive treatment because their GPs are unaware of the depressive symptomatology. GPs should keep in mind that depressive symptomatology is common in HF patients and, consequently, should pay special attention to HF patients' potentially depressive symptomatology in order to avoid an undersupply of depression treatment. Due to the potentially harmful cardiac sideeffects of antidepressants (eg, described by *Rustard* et al. [41]) and the actual efforts to reduce polypharmacy, the type of treatment should be chosen carefully whilst considering non-pharmacologic treatment strategies for depression; exercise [55], cognitive behavioural therapy [22], and collaborative care [56] are beneficial in improving depressive symptoms in HF patients.

In general, we have to keep in mind that, just like the severity of HF, comorbid depression seems to considerably reduce CFH patients' HRQOL. Therefore, if they have not already done so, GPs have to discuss with their patients the types of measures available to improve their HRQOL in addition to standard HF and depression therapy.

Conclusion

If GPs knew of their patients' depressive symptomatology, there were various GP-initiated treatments of depressive symptomatology in HF patients far exceeding pharmacotherapy or referrals to psychotherapists. Those data are not necessarily represented in routine data. In general practice, GPs should be aware of the gap between GP-initiated and patient-utilised depression treatments in patients with chronic HF, which might lead to a undersupply of depression treatment. Patients whose GP was unaware of their depressive symptomatology had a lower chance of receiving antidepressants, but surprisingly neither the GP's awareness of depressive symptomatology nor depression treatment was significantly associated with the patients' HRQOL. The authors hypothesise, that GPs might have been aware of HF patients with more severe depressive symptomatology resulting in a reduced HRQOL. GPs might have overseen depressive symptomatology without significant impairment of the patients' HRQOL. Therefore, in the end, both groups of patients might have displayed comparable levels of HRQOL; the former patients with ongoing depression treatment and the latter without. This could explain the missing association between GPs' awareness of depressive symptomatology and their patients' HRQOL. This hypothesis will have to be further investigated in qualitative as well as longitudinal studies.

Abbreviations

GP: General Practitioner; HF: Chronic heart failure; HRQOL: Health-related quality of life

Acknowledgements

We thank all participating GPs and patients for their good collaboration.
Members of RECODE-HF Study Group:
Winfried Adam, Cassandra Behrens, Eva Blozik, Sigrid Boczor, Marion Eisele, Malte Harder, Christoph Herrmann-Lingen, Agata Kazek, Dagmar Lühmann, Anja Rakebrandt, Koosje Roeper, Martin Scherer, Stefan Störk, Jens-Martin Träder.

Funding
The study was funded by the German Federal Ministry of Education and Research (grant numbers 01GY1150 and 01EO1004).

Availability of data and materials
The data from this study is not available for public use, as the data is owned by the RECODE-HF Study Group and the authors are not allowed to share this information with third parties.

Authors' contributions
ME drafted the manuscript, made substantial contributions to the study's conception and design, coordinated the research project and was involved in data analysis and interpretation; SB made substantial contributions to the study's conception and design, was involved in data analysis and interpretation and critically revised the manuscript; AR made substantial contributions to the study's conception and design, was involved in data acquisition, analysis and interpretation and critically revised the manuscript, EB made substantial contributions to the study's conception and design and critically revised the manuscript; JMT made substantial contributions to the study's conception and design and critically revised the manuscript; SS is the principal investigator of the Würzburg study center, made substantial contributions to the study's conception and design, and critically revised the manuscript; CHL is the principal investigator of the Göttingen sub-study center, made substantial contributions to the study's conception and design, and critically revised the manuscript; MS is the principal investigator of the entire study, acquired funding for and designed the study, and critically revised the manuscript. All authors read and approved the final manuscript.

Consent for publication
Not applicable.

Competing interests
CHL receives royalties fom Hogrefe Huber publishers for the German HADS version. SB received fees for part-time lecturing/statistical consulting from Asklepios Medical School GmbH. EB is employed at Helsana Health Insurances, Zürich, Switzerland. All other authors declare that they have no competing financial interests.
Non-financial competing interests: ME and EB are members of the German College of General Practitioners and Family Physicians. MS is vice president of the German College of General Practitioners and Family Physicians. CHL chairs the working group on Psychosomatics in Cardiology at the German College of Psychosomatic Medicine and is the current president of the American Psychosomatic Society. All other authors declare that they do not have any competing non-financial interests.

Author details
[1]Department of Primary Medical Care, Center for Psychosocial Medicine, University Medical Center Hamburg-Eppendorf, Martinistraße 52, 20246 Hamburg, Germany. [2]Department of Primary Medical Care, University of Luebeck, Ratzeburger Allee 160, 23538 Luebeck, Germany. [3]Comprehensive Heart Failure Center Würzburg, University and University Hospital Würzburg, Straubmühlweg 2a, 97078 Würzburg, Germany. [4]University of Göttingen Medical Center, and German Center for Cardiovascular Research, partner site Göttingen, von-Siebold-Str. 5, D-37099 Göttingen, Germany.

References

1. Global, regional, and national incidence, prevalence, and years lived with disability for 301 acute and chronic diseases and injuries in 188 countries, 1990–2013: a systematic analysis for the Global Burden of Disease Study 2013. The Lancet. 2015 [cited 2015 Aug 24]; Available from: http://linkinghub.elsevier.com/retrieve/pii/S0140673615606924
2. Hunt SA, Abraham WT, Chin MH, Feldman AM, Francis GS, Ganiats TG, et al. ACC/AHA 2005 guideline update for the diagnosis and management of chronic heart failure in the adult a report of the American College of Cardiology/American Heart Association task force on practice guidelines (writing committee to update the 2001 guidelines for the evaluation and management of heart failure): developed in collaboration with the American College of Chest Physicians and the International Society for Heart and Lung Transplantation: endorsed by the Heart Rhythm Society. Circulation 2005 [cited 2013 Jun 18];112:e154–e235. Available from: http://circ.ahajournals.org/content/112/12/e154
3. Moraska AR, Chamberlain AM, Shah ND, Vickers KS, Rummans TA, Dunlay SM, et al. Depression, healthcare utilization, and death in heart failure a community study. Circ Heart Fail. 2013 [cited 2015 Aug 26];6:387–394. Available from: http://circheartfailure.ahajournals.org/content/6/3/387
4. Hunt SA. ACC/AHA 2005 guideline update for the diagnosis and management of chronic heart failure in the adult: a report of the American College of Cardiology/American Heart Association task force on practice guidelines (writing committee to update the 2001 guidelines for the evaluation and management of heart failure). J Am Coll Cardiol 2005;46:e1–82.
5. Juenger J, Schellberg D, Kraemer S, Haunstetter A, Zugck C, Herzog W, et al. Health related quality of life in patients with congestive heart failure: comparison with other chronic diseases and relation to functional variables. Heart. 2002 [cited 2016 Feb 18];87:235–241. Available from: http://heart.bmj.com/content/87/3/235
6. Masoudi FA, Rumsfeld JS, Havranek EP, House JA, Peterson ED, Krumholz HM, et al. Age, functional capacity, and health-related quality of life in patients with heart failure. J Card Fail. 2004;10:368–73.
7. Joynt KE, Whellan DJ, O'connor CM. Why is depression bad for the failing heart? A review of the mechanistic relationship between depression and heart failure. J Card Fail. 2004 [cited 2013 Mar 25];10:258–271. Available from. http://www.sciencedirect.com/science/article/pii/S1071916403007176
8. Bekelman DB, Havranek EP, Becker DM, Kutner JS, Peterson PN, Wittstein IS, et al. Symptoms, depression, and quality of life in patients with heart failure. J Card Fail. 2007;13:643–8.
9. Ponikowski P, Voors AA, Anker SD, Bueno H, Cleland JGF, Coats AJS, et al. 2016 ESC guidelines for the diagnosis and treatment of acute and chronic heart failure: The task force for the diagnosis and treatment of acute and chronic heart failure of the European Society of Cardiology (ESC)developed with the special contribution of the heart failure association (HFA) of the ESC. Eur Heart J. 2016;37:2129–2200. [cited 2017 Aug 23] Available from: https://academic.oup.com/eurheartj/article/37/27/2129/1748921.
10. Bundesärztekammer (BÄK), Kassenärztliche Bundesvereinigung (KBV), Arbeitsgemeinschaft der Wissenschaftlichen Medizinischen Fachgesellschaften (AWMF). Nationale VersorgungsLeitlinie Chronische Herzinsuffizienz-Langfassung [Internet]. Version 2. 2017 [cited 2017 Jan 18]. Available from: http://www.leitlinien.de/mdb/downloads/nvl/herzinsuffizienz/herzinsuffizienz-2aufl-vers2-lang.pdf
11. Cully JA, Jimenez DE, Ledoux TA, Deswal A. Recognition and treatment of depression and anxiety symptoms in heart failure. Prim Care Companion J Clin Psychiatry. 2009 [cited 2015 Aug 25];11:103–109. Available from: http://www.ncbi.nlm.nih.gov/pmc/articles/PMC2708006/
12. Koenig HG. Recognition of depression in medical patients with heart failure. Psychosomatics. 2007 [cited 2013 Jun 12];48:338–347. Available from: http://www.sciencedirect.com/science/article/pii/S0033318207710289
13. Eisele M, Blozebrandt A, Boczor S, Kazek A, Pohontsch N, Okolo-Kulak M, et al. Factors associated with general practitioners' awareness of depression in primary care patients with heart failure: baseline-results from the observational RECODE-HF study. BMC Fam Pract. 2017 [cited 2017 Jun 12]; 18:71. Available from: https://doi.org/10.1186/s12875-017-0641-1
14. Crystal S, Sambamoorthi U, Walkup JT, Akıncıgil A. Diagnosis and treatment of depression in the elderly Medicare population: predictors, disparities, and trends. J Am Geriatr Soc. 2003 [cited 2016 Feb 9];51:1718–1728. Available from: http://onlinelibrary.wiley.com/doi/10.1046/j.1532-5415.2003.51555.x/abstract
15. Hunt SA, Abraham WT, Chin MH, Feldman AM, Francis GS, Ganiats TG, et al. 2009 focused update incorporated into the ACC/AHA 2005 guidelines for the diagnosis and management of heart failure in adults: a report of the American College of Cardiology Foundation/American Heart Association Task Force on Practice Guidelines: developed in collaboration with the International Society for Heart and Lung Transplantation. Circulation. 2009; 119:e391–479.

16. Heart Failure Society of America. Executive summary: HFSA 2010 comprehensive heart failure practice guideline. J Card Fail. 2010 [cited 2013 Jun 12];16:475–539. Available from: http://www.onlinejcf.com/article/S1071-9164(10)00174-0/abstract
17. National Clinical Guideline Centre. Chronic heart failure: the management of chronic heart failure in adults in primary and secondary care. London: National Clinical Guideline Centre. 2010 [cited 2017 Jan 12]. Available from: http://guidance.nice.org.uk/CG108/Guidance/pdf/English.
18. McMurray JJV, Adamopoulos S, Anker SD, Auricchio A, Böhm M, Dickstein K, et al. ESC guidelines for the diagnosis and treatment of acute and chronic heart failure 2012: the task force for the diagnosis and treatment of acute and chronic heart failure 2012 of the European Society of Cardiology. Developed in collaboration with the heart failure association (HFA) of the ESC. Eur Heart J. 2012;33:1787–847.
19. Angermann CE, Gelbrich G, Störk S, Gunold H, Edelmann F, Wachter R, et al. Effect of Escitalopram on all-cause mortality and hospitalization in patients with heart failure and depression: the MOOD-HF randomized clinical trial. JAMA. 2016 [cited 2017 Aug 28];315:2683–2693. Available from: http://jamanetwork.com/journals/jama/fullarticle/2530538
20. O'Connor CM, Jiang W, Kuchibhatla M, Silva SG, Cuffe MS, Callwood DD, et al. Safety and efficacy of Sertraline for depression in patients with heart failure: results of the SADHART-CHF (Sertraline against depression and heart disease in chronic heart failure) trial. J Am Coll Cardiol. 2010 [cited 2013 Jun 12];56:692–699. Available from: http://www.sciencedirect.com/science/article/pii/S0735109710022382
21. Fraguas R, da Silva Telles RM, Alves TCTF, Andrei AM, Rays J, Iosifescu DV, et al. A double-blind, placebo-controlled treatment trial of citalopram for major depressive disorder in older patients with heart failure: the relevance of the placebo effect and psychological symptoms. Contemp Clin Trials. 2009;30:205–211. [cited 2017 Apr 24] Available from: http://www.sciencedirect.com/science/article/pii/S1551714409000081.
22. Freedland KE, Carney RM, Rich MW, Steinmeyer BC, Rubin EH. Cognitive behavior therapy for depression and self-Care in Heart Failure Patients: a randomized clinical trial. JAMA Intern Med. 2015;175:1773–82. [cited 2017 Aug 28] Available from: http://www.ncbi.nlm.nih.gov/pmc/articles/PMC4712737/.
23. Eisele M, Blozik E, Störk S, Träder J-M, Herrmann-Lingen C, Scherer M. Recognition of depression and anxiety and their association with quality of life, hospitalization and mortality in primary care patients with heart failure - study protocol of a longitudinal observation study. BMC Fam Pract. 2013;14:180.
24. Bjelland I, Dahl AA, Haug TT, Neckelmann D. The validity of the hospital anxiety and depression scale. An updated literature review. J Psychosom Res. 2002;52:69–77.
25. Herrmann-Lingen C, Buss U, Snaith R. HADS-D-hospital anxiety and depression scale-deutsche version: Deutsche adaptation der Hospital anxiety and depression scale (HADS), 2. Auflage. Bern: Huber; 2005.
26. Spitzer RL, Kroenke K, Williams JB. Validation and utility of a self-report version of PRIME-MD: the PHQ primary care study. Primary care evaluation of mental disorders. Patient health questionnaire. JAMA J Am Med Assoc. 1999;282:1737–44.
27. Kroenke K, Spitzer RL, Williams JBW. The PHQ-9. J Gen Intern Med. 2001;16: 606–13. Available from: http://www.ncbi.nlm.nih.gov/pmc/articles/PMC1495268/
28. Löwe B, Gräfe K, Zipfel S, Witte S, Loerch B, Herzog W. Diagnosing ICD-10 depressive episodes: superior criterion validity of the patient health questionnaire. Psychother Psychosom. 2004;73:386–90.
29. Pilkonis PA, Choi SW, Reise SP, Stover AM, Riley WT, Cella D. Item banks for measuring emotional distress from the patient-reported outcomes measurement information system (PROMIS®): depression, anxiety, and anger. Assessment. 2011 [cited 2013 Mar 13];18:263–283. Available from: http://asm.sagepub.com/content/18/3/263
30. Choi SW, Reise SP, Pilkonis PA, Hays RD, Cella D. Efficiency of static and computer adaptive short forms compared to full-length measures of depressive symptoms. Qual Life Res Int J Qual Life Asp Treat Care Rehabil. 2010;19:125–36.
31. Janssen MF, Pickard AS, Golicki D, Gudex C, Niewada M, Scalone L, et al. Measurement properties of the EQ-5D-5L compared to the EQ-5D-3L across eight patient groups: a multi-country study. Qual Life Res Int J Qual Life Asp Treat Care Rehabil. 2012;22(7):1717-27.
32. Schäfer I, Hansen H, Schön G, Höfels S, Altiner A, Dahlhaus A, et al. The influence of age, gender and socio-economic status on multimorbidity patterns in primary care. First results from the multicare cohort study. BMC Health Serv Res. 2012 [cited 2016 Mar 10];12:89. Available from: https://doi.org/10.1186/1472-6963-12-89
33. Coelho R, Ramos S, Prata J, Bettencourt P, Ferreira A, Cerqueira-Gomes M. Heart failure and health related quality of life. Clin Pract Epidemiol Ment Health CP EMH. 2005 [cited 2017 Mar 15];1:19. Available from: http://www.ncbi.nlm.nih.gov/pmc/articles/PMC1274338/
34. Peters-Klimm F, Kunz CU, Laux G, Szecsenyi J, Müller-Tasch T. Patient- and provider-related determinants of generic and specific health-related quality of life of patients with chronic systolic heart failure in primary care: a cross-sectional study. Health Qual Life Outcomes. 2010 [cited 2014 Jan 3];8:98. Available from: http://www.hqlo.com/content/8/1/98/abstract
35. Creed F, Morgan R, Fiddler M, Marshall S, Guthrie E, House A. Depression and anxiety impair health-related quality of life and are associated with increased costs in general medical inpatients. Psychosomatics. 2002;43:302–9.
36. Bush DE, Ziegelstein RC, Tayback M, Richter D, Stevens S, Zahalsky H, et al. Even minimal symptoms of depression increase mortality risk after acute myocardial infarction. Am J Cardiol. 2001 [cited 2017 Jul 12];88:337–341. Available from: http://www.sciencedirect.com/science/article/pii/S0002914901016757
37. Mitchell J, Trangle M, Degnan B, Gabert T, Haight B, Kessler D, Mack N, Mallen E, Novak H, Rossmiller D, Setterlund L, Somers K, Valentino N, Vincent S. Institute for Clinical Systems Improvement. Adult Depression in Primary Care. 2013. [cited 2015 Dec 22]; Available from: https://www.icsi.org/guidelines__more/catalog_guidelines_and_more/catalog_guidelines/catalog_behavioral_health_guidelines/depression/.pdf
38. Deutsche Gesellschaft für Psychiatrie, Psychotherapie und Nervenheilkunde (DGPPN), Ärztliches Zentrum für Qualität in der Medizin (ÄZQ). S3-Leitlinie/Nationale VersorgungsLeitlinie Unipolare Depression-Langfassung, 2. Auflage. 2015 [cited 2015 Dec 22]; Available from: https://doi.org/10.6101/AZQ/000266
39. Depression in adults: recognition and management | 1-recommendations | Guidance and guidelines | NICE [Internet]. [cited 2015 Dec 22]. Available from: http://www.nice.org.uk/guidance/cg90/chapter/1-recommendations#step-2-recognised-depression-persistent-subthreshold-depressive-symptoms-or-mild-to-moderate
40. Nutting PA, Rost K, Dickinson M, Werner JJ, Dickinson P, Smith JL, et al. Barriers to initiating depression treatment in primary care practice. J Gen Intern Med. 2002 [cited 2016 Feb 3];17:103–111. Available from: http://onlinelibrary.wiley.com/doi/10.1046/j.1525-1497.2002.10128.x/abstract
41. Rustad JK, Stern TA, Hebert KA, Musselman DL. Diagnosis and treatment of depression in patients with congestive heart failure: a review of the literature. Prim Care Companion CNS Disord. 2013 [cited 2016 Feb 10];15. Available from: http://www.ncbi.nlm.nih.gov/pmc/articles/PMC3869617/
42. Weel C van, Weel-Baumgarten E van, Rijswijk E van. Treatment of depression in primary care. BMJ. 2009 [cited 2016 Feb 9];338:b934. Available from: http://www.bmj.com/content/338/bmj.b934
43. Iqbal J, Francis L, Reid J, Murray S, Denvir M. Quality of life in patients with chronic heart failure and their carers: a 3-year follow-up study assessing hospitalization and mortality. Eur J Heart Fail. 2010 [cited 2016 Feb 8];12:1002–1008. Available from: http://onlinelibrary.wiley.com/doi/10.1093/eurjhf/hfq114/abstract
44. Hobbs FDR, Kenkre JE, Roalfe AK, Davis RC, Hare R, Davies MK. Impact of heart failure and left ventricular systolic dysfunction on quality of life: a cross-sectional study comparing common chronic cardiac and medical disorders and a representative adult population. Eur Heart J. 2002;23:1867–76.
45. Wei W, Sambamoorthi U, Olfson M, Walkup JT, Crystal S. Use of psychotherapy for depression in older adults. Am J Psychiatry. 2005 [cited 2016 Feb 16];162:711–717. Available from: http://www.ncbi.nlm.nih.gov/pmc/articles/PMC2921918/
46. Kendrick T, Dowrick C, McBride A, Howe A, Clarke P, Maisey S, et al. Management of depression in UK general practice in relation to scores on depression severity questionnaires: analysis of medical record data. BMJ. 2009 [cited 2016 Feb 23];338:b750. Available from: http://www.bmj.com/content/338/bmj.b750
47. Eisele M, Kaduszkiewicz H, Konig H-H, Lange C, Wiese B, Prokein J, et al. Determinants of health-related quality of life in older primary care patients: results of the longitudinal observational AgeCoDe study. Br J Gen Pract. 2015 [cited 2015 Nov 6];65:e716–e723. Available from: http://bjgp.org/cgi/doi/10.3399/bjgp15X687337
48. Brettschneider C, Leicht H, Bickel H, Dahlhaus A, Fuchs A, Gensichen J, et al. Relative impact of multimorbid chronic conditions on health-related quality of life–results from the MultiCare cohort study. PLoS One. 2013;8:e66742.

49. Eurich DT, Johnson JA, Reid KJ, Spertus JA. Assessing responsiveness of generic and specific health related quality of life measures in heart failure. Health Qual Life Outcomes. 2006 [cited 2016 Feb 8];4:89. Available from: https://doi.org/10.1186/1477-7525-4-89
50. Comin-Colet J, Lainscak M, Dickstein K, Filippatos GS, Johnson P, Lüscher TF, et al. The effect of intravenous ferric carboxymaltose on health-related quality of life in patients with chronic heart failure and iron deficiency: a subanalysis of the FAIR-HF study. Eur Heart J. 2013 [cited 2016 Feb 8];34:30–38. Available from: http://eurheartj.oxfordjournals.org/content/34/1/30
51. Rivas B de, Permanyer-Miralda G, Brotons C, Aznar J, Sobreviela E. Health-related quality of life in unselected outpatients with heart failure across Spain in two different health care levels. Magnitude and determinants of impairment: the INCA study. Qual Life Res. 2008 [cited 2016 Feb 8];17:1229–1238. Available from: http://link.springer.com/article/10.1007/s11136-008-9397-3
52. Schowalter M, Gelbrich G, Störk S, Langguth J-P, Morbach C, Ertl G, et al. Generic and disease-specific health-related quality of life in patients with chronic systolic heart failure: impact of depression. Clin Res Cardiol. 2012 [cited 2016 Feb 18];102:269–278. Available from: http://link.springer.com/article/10.1007/s00392-012-0531-4
53. Thombs BD, de Jonge P, Coyne JC, Whooley MA, Frasure-Smith N, Mitchell AJ, et al. Depression screening and patient outcomes in cardiovascular care: a systematic review. JAMA J Am Med Assoc. 2008;300:2161–71.
54. Thombs BD, Roseman M, Coyne JC, de Jonge P, Delisle VC, Arthurs E, et al. Does evidence support the American Heart Association's recommendation to screen patients for depression in cardiovascular care? An updated systematic review. PLoS One. 2013;8:e52654.
55. Blumenthal JA, Babyak MA, O'Connor C, Keteyian S, Landzberg J, Howlett J, et al. Effects of exercise training on depressive symptoms in patients with chronic heart failure: the HF-ACTION randomized trial. JAMA J Am Med Assoc. 2012 [cited 2017 Aug 28];308:465–474. Available from: http://www.ncbi.nlm.nih.gov/pmc/articles/PMC3953459/
56 Bekelman DB, Plomondon ME, Carey EP, Sullivan MD, Nelson KM, Hattler B, et al. Primary results of the patient-centered disease management (PCDM) for heart failure study: a randomized clinical trial. JAMA Intern Med. 2015 [cited 2017 Aug 28];175:725–732. Available from: http://jamanetwork.com/journals/jamainternalmedicine/fullarticle/2210885

11

'Doing the right thing': factors influencing GP prescribing of antidepressants and prescribed doses

Chris F. Johnson[1*], Brian Williams[2], Stephen A. MacGillivray[3], Nadine J. Dougall[2] and Margaret Maxwell[4]

Abstract

Background: Antidepressant prescribing continues to increase, with 5-16% of adults receiving antidepressants annually. Total prescribing growth is due in part to increased long-term use, greater selective serotonin re-uptake inhibitor (SSRI) use and the use of higher SSRI doses. Evidence does not support routine use of higher SSRI doses for depression treatment, and factors influencing the use of such doses are not well known. The aim of this study was to explore factors influencing GPs' use of antidepressants and their doses to treat depression.

Methods: Semi-structured interviews with a purposive sample of 28 practising GPs; sampled by antidepressant prescribing volume, practice size and deprivation level. A topic guide drawing on past literature was used with enough flexibility to allow additional themes to emerge. Interviews were audio-recorded and transcribed verbatim. Framework analysis was employed. Constant comparison and disconfirmation were carried out across transcripts, with data collection being interspersed with analysis by three researchers. The thematic framework was then systematically applied to the data and conceptualised into an overarching explanatory model.

Results: Depression treatment involved ethical and professional imperatives of 'doing the right thing' for individuals by striving to achieve the 'right care fit'. This involved medicalised and non-medicalised patient-centred approaches. Factors influencing antidepressant prescribing and doses varied over time from first presentation, to antidepressant initiation and longer-term treatment. When faced with distressed patients showing symptoms of moderate to severe depression GPs were confident prescribing SSRIs which they considered as safe and effective medicines, and ethically and professionally appropriate.
Many GPs were unaware that higher doses lacked greater efficacy and onset of action occurred within 1-2 weeks, preferring to wait 8-12 weeks before increasing or switching. Ongoing pressures to maintain prescribing (e.g. fear of depression recurrence), few perceived continuation problems (e.g. lack of safety concerns) and lack of proactive medication review (e.g. patients only present in crisis), all combine to further drive antidepressant prescribing growth over time.

Conclusions: GPs strive to 'do the right thing' to help people. Antidepressants are only a single facet of depression treatment. However, increased awareness of drug limitations and regular proactive reviews may help optimise care.

Keywords: General practice, Primary health care, Depression, Antidepressive agents, Doctor-patient relationship, Qualitative research

* Correspondence: c.johnson2@nhs.net
[1]Pharmacy and Prescribing Support Unit, NHS Greater Glasgow and Clyde, 2nd Floor, Main Building, West Glasgow Ambulatory Care Hospital, Dalnair Street, Yorkhill, Glasgow G3 8SJ, UK
Full list of author information is available at the end of the article

Background

Antidepressant prescribing has increased substantially across Western societies over the last 40 years [1–3], attracting much discussion, debate, concern and controversy [1, 4, 5]. The issues are wide and varied: whether antidepressants are overprescribed or not [4, 5]; whether antidepressants are effective or ineffective in treating depression [6]; Westernised societies' expected right to happiness and consequential medicalisation of unhappiness [7, 8]; the direct/indirect role which the pharmaceutical industry may have in influencing the definition of depressive disorder [9, 10]; promoting simple marketing models of depressive illness [11]; 'ghostwriting' antidepressant studies [9, 10]; and more controversially, reporting bias, missing data [12], and antidepressant associated self-harm [13]. Despite these debates and controversies, depression remains a common, recurrent, debilitating and potentially fatal condition with antidepressants being only one of the many components of depression treatment which have been shown to be effective [14–17].

Although prescribing continues to increase, there has been no corresponding increase in depression incidence or prevalence [18, 19]. Most antidepressants are prescribed by general practitioners (GPs) with the majority (60-85%) of adults receiving them for the treatment of depression [20–22] and a minority receiving them for other conditions [23], with an estimated 5-16% of adults receiving antidepressants in Europe and USA annually [24, 25]. Factors that have contributed to prescribing growth include: the introduction of tricyclic antidepressants (TCAs) in the late 1960s [1], then the addition of selective serotonin re-uptake inhibitors (SSRIs) in the 1980s [26]; increased long-term prescribing in the 1990s and 2000s [19]; lack of regular review [27]; and more recently the use of higher doses [21, 28, 29].

SSRIs are of particular interest as they account for the majority of antidepressant prescriptions, dominating antidepressant volumes across Western Societies [24, 25], and are routinely prescribed at higher doses than previously reported in the literature in the UK and New Zealand [21, 29]. In one study, higher than standard SSRI doses were associated with the practice which the patient attended; long-term use of SSRIs; and co-prescribing of SSRI with long-term benzodiazepines and/or z-hypnotics (B&Zs) [22]. However, current evidence does not support the routine use of higher licensed doses as they lack greater efficacy [17, 30, 31]. Higher doses are also associated with more adverse effects including anxiety, agitation and insomnia [30] which may lead to co-prescribing of sedating drugs such as B&Zs, antipsychotics and other antidepressants such as trazodone. Such combinations of high dose SSRI and sedating antidepressant use may also influence the large variations in antidepressant volumes prescribed between practices [32]. There is a need to understand these variations in prescribing practice.

Methods

Aim

The aim of this study was to explore factors influencing GPs' use of antidepressants and their doses to treat depression.

Design and setting

Quantitative methods can be limited in providing depth of clarity on this issue, therefore qualitative methods were used to enable an in-depth understanding of GPs' perspectives and rationale for prescribing. Focus groups were considered inappropriate as it was expected that predominant voices may drown out more moderate voices, and impractical for busy GPs to attend within normal working hours. Therefore we captured in-depth GP perspectives on their practical experience and opinions of what influences their antidepressant prescribing through one-to one, face-to-face, interviews conducted in each GP's office.

Sampling and recruitment

We recruited 28 GPs working in general practices across the National Health Service Greater Glasgow and Clyde (NHSGG&C) region in Scotland. NHSGG&C provides taxpayer funded healthcare services for a diverse population of 1.2 million people across a varied urban region containing 260 general practices.

In order to achieve information-rich cases and diverse perspectives, a purposive sample was sought by allocating all general practices in NHSGG&C to a sampling frame using practice characteristics: volume of antidepressants prescribed; number of GPs; and practice deprivation score. We aimed to recruit 30 GPs from across NHSGG&C with an equal number of male and female GPs, and a proportion of GPs partners working in the same practice (7 practices).

Antidepressant prescribing data for the 260 practices was obtained from the Prescribing and Information System for Scotland for year to March 2014, as previously described [22]. The 260 practices were first ranked from lowest to highest antidepressant prescribers, and then categorised as low, medium and high prescribers based on the number of defined daily doses (DDDs)/1000 patients. These were then subcategorised as small (single handed GP), medium (2-3 GPs) and large (≥4 GPs) by the number of GPs contracted to individual practices, as recorded in April 2014 [33]. Finally, practices were ranked by Scottish Index of Multiple Deprivation rank derived from each practice's postcode [34], and categorised as being in areas of low, medium and high deprivation.

Between August 2014 and December 2015, GPs matching the sampling frame were initially contacted by letter and followed up by telephone within 2 weeks by administrative staff. In total 188 GPs were written to, in groups of 30 to 40, during the study period. GPs were informed about the aims of the study, that study findings would be used to support appropriate antidepressant use within NHSGG&C, and that previous NHSGG&C work had identified the routine use of higher SSRI doses [21, 22]. Potential participants showing interest were then contacted by CFJ to arrange interviews at their offices'. Prior to interviews starting, CFJ discussed the study and sought participant's consent for inclusion in the study. GPs were not incentivised to participate in any way. A total of 28 GPs participated, 14 male and 14 female, see Table 1.

Data collection

One-to-one, face-to-face, semi-structured interviews were carried out by one researcher, a prescribing support pharmacist (CFJ), at the GP's office. Interviews lasted between 15 and 55 min with most lasting approximately 30 min. Although an initial topic guide was developed using previous literature, it was flexible enough to allow additional topics to emerge (see Additional file 1: Topic guide for first interview (v6) and final version of topic guide (v14)). Interviewees were also asked for their perspectives on factors associated with higher SSRI dose use for depression treatment as previously identified [22]. Early interviews and subsequent interviews informed the refinement of subsequent topic guides and the inclusion of emergent themes expressed as GPs' views and experiences at interview. Interviews were audio-recorded and transcribed verbatim.

Analysis

Data analysis was inductive and continuous, and began from the start of data collection. Constant-comparative technique was used [35] while adopting Framework analysis [36] as the broad structure for the analytical procedure. Familiarisation with, and constant-comparison between transcripts permitted additional important themes to emerge. Transcripts were initially read and emerging themes and patterns discussed by three authors (CFJ, BW and MM) to identify a thematic framework. Constant-comparison and disconfirmation were then carried out repeatedly and systematically (by CFJ) between transcripts to enhance and confirm the thematic framework. Data collection was interspersed with analysis, with findings informing subsequent interviews, allowing interviewees to explain and/or expand on key themes. As CFJ was aware that being a prescribing support pharmacist may influence GPs' responses, interviewees were asked if this could have affected their responses. The thematic framework was then systematically applied to the data which were indexed and summarised in charts, by CFJ. Broad themes and patterns (mapping), both within and across interviews were identified. NVivo 11 was used to store and organise data.

From this process, an understanding of the factors influencing GPs decision-making regarding the use of antidepressants and their doses emerged, and were conceptualised into an overarching explanatory model of factors influencing prescribing.

Ethical approval

The study was approved by the Ethics Committee of the School of Health Sciences, University of Stirling 21st April 2014.

Table 1 Individual GP and practice characteristics

Individual GP Characteristics (n = 28)			
Female (%)			14 (50)
Median age (range)			43 (33 to 60)
Years since qualified as doctor, median (range)			19 (10 to 37)
Years as a GP median (range)			12 (2 to 33)
Number of GPs with psychiatry training as part of GP training rotation (%)			19 (68)
Number of GPs with extra psychiatric training/experience as locum or psychiatry trainee (%)			4 (14)
Individual practice characteristics (n = 20)			
Antidepressant volumes in DDD/1000 patients, n (GPs)	Low = 9 (10)	Medium = 4 (6)	High = 7 (12)
Number of GP partners, n (GPs)	Small (single handed) = 1 (1)	Medium (2-3 GPs) = 10 (13)	Large (≥4 GPs) = 9 (14)
Deprivation, n (GPs)	Low = 6 (6)	Medium = 5 (7)	High = 9 (15)
Training practice, n (GPs)	Yes = 10 (16)	No = 10 (12)	

DDD defined daily doses. DDDs are units of measurement defined by the World Health Organization as 'the assumed average maintenance dose per day for a drug used for its main indication in adults'. DDDs do not necessarily reflect the recommended or prescribed daily dose but allow a convenient method to compare prescribing volumes between organisations [59]

Results

Analysis revealed that depression treatment involved two key overarching concepts of 'doing the right thing' and achieving the 'right care fit' for individuals. This involved medicalised and non-medicalised patient-centred approaches with antidepressants only being a single facet of treatment. However, factors influencing antidepressant prescribing and prescribed doses varied over time from first presentation and the beginning of treatment, to antidepressant initiation and longer-term treatment (Fig. 1). Seven interwoven factors influenced antidepressant prescribing. Five of these factors can be described as strongly influential: 1) Depression diagnosis and management; 2) Patients' expectations and characteristics; 3) GP's experience and relationships; 4) Antidepressant use: safety, risk management and effectiveness; 5) Review frequency. Two were moderately influential: 6) Local prescribing resources and 7) Mental health services. As outlined below with illustrative quotes, also see Additional file 2: Supplementary quotes.

The magnitude of the influence exerted by these factors varied with time. For example, review frequency was high and highly influential at the beginning of treatment in supporting and increasing appropriate antidepressant use for more severe illness, whereas in the intermediate period following the first few months of antidepressant treatment, review frequency decreased, thereby reducing the potential for appropriate continuation or discontinuation. In the longer-term, reviews became more infrequent and coupled with some patients presenting in crisis further increased cumulative prescribing (Fig. 1).

When faced with patients showing symptoms of moderate to severe depression, GPs were confident prescribing SSRIs, which they considered safe and effective medicines. Prescribing was seen ethically and professionally as 'doing the right thing' for the patient in the face of distress. However, many were unaware higher doses lacked greater efficacy and onset of action occurred within 1-2 weeks, preferring to wait 8-12 weeks before increasing or switching. The ongoing pressures to maintain prescribing (e.g. patient wishes, fear of depression recurrence), few perceived continuation problems (e.g. lack of safety concerns) and the lack of proactive medication reviews (e.g. patients only present in crisis) contributed to further antidepressant prescribing growth over time (Fig. 1).

Depression diagnosis and management

Diagnosing depression

Across the sampling frame diagnosing depression was rarely seen as a simple task or process. This was due to a

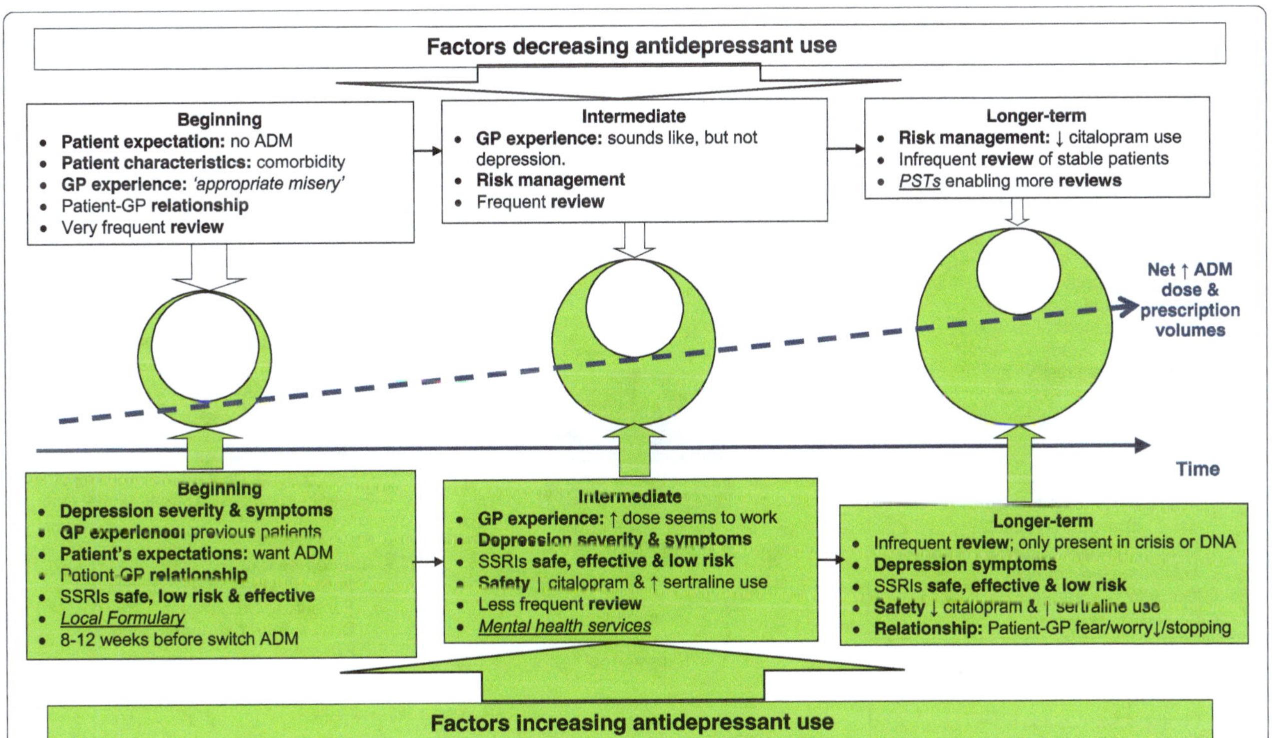

Fig. 1 Factors increasing and decreasing antidepressant prescribing for depression treatment. Factors strongly influencing antidepressant prescribing bold and moderately influential factors in italics and underlined. ADM: antidepressant. DNA: do not attend. PST: Prescribing Support Teams. SSRI: selective serotonin re-uptake inhibitor

variety of issues and complex interactions involving: normal life events; relationship problems; social and environmental issues; patients' expectations of happiness; duration of symptoms; mixed anxiety and depressive symptoms; co-morbidities; and the risk of medicalising normal and *"appropriate misery" (D21,18p3)* due to life events. However, time well spent in this initial presentation period – regularly reviewing patients – was seen as an important part of the biopsychosocial assessment. Some practitioners routinely used depression rating scales to quantify depression severity or as a tool to support discussions with patients, whereas others found rating scales hampered assessment, or were not used as they lacked a social domain. Patient information was used to ascertain and balance how well signs, symptoms and subjective assessment fitted with standardised concepts of clinical depression and severity to achieve the best treatment 'fit' (Fig. 2).

> *...the bottom line for GPs is that we want to help, we want to offer something that we think will help. D12,8*

> *You also want to look at the person as a whole and find out where they are in their life. You have to assess the actual severity of the situation before determining what kind of treatment would be appropriate for them. Then, we would go down the route of discussing what sort of therapies we could offer them. D25,6*

In general, GPs rarely prescribed antidepressants at the first presentation, unless patients had a recurrent depressive episode where antidepressants were previously effective, as a large proportion of patients presented in crisis and were experiencing an acute reaction to life events or stressors. GPs in our study viewed it as more important to listen to patients and discuss issues in the first instance, especially for mild to moderate forms of depression where patients needed someone to talk to, not prescribe. Allowing a period of 'watch and wait' where depressive symptoms would remit.

> *...for a lot of people with a mild to moderate depressive illness, is to say, "you might not need anything here. You might just need, someone to talk to you about it and some support and things might improve on their own." D12,96*

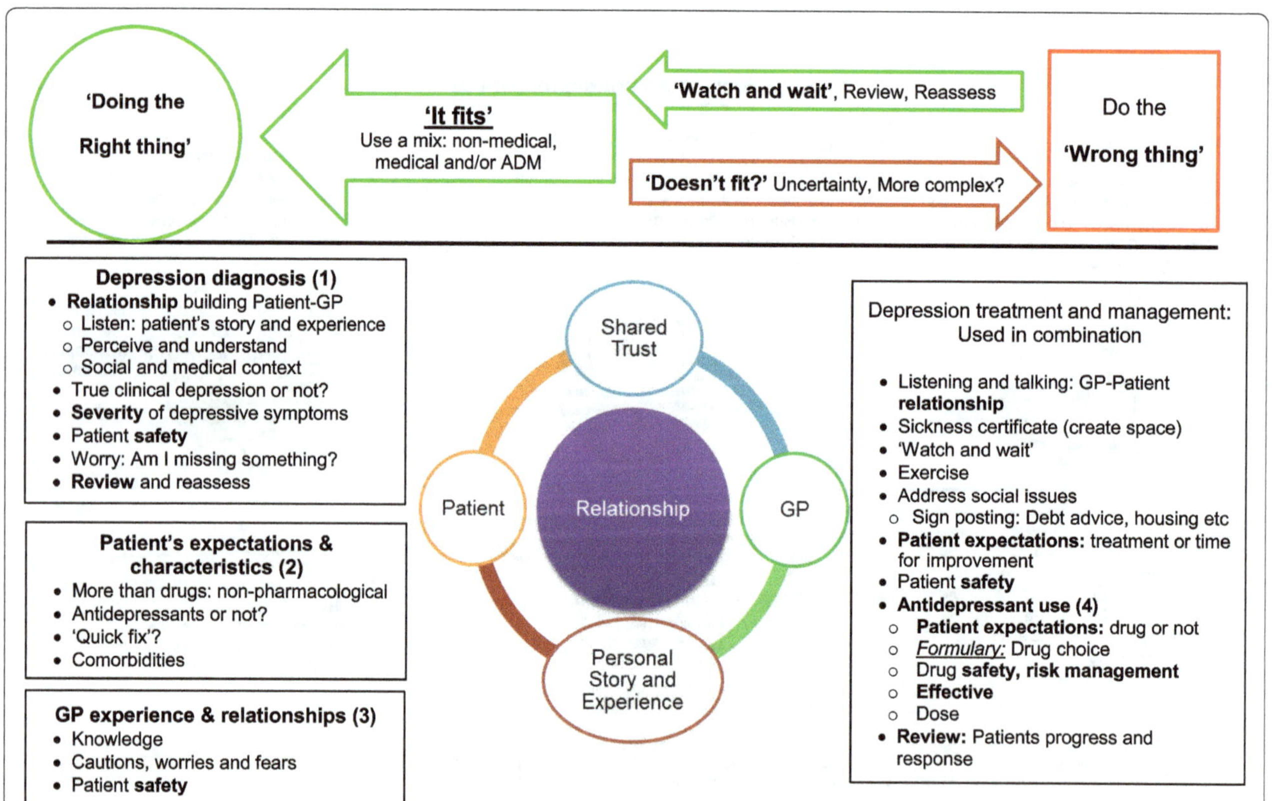

Fig. 2 Balancing treatment and management options. Factors strongly influencing antidepressant prescribing bold and moderately influential factors are in italics and underlined

Although for some patients, there was an expectation about receiving something.

> *They think they're coming here [pause] for me to do something for them [empathetically said]. And that, they almost feel as if there needs to be a physical display of that, like the prescription or whatever. D2,14*

For more severe cases, and for patients that GPs knew well, they would consider prescribing at the first presentation if symptoms were sufficiently severe to warrant an antidepressant. However, this was not routine practice. Referral to specialist Community Mental Health Teams (CMHTs) was also considered for people with more severe symptoms.

More than drugs

Treatment involved more than drugs. As already identified, GPs considered listening, talking and allowing patients time for spontaneous remission as an important core part of appropriate care, treatment and management. For all severities of depression, and where patients preferred not to take antidepressants for moderate to more severe depression due to stigma or personal choice, GP's embraced, supported and used multiple options to manage and treat signs and symptoms in line with the patient's preferences. This included a varied array of medical and non-medicalised approaches: creating space for patients by using sickness certification; exercise and exercise referrals to local council gyms; counselling; signposting to information sources e.g. Links-workers to address money worries; bibliotherapy in libraries; online cognitive behavioural therapy e.g. Moodgym; talking therapies via NHS and non-NHS providers in combination with or without antidepressants. A multifactorial interwoven approach was thus created in achieving the 'right care fit' and 'doing the right thing', with drug treatment being only one of many therapeutic approaches.

> *I explain to them that, "You have to look at this [responding to an antidepressant] in conjunction with other things." So, it's always going to be a multifactorial approach. It's never going to be just one thing [an antidepressant]. D28,28.*

Patients' expectations and characteristics

Data indicated that GPs' prescribing was not overtly influenced by patients' expectations of receiving an antidepressant. The need for a clear benefit to the patient was still the main influence, assessed on the basis of knowing the patient's history, comorbidities and social context. However, it was acknowledged that time pressures could play a role, as it was difficult to discuss and encourage the use of non-antidepressant alternatives if clinics were running late.

> *I think most of my colleagues here wouldn't prescribe unless they felt somebody was going to get benefit from them [antidepressants]. We all kind of have roughly the same sense of what's bad and what's good. D4,24*

Many GPs felt that some patients were looking for 'a quick fix', and that this was rooted in wider societal expectations that problems could and should be solved medically. However, it was usually those with milder symptoms that had greater expectations of 'a quick fix'. As they presented in crisis there was an expectation to do something to solve the problem; a physical display with a prescription, which was sometimes driven by family members more than patients. For some the 'quick fix' was short-term antidepressant use, which stopped within a couple of months of starting, while others did not expect 'a quick fix' and wanted to avoid antidepressants altogether.

> *I think there's an expectation generally, that if there is a problem perhaps you know there is a pill for it. I think that is an expectation that's held by a lot of people. Other people are very resistant to the idea of taking antidepressants. D18,6*

GP experience and relationships

Experiential learning significantly influenced how GPs prescribed antidepressants. This cumulative knowledge was gained through a mixture of formal training, such as general practice training schemes and acute psychiatric experience, and informal reflective practice - seeing improvements in one patient and repeating the same intervention with others. However, with time and greater experience prescribers formulated their own ideas about depression management, becoming more *"idiosyncratic"* to achieve the 'best care fit' such as using mirtazapine rather than fluoxetine, where insomnia was a significant issue, or sertraline instead of citalopram for patients with cardiac disease.

> *I think initially absolutely with guidelines and I guess, as I alluded to before, the more experienced I've got, the more idiosyncratic I've got. It tends to be how a patient's presenting, so it might be side-effects or likely side-effects or beneficial side-effects that may guide me on where I would go [with treatment]. D24,20*

National and local guidelines were considered by GPs to weakly influence antidepressant prescribing, with some specialist resources being helpful in specific situations e.g. switching drugs. However, local prescribing resources, namely the formulary and prescribing support teams, did influence drug choices and cost effective prescribing decisions.

We've got our in-house pharmacist, and it's fantastic, 'cause we sit down and talk about these things... For example, with venlafaxine slow release people, we've changed all of them [to lower cost ordinary release], and we resisted pressure from secondary care and patients as well. So that's definitely a positive influence. Because we're not pharmacists, and we don't know nearly as much about pharmacology as pharmacists do. D26,129

Most GPs indicated they prescribed within formulary guidance whereas psychiatrists and other specialists tended to prescribe third or fourth line agents which were outwith formulary guidance. This sometimes caused friction, especially with children and adolescents where the evidence is weaker; there were potentially greater safety concerns and risks; and shared care structures were lacking or not considered robust enough, thus providing a 'poor care fit' and raising potential medico-legal issues.

The other issue is prescribing antidepressants in young people. We won't prescribe antidepressants that are unlicensed in young people. We won't prescribe them in people under the age of 18 because there is no shared-care protocol. Unfortunately, without the support of shared-care protocol we don't feel really we have the specialist knowledge to be prescribing it much for [children and adolescents]. D25,29 We've been asked to prescribe sertraline and fluoxetine, I think, in people around about age 15. Both of which we've refused. We've refused all of them. The issue then is that they feel that once they've initiated it we should take over the prescription. But because there's no shared-care protocol it still leaves us fairly vulnerable. So, we have still decided as a partnership that we won't be involved in that...D25,31

However, these frictions were partly overcome where there was good communication, supportive structures and good relationships.

Pharmaceutical companies were considered not to influence prescribing as GPs avoided seeing company representatives for a variety of reasons e.g. anger about 'me-too' drugs, promotion of active isomers of cheaper older drugs sold at a premium price. However, GPs acknowledged that companies had subtle influences on depression management.

Well... escitalopram really pissed me off, I hate that sort of carry on, it was like loratadine and desloratadine, I just hate that! I mean 'me-too' drugs that happen to appear just as patents are running out and are another way of creaming money out of the unsuspecting public,... D21,70

...there was the Defeat Depression campaign and that was the Royal College. But the Royal College and GPs really got into tow I think with pharma in a big way, and I think actually that was probably fairly influential but,... pharma were probably being very very clever there, and more subtle than usual. I would say...people get quite well develop antibodies to pharma now. So they actually probably have to work harder to convince me... But they are more subtle, and they have subtle links. D18,23

In general the media was considered not to influence prescribing, but some GPs were aware of previous media articles regarding fluoxetine and adolescent suicide, which had changed prescribing habits. The media was thought to influence patients' attitudes and expectations regarding depression treatment, although this was often presented in a confused ambiguous manner.

I think that the media give quite a muddled view on things. They all seem to be reporting the celebrities who are getting treatment or counselling for this, that and the other. And, then, on the other hand, they bash GPs for overprescribing antidepressants like sweeties.D3,20

Antidepressant use: safety, risk management and effectiveness

Drug choice

Across the sampling frame prescribing was influenced by GP's prior clinical experience, severity of patient's depressive symptoms and needs, along with age and comorbidities. Treatment options were agreed through GP-patient discussions.

You aim to certainly do it [prescribe] in partnership with the patient. At the end of the day, if you don't do it in partnership with them and you prescribed it, then they won't take it anyway, so you do it in partnership with the patient. ...based on advice, guidelines. I think there is an element of doing what you believe is the right thing from your own experience. D8,22

SSRIs were seen as being effective, well tolerated and a safe choice, especially when compared to TCAs. Consideration was also given to the slight differences between SSRIs with fluoxetine seen by some as more stimulating and appropriate for depression, whereas sertraline and citalopram were considered more appropriate for mixed depression anxiety symptoms and better tolerated. The Medicines and Healthcare products Regulatory Agency (MHRA) safety warning regarding citalopram and escitalopram causing dose dependent QT interval prolongation, which is associated with ventricular tachycardia and sudden cardiac death [37], had influenced prescribers who were now using less citalopram and more sertraline.

> *They're safer. So, no one in their right mind now is going to give an MAOI if you're a GP. There's no good reason to start a tricyclic rather than an SSRI unless you'd been through a few of them [antidepressants] already. You know, there's far less risk from a GP's point of view in terms of overdosing, in terms of side effects from the medication. D22,33*

Mirtazapine's side effects were considered beneficial for some patients, with weight gain being positive for underweight patients while the sedative effects alleviated insomnia and anxiety symptoms for some. Low dose mirtazapine was being used in preference to more traditional low dose trazodone or as a safer non-addictive alternative to avoid B&Zs.

> *...well I know that it's a funny drug [mirtazapine], because it's supposed to be only sedating at low dose, because it has the antihistamine effect. We use it a lot at 15mg just for the sedating effects, as a non-addictive sleeping pill, really. D26,39*

Opinion was split when using mirtazapine to treat depression - some quickly increased to therapeutic doses while others maintained people on 15 mg subtherapeutic doses. In part this may have been influenced by CMHTs and Addictions Teams use of low dose mirtazapine as a single agent or in combination with other antidepressants. A small minority of GPs acknowledged that they rarely added another antidepressant to augment current treatment, e.g. adding mirtazapine to an SSRI, and considered their practice to be influenced by CMHTs as only a minority of these GPs had extensive psychiatric training. Others, however, questioned the appropriateness of combining antidepressants without specialist input and considered it as the specialist's domain, as with other psychotropics e.g. antipsychotic augmentation with quetiapine. Although, most were comfortable initiating low dose amitriptyline for neuropathic pain for patients already receiving an antidepressant for depression.

> *Well that's one of the places I have been influenced by secondary care. Because a lot of the psychiatrists say, we're going to add this to augment the effect of this. It's usually mirtazapine and citalopram together. And I actually do think that works, I'm not quite sure the biochemistry behind that. But... erm, I now do that sometimes myself. It's often for the poor sleepers. D26,65*

SSRI efficacy: time to effect and dose response

All GPs reported that they prescribed standard therapeutic SSRI doses: 20 mg daily for citalopram, fluoxetine and paroxetine, or 50 mg daily for sertraline. Half considered that SSRIs were effective within 2 to 4 weeks, with some indicating that some patients respond well within the first 2 weeks of treatment. The remaining half considered efficacy was achieved within 6 to 8 weeks. When SSRIs taken at therapeutic doses were ineffective or partially effective, a large proportion of GPs would wait 8 to 12 weeks before increasing the dose or changing antidepressants. Most of these prescribers were female and had completed GP psychiatric or extra psychiatry training but did not differ in other characteristics to GPs that increased or changed sooner. In part, persevering with one antidepressant for a longer period may have been due to concerns about giving people an adequate trial and fears of running out of pharmacological treatment options.

> *Keep them on... probably quite some time, 2 or 3 months, and if they weren't responding, then change. D17, 50*

From experience, a minority of GPs thought that standard SSRI doses provided maximum efficacy, with higher doses lacking greater benefits, so rarely increased or 'pushed doses' up. In contrast the majority considered higher SSRI doses were more efficacious with sertraline being routinely increased. There were no differences in characteristics between the two groups, with both acknowledging that psychiatrists routinely 'pushed the dose' of SSRIs. However when discussed as part of the MHRA advice restricting citalopram to lower doses, most observed that a few patients' depressive symptoms worsened while most remained well controlled on lower doses.

> *As we know the response to higher doses doesn't grow, you know, parallel to the increasing dose. So, if we get a good response to the first dose... doubling the dose to, a higher dose doesn't always make a big difference. That's our clinical experience. D6,44*

Some prescribers acknowledged being drawn into responding to a patient's distress by 'doing something' although they were aware the intervention may have limited or negligible benefits. Some considered this to be less than an ideal care 'fit' even though it provided patients with hope, demonstrated that patients had been listened to, and that all options were being tried.

> *...when you've got a patient, a desperate patient in front of you wanting something to be done, it's the temptation is to crank up the dose. Again, one of my colleagues will go up to much higher doses of fluoxetine than, than perhaps the rest of us would. D3,60*

SSRI efficacy: use of higher SSRI doses for depression treatment

GPs' opinions were sought regarding previous observations that higher SSRI doses were routinely being prescribed [21, 28, 29] and that higher than standard SSRI doses for the treatment of depression were associated with the practice the patient attended, long-term use (receiving the same antidepressant for ≥2 years), and co-prescribing of long-term (≥8 weeks) B&Zs [22].

GPs considered that practice factors associated with higher SSRI doses may be due to more aggressive prescribers 'pushing the dose', but was in part due to prescriber's experience, what worked with previous patients and/or if GPs had psychiatry training. Although GPs admitted to being more comfortable prescribing antidepressants and patients were more comfortable taking antidepressants, most practitioners considered that their prescribing was similar to their colleagues. Only two GPs considered that they prescribed more, one due to being female and seeing more female patients and the other because he prescribed lots of everything.

A few GPs highlighted differences in management styles between them and their colleagues relating to: frequency of review and follow up, use of alternatives, and again that a minority were happier prescribing antidepressant combinations for depression, whereas the majority were not.

> *I think there's two of us in the practice seeing more people who have got psychological problems. I would then however suspect that others might prescribe more antidepressants per head if you know what I mean. Whereas I would be more interested in trying alternatives to antidepressants. D18,26*

Higher doses associated with long-term SSRI use were considered to be due to a combination of factors, greater depression severity with more refractory symptoms and dose escalation over the years for those prescribed SSRIs in response to crises, as previous dose increases were considered effective. However, the dose may not have been reviewed and reduced at a later date, and then further increased with subsequent crises, with colleagues within the practice not feeling comfortable reducing and/or stopping medication because they had not increased the dose. As patients presented in crisis, and not when they are well, there were challenges in ensuring proactive routine antidepressant reviews and opportunities to appropriately reduce prescribing. GPs did however acknowledge that most patients who were proactively reviewed due to the MHRA citalopram warning were able to reduce or stop citalopram without any significant problems.

Patient and GP fears of relapse due to reducing or stopping antidepressants – causing more harm than good – were also discussed by some prescribers. Especially for patients with chronic depression, creating challenges for restarting, optimising and stabilising individuals.

> *I suppose if you've got somebody that goes through crisis and they're on a drug anyway for a long time, every time they have a crisis the dose might be bumped up and then not reduced. So, I wonder if there's an element of just not reducing the drug when it's appropriate... and patients psychologically seem to be quite dependent on these drugs as well. So, they might want that increased dose too. D10,93*

Higher SSRI doses associated with long-term B&Z treatment were considered to be linked with patients being more complicated, possibly having greater psychiatric multimorbidity as well as underlying social and personal issues not being addressed but medicated instead. Patients were generally more willing to engage and seek pharmacological treatment and resisted reductions. However, clinicians rarely consider adverse effects with higher SSRI doses increasing anxiety or B&Z's lowering mood.

> *...it is probably if you've got somebody who's on long-term benzos it suggests they're not very well. There's long-term issues there. ...probably most of those issues are not going to be dealt with by a drug. D24,74*

Finally, in summarising the factors influencing antidepressant prescribing and dose used, data indicated that 'doing the right thing' and appropriately initiating antidepressants where there was a clear need increased antidepressant prescribing growth, Fig. 1. However, after patients were established on antidepressants and with increasing treatment duration, there were fewer and fewer factors over time which provided counterbalances to reduce prescribing and use, thus explaining the phenomenon sustaining and driving net antidepressant prescribing growth over time.

Discussion

Summary

Diagnosising and treating depression was rarely seen as a simple task or process by GPs due to the complex interaction of normal life events, relationships, social and environmental pressures. Treatment involved ethical and professional imperatives expressed as two overarching concepts of 'doing the right thing' and achieving the 'right care fit' for individuals. This involved medicalised and non-medicalised patient-centred approaches, with antidepressants only being a single facet of individualised care (Fig. 2).

Five factors were strongly influential: 1) Depression diagnosis and management; 2) Patients' expectations and characteristics; 3) GP's experience and relationships; 4) Antidepressant use: safety, risk management and effectiveness; and 5) Review frequency. The magnitude of the influence exerted by these factors varied with the individual's needs; treatment options; antidepressants prescribed and doses used over time, from first presentation, to antidepressant initiation and longer-term treatment. Many GPs were unaware that onset of action occurred within 1-2 weeks, preferring to wait 8-12 weeks before increasing or switching.

When faced with distressed patients showing symptoms of moderate to severe depression, GPs were confident prescribing SSRIs which they considered as safe and effective medicines, as well as ethically and professionally appropriate. However, individual patient comorbidities, national safety warnings and use of sedating antidepressants as non-addictive alternatives to B&Zs influenced drug choice for managing risks, optimising patient safety and benefit.

Many GPs were also unaware that higher SSRI doses lacked greater efficacy. This lack of awareness was accompanied by: ongoing pressures to maintain prescribing (e.g. patient wishes, fear of depression recurrence); few perceiving continuation as problematic (e.g. lack of safety concerns); and the lack of proactive medication reviews (e.g. patients only present in crisis), all combining to further drive antidepressant prescribing growth over time (Fig. 1).

Strengths and limitations

Strengths: The main strength of this study was the sampling frame used which ensured the views of a wide variety of working GPs' experiences were captured from a large urban region with the same formulary, prescribing support team and local depression guidelines. This study also sought local GP perspectives on previous research findings from other general practices within their urban region [22], thereby allowing GPs to use their unique insight in considering local and national contextual issues contributing to the use of higher SSRI doses, as seen elsewhere [28, 29]. Another advantage was that during the study period there were no changes to the local formulary, prescribing support team activities or depression guidelines, although in May 2015 the British Association of Psychopharmacology issued new guidelines [17]. This was assessed as having negligible effects on GPs' responses, as most acknowledged guidance was a weak influencing factor on prescribing. Finally, as GPs acknowledged that prescribing support teams did influence their prescribing, they were asked if the interviewer (CFJ) being a prescribing support pharmacist had influenced their responses, to which they indicated that this had not.

Limitations: As GPs were not incentivised to participate we suspect that participants may have been more interested in mental health and psychotropic prescribing, and more willing to openly share experience and reflect on practice. Some potential participants acknowledged that a lack of time and work pressure prohibited study participation when contacted by telephone. Emergent themes were discussed as part of the interview, however these themes were not overtly checked for trustworthiness with future interviewees. The variety and availability of medicalised and non-medicalised support services did vary within the region which may have influenced prescribing, however GPs acknowledged that these were only one aspect of patient care and support, and such variation in support services will also be the case in other urban regions. Finally, although data collected from one large urban region may also be considered a limitation as rurality and regional variations are associated with prescribing variations [32], the findings are of interest to others working in similar urban practices.

Comparison and links with literature

Safety and risk management were recurring features of this study. Other studies have highlighted that GPs were confident using SSRIs due to perceived and actual safety benefits when compared with other antidepressants [38, 39]. This study highlights that national safety warnings have changed SSRI prescribing practice, reducing citalopram use and increasing sertraline use which is traditionally prescribed at higher doses [21]. It also highlights prescribers' preference for low dose mirtazapine or trazodone instead of more risky B&Zs. However as with B&Zs, tolerance develops to antidepressant sedative effects within a short period of time [40, 41].

Experience, training and individual patient characteristics influenced drug choice and use, as reported elsewhere [42, 43], however some GPs indicated that prescribing became more *"idiosyncratic"*, using learned experience and habits to achieve the 'best care fit' for individuals. In one systematic review such experience was identified as a barrier to the use of evidence-based medicine in practice [44]. However, in contrast to our study, they did not consider the role of specialist services affecting GPs' treatment decisions, whether that consisted of shared experience and good working relationships, or conversely, a lack of robust support structures and fractured care [45]. In part, some of these idiosyncrasies and experiences may contribute to variations in antidepressant prescribing as one partner within a practice can skew the prescribing figures [46].

Unexpectedly, prescriber preference for waiting as long as 8 to 12 weeks before increasing or switching antidepressants links with a previous quantitative study demonstrating an 8 week lag in drug optimisation [47]. Together these identify a new potential factor which may influence early antidepressant discontinuation, possibly linking with perceived inertia and service dissatisfaction as previously identified [48, 49]. Prescribers also demonstrated that antidepressants were only one of many treatment modalities, and that the GPs themselves had a therapeutic function as listener, counsellor and facilitator [49–51], as well as creating space through use of sickness certificates [52]. As with other studies, GPs rarely saw depression diagnosis and management as a simple task or process. This was due to the complex interplay of social, environmental and comorbidity issues, as well as individuals' expectations of happiness and unvoiced agendas [38, 53]. Although GPs did not readily take the perceived easy option to prescribe antidepressants, preferring instead to 'watch and wait,' they would consider prescribing earlier if depressive symptoms were more severe and/or they knew the patient well [42, 50]. Unlike other studies identifying patients' expectations of antidepressants being a 'quick fix' [38, 49], GPs in this study were clear in viewing this as not being unique to depression treatment, but reflecting wider societal expectations.

Implications for practice

The main implications for practitioners are to be more aware of SSRI dose limitations; higher doses lacking greater efficacy, and time to effect when treating depression [17, 30, 31]. This would potentially have direct and indirect effects on reducing unnecessary prescribing and adverse drug effects, e.g. anxiety and insomnia which might be mistaken for residual depressive symptoms. As well as reducing the co-prescribing of sedating antidepressants, and antipsychotics or B&Zs with their respective cardiometabolic [54] and mood lowering effects [55, 56]. Another dosing concern is the routine use of subtherapeutic mirtazapine doses which may help anxiety and/or insomnia symptoms in the short-term for individuals with mixed depression anxiety but does not optimise depression treatment in line with current evidence [57].

An 8-12 week delaying in drug optimisation potentially slows patient recovery, and when doses and/or drugs are changed it might be harder to differentiate true antidepressant response from spontaneous remission, as 50% of patients recover within 12 weeks [58]. Therefore, in order appropriately optimise antidepressant use for depression treatment it is important that prescribers are more aware that the greatest response occurs within the first 2 weeks of treatment [17, 31].

Finally, a major challenge is creating time to proactively review patients and their antidepressants when individuals are not in a crisis and expecting *"something to be done"*. This is easier said than done, as service pressures, demands and staffing issues limit capacity for proactive reviews. However, where there are safety concerns e.g. MHRA citalopram/escitalopram warning, or as part of a local initiative [21], unnecessary treatment can be reduced or stopped through proactive review.

Future research

Treatment decisions involving complex ethical and moral processes and judgements to achieve the 'right care fit' and to 'to do the right thing' for patients which may also be relevant to other areas of prescribing such as antibiotic use and minimisation. Future studies should consider the patients' perspective and expectations about depression treatment and management and drug limitations. The greater use of antipsychotics, with their known detrimental metabolic effects, to treat depression and/or concomitant insomnia and anxiety is also an area for concern with significant resource implications. Therefore, future studies should consider monitoring and assessing the short and long-term impact of such strategies in primary care.

Conclusion

GPs strive to 'do the right thing' to help people. Antidepressants are only a single facet of depression treatment. However, increased awareness of drug limitations, time to effect, more rapid switching and regular proactive reviews may help optimise care and appropriately minimise antidepressant prescribing.

Abbreviations

ADM: Antidepressant medicines; B&Zs: Benzodiazepines and/or z-hypnotics; CMHT: Community Mental Health Teams; DDD: Defined daily dose; DNA: Do not attend; GP: General practitioner; MAOI: Monoamine oxidase inhibitor; MHRA: Medicines and Healthcare products Regulatory Agency; NHSGG&C: NHS Greater Glasgow and Clyde; PST: Prescribing support team; SIMD: Scottish Index of Multiple Deprivation; SSRI: Selective serotonin re-uptake inhibitor; TCA: Tricyclic antidepressant

Acknowledgements

Special thanks to all GP practices and prescribing support teams for their support, and the Chief Scientist Office of the Scottish Government for support through the Nursing, Midwifery and Allied Health Professions Research Unit.

Funding

This project was funded by NHSGG&C and an educational bursary from NHS Scotland. This work is independent of the funders and does not necessarily represent their view.

Authors' contributions

CFJ identified the evidence gap in the literature, conceptualised the study, recruited and interviewed GPs. CFJ, BW, SAM, and MM worked jointly on data analysis. CFJ primarily wrote the manuscript with input from BW, SAM, NJD and MM. All authors read and approved the final manuscript.

Authors' information

CFJ is a senior prescribing support and antidepressant specialist pharmacist, and honorary lecturer in clinical pharmacy.
BW is professor of behavioural and health services research.
SAM is a senior lecturer in evidence synthesis specialising in the assessment of healthcare technologies for depression.
NJD is an associate professor of health statistics and mental health research.
MM is professor of health services and mental health research, and Director of the Chief Scientist Office funded Nursing, Midwifery and Allied Health Professions Research Unit.

Competing interests

The authors declare they have no competing interests.

Consent for publication

Participants gave written consent for annonymised study data to be published.

Author details

[1]Pharmacy and Prescribing Support Unit, NHS Greater Glasgow and Clyde, 2nd Floor, Main Building, West Glasgow Ambulatory Care Hospital, Dalnair Street, Yorkhill, Glasgow G3 8SJ, UK. [2]School of Health and Social Care, Edinburgh Napier University, Sighthill Court, Edinburgh EH11 4BN, UK. [3]School of Nursing and Health Sciences, University of Dundee, Airlie Place, Dundee DD1 4HN, UK. [4]Nursing Midwifery and Allied Health Professionals Research Unit, University of Stirling, Unit 13 Scion House, Stirling University Innovation Park, Stirling FK9 4NF, UK.

References

1. Parish PA. The prescribing of psychotropic drugs in general practice. J R Coll Gen Pract. 1971;21(92 Suppl 4):1–77.
2. Knapp M, McDaid D, Mossialos E, Thornicroft G. Mental health policy and practice across Europe: the future direction of mental health care. Maidenhead: McGraw-Hill, Open University Press; 2007.
3. Chen Y, Kelton CM, Jing Y, Guo JJ, Li X, Patel NC. Utilization, price, and spending trends for antidepressants in the US Medicaid program. Res Soc Adm Pharm. 2008;4(3):244–57.
4. Reid IC. Are antidepressants overprescribed? No. BMJ. 2013;346:f190.
5. Spence D. Are antidepressants overprescribed? Yes. BMJ. 2013;346:f191.
6. Pies R. Antidepressants: conundrums and compexities of efficacy studies. J Clin Psychopharmacol. 2015;36(1):1–4.
7. Pilgrim D, Bentall R. The medicalisation of misery: a critical realist analysis of the concept of depression. J Mental Health. 1999;8(3):261–74.
8. Dowrick C, Frances A. Medicalising unhappiness: new classification of depression risks more patients being put on drug treatment from which they will not benefit. BMJ. 2013;347:f7140.
9. Horwitz AV, Wakefield JC. The loss of sadness: how psychiatry transformed normal sorrow into depressive disorder. Oxford: Oxford University Press; 2007. p. 182.
10. Cosgrove L, Wheeler EE. Drug firms, the codification of diagnostic categories, and bias in clinical guidelines. J Law, Medicine & Ethics. 2013;41(3):644–53.
11. Shorter E. The 25th anniversary of the launch of Prozac gives pause for thought: where did we go wrong? Br J Psychiatry. 2014;204:331–2.
12. Turner EH, Matthews AM, Linardatos E, Tell RA, Rosenthal R. Selective publication of antidepressant trials and its influence on apparent efficacy. N Engl J Med. 2008;358(3):252–60.
13. Miller M, Swanson SA, Azrael D, Pate V, Stürmer T. Antidepressant dose, age, and the risk of deliberate self-harm. JAMA Intern Med. 2014;174(6):899–909.
14. Kirsch I, Deacon BJ, Huedo-Medina TB, Scoboria A, Moore TJ, Johnson BT. Initial severity and antidepressant benefits: a meta-analysis of data submitted to the Food and Drug Administration. PLoS Med. 2008;5(2):e45.
15. Wiles N, Thomas L, Abel A, Ridgway N, Turner N, Campbell J, et al. Cognitive behavioural therapy as an adjunct to pharmacotherapy for primary care based patients with treatment resistant depression: results of the CoBalT randomised controlled trial. Lancet. 2013;381(9864):375–84.
16. National Collaborating Centre for Mental Health. Depression. The treatment and management of depression in adults (update). Leicester: British Psychological Society and the Royal College of Psychiatrists; 2009.
17. Cleare A, Pariante CM, Young AH, Anderson IM, Christmas D, Cowen PJ, et al. Evidence-based guidelines for treating depressive disorders with antidepressants: a revision of the 2008 British Association for Psychopharmacology guidelines. J Psychopharmacol. 2015;29(5):459–525.
18. Munoz-Arroyo R, Sutton M, Morrison J. Exploring potential explanations for the increase in antidepressant prescribing in Scotland using secondary analyses of routine data. Br J Gen Pract. 2006;56(527):423–8.
19. Moore M, Yuen H, Dunn N, .Mullee MA, Maskell J, Kendrick T. Explaining the rise in antidepressant prescribing: a descriptive study using the general practice research database. BMJ 2009;339(7727):956.
20. Petty DR, House A, Knapp P, Raynor T, Zermansky A. Prevalence, duration and indications for prescribing of antidepressants in primary care. Age & Ageing. 2006;35(5):523–6.
21. Johnson CF, Macdonald HJ, Atkinson P, Buchanan AI, Downes N, Dougall N. Reviewing long-term antidepressants can reduce drug burden: a prospective observational cohort study. Br J Gen Pract. 2012;62(604):e773–9.
22. Johnson CF, Dougall NJ, Williams B, Macgillivray SA, Buchanan AI, Hassett RD. Patient factors associated with SSRI dose for depression treatment in general practice: a primary care cross sectional study. BMC Fam Pract. 2014;15:210.
23. Joint Formulary Committee. British national formulary. 67th ed. London: BMJ Group and Pharmaceutical Press; 2014.
24. Prieto-Alhambra D, Petri H, Goldenberg JSB, Khong TP, Klungel OH, Robinson NJ, et al. Excess risk of hip fractures attributable to the use of antidepressants in five European countries and the USA. Osteoporosis Int. 2014;25(3):847–55.
25. Information Services Division Scotland. Medicines used in Mental Health, Years 2004/05 - 2014/15. http://www.isdscotland.org/Health-Topics/Prescribing-and-Medicines/Publications/index.asp. Accessed 13 June 2017.
26. Middleton N, Gunnell D, Whitley E, Dorling D, Frankel S. Secular trends in antidepressant prescribing in the UK, 1975-1998. J Public Health Med. 2001;23(4):262–7.
27. Sinclair JE, Aucott LS, Lawton K, Reid IC, Cameron IC. The monitoring of long term prescriptions if antidepressants: observational study in a primary care setting. Fam Pract. 2014;31(4):419–26.
28. Lockhart P, Guthrie B. Trends in primary care antidepressant prescribing 1995–2007: a longitudinal population database analysis. Br J Gen Pract. 2011;61(590):e565–72.
29. Ministry of Health. Patterns of antidepressant drug prescribing and intentional self-harm outcomes in New Zealand: an ecological study. Wellington: Ministry of Health; 2007. p. 15.
30. Adli M, Baethge C, Heinz A, Langlitz N, Bauer M. Is dose escalation of antidepressants a rational strategy after a medium-dose treatment has failed? A systematic review. Eur Arch Psychiatry & Clin Neurosci. 2005;255(6):387–400.
31. Taylor D, Paton C, Kapur S. The Maudsley prescribing guidelines in psychiatry. 12th Edition. Chichester: Wiley Blackwell; 2015.
32. Morrison J, Anderson MJ, Sutton M, Munoz-Arroyo R, McDonald S, Maxwell M, et al. Factors influencing variation in prescribing of antidepressants by general practices in Scotland. Br J Gen Pract. 2009;59(559):e25–31.
33. Information Services Division Scotland. GP workforce and practice populations. 2014. http://www.isdscotland.org/Health-Topics/General-Practice/Publications/data-tables.asp?id=1350#1350. Accessed 13 June 2017.
34. Scottish Index of Multiple Deprivation. Background and Methodology. 2012. http://www.gov.scot/Topics/Statistics/SIMD/BackgroundMethodology. Accessed 13 June 2017.
35. Silverman D. Interpreting qualitative data: methods for analysing talk, text and interaction. London: Sage; 1993.
36. Ritchie J, Spencer L. Qualitative data analysis for applied policy research. In: Huberman AM, Miles MB, editors. The qualitative researcher's companion. London: Sage Publications; 2002. p. 305–29.

37. Medicines and Healthcare products Regulatory Agency. Citalopram and escitalopram: QT interval prolongation—new maximum daily dose restrictions (including in elderly patients), contraindications, and warnings. Drug Safety Update. 2011;5(5):A1. http://www.mhra.gov.uk/Safetyinformation/DrugSafetyUpdate/CON137769. Accessed 13 June 2017.
38. Macdonald S, Morrison J, Maxwell M, Munoz-Arroyo R, Power A, Smith M, et al. A coal face option': GPs' perspectives on the rise in antidepressant prescribing. Br J Gen Pract. 2009;59(566):e299–307.
39. Koski A, Vuori E, Ojanpera I. Newer antidepressants: evaluation of fatal toxicity index and interaction with alcohol based on Finnish postmortem data. Int J Legal Med. 2005;119(6):344–8.
40. Nutt DJ. Tolerability and safety aspects of mirtazapine. Hum Psychopharmacol. 2002;17(Suppl 1):S37–41.
41. Mendelson WB. A review of the evidence for the efficacy and safety of trazodone in insomnia. J Clin Psychiatry. 2005;66(4):469–76.
42. Bradley CP. Factors which influence the decision whether or not to prescribe: the dilemma facing general practitioners. Br J Gen Pract. 1992; 42(364):454–8.
43. Zimmerman M, Posternak M, Friedman M, Attiullah N, Baymiller S, Boland R, et al. Which factors influence psychiatrists' selection of antidepressants? Am J Psychiatry. 2004;161(7):1285–9.
44. Zwolsman S, Te Pas E, Hooft L, WieringaDe WM, Van Dijk N. Barriers to GPs' use of evidence-based medicine: a systematic review. Br J Gen Pract. 2012; 62(600):e511–21.
45. Sampson R, Barbour R, Wilson P. The relationship between GPs and hospital consultants and the implications for patient care: a qualitative study. BMC Fam Pract. 2016;17:45.
46. Guthrie B, Donnan PT, Murphy DJ, Makubate B, Dreischulte T. Bad apples or spoiled barrels? Multilevel modelling analysis of variation in high-risk prescribing in Scotland between general practitioners and between the practices they work in. BMJ Open. 2015;5:e008270.
47. Saragoussi D, Chollet J, Bineau S, Chalem Y, Milea D. Antidepressant switching patterns in the treatment of major depressive disorder: a general practice research database (GPRD) study. Int J Clin Pract. 2012;66(11):1079–87.
48. Jaffray M, Cardy AH, Reid IC, Cameron IM. Why do patients discontinue antidepressant therapy early? A qualitative study. Eur J Gen Pract. 2014;20(3):167–73.
49. Schofield P, Crosland A, Waheed W, Aseem S, Gask L, Wallace A, et al. Patients' views of antidepressants: from first experiences to becoming expert. Br J Gen Pract. 2011;61(585):142–8.
50. Hyde J, Calnan M, Prior L, Lewis G, Kessler D, Sharp D. A qualitative study exploring how GPs decide to prescribe antidepressants. Br J Gen Pract. 2005;55(519):755–62.
51. Balint M. The pyramid and the psychotherapeutic relationship. Lancet. 1961;278(7211):1051–4.
52. Macdonald S, Maxwell M, Wilson P, Smith M, Whittaker W, Sutton M, et al. A powerful intervention: general practitioners'; use of sickness certification in depression. BMC Fam Pract. 2012;13:82.
53. Malpass A, Kessler D, Sharp D, Shaw A. I didn't want her to panic': unvoiced patient agendas in primary care consultations when consulting about antidepressants. Br J Gen Pract. 2011;61(583):e63–71.
54. Laugharne J, Waterreus AJ, Castle DJ, Dragovic M. Screening for the metabolic syndrome in Australia: a national survey of psychiatrists' attitudes and reported practice in patients prescribed antipsychotic drugs. Australas Psychiatry. 2016;24(1):62–6.
55. Ashton H. Toxicity and adverse consequences of benzodiazepine use. Psychiatr Ann. 1995;25(3):158–65.
56. Kripke DF. Greater incidence of depression with hypnotic use than with placebo. BMC Psychiatry. 2007;7:42.
57. Benkert O, Muller M, Szegedi A. An overview of the clinical efficacy of mirtazapine. Hum Psychopharmacol. 2002;17(Suppl 1):S23–6.
58. Spijker J, de Graaf R, Bijl RV, Beekman AT, Ormel J, Nolen WA. Duration of major depressive episodes in the general population: results from The Netherlands mental health survey and incidence study (NEMESIS). Br J Psychiatry. 2002;181:208–13.
59. World Health Organisation. Definition and general considerations of defined daily doses. https://www.whocc.no/ddd/definition_and_general_considera/. Accessed 13 June 2017.

12

The perceived impact of family physicians on the district health system in South Africa

Klaus B. von Pressentin[1*], Robert J. Mash[1], Laurel Baldwin-Ragaven[2], Roelf Petrus Gerhardus Botha[3], Indiran Govender[4], Wilhelm Johannes Steinberg[5] and Tonya M. Esterhuizen[6]

Abstract

Background: Evidence from first world contexts support the notion that strong primary health care teams contain family physicians (FPs). African leaders are looking for evidence from their own context. The roles and scope of practice of FPs are also contextually defined. The South African family medicine discipline has agreed on six roles. These roles were incorporated into a family physician impact assessment tool, previously validated in the Western Cape Province.

Methods: A cross-sectional study design was used to assess the perceived impact of family physicians across seven South African provinces. All FPs working in the district health system (DHS) of these seven provinces were invited to participate. Sixteen respondents (including the FP) per enrolled FP were asked to complete the validated 360-degree assessment tool.

Results: A total number of 52 FPs enrolled for the survey (a response rate of 56.5%) with a total number of 542 respondents. The mean number of respondents per FP was 10.4 (SD = 3.9). The perceived impact made by FPs was high for five of the six roles. Co-workers rated their FP's impact across all six roles as higher, compared to the other doctors at the same facility. The perceived beneficial impact was experienced equally across the whole study setting, with no significant differences when comparing location (rural vs. metropolitan), facility type or training model (graduation before and ≥ 2011).

Conclusions: The findings support the need to increase the deployment of family physicians in the DHS and to increase the number being trained as per the national position paper.

Keywords: Family physicians, District health system, Perceived impact, Primary health care, Cross-sectional study

Background

Strong primary health care (PHC) systems lead to better health outcomes for the population they serve [1, 2]. The 2008 World Health Report "Primary Health Care - Now More Than Ever" defines strong PHC systems as those systems which offer first contact care that is patient-centred with an orientation to the patient's family and community context, embedded in a service that is comprehensive, integrated, continuous, and community-orientated, and in which patient-care is well co-ordinated [1]. This report warned against oversimplified approaches to PHC in developing countries, which only focus on priority diseases or rely on unsupported health workers who are poorly equipped for the complexity of PHC. The World Health Assembly supports the report's recommendation that PHC should be offered by a multidisciplinary team that includes a family physician (FP) [3–6].

The contribution of family medicine to health system improvement has been supported by empirical research evidence, policy documents and public statements from global health leaders [7–11]. The research evidence base, however, arises mainly from high income settings, in which communities and health systems are different

* Correspondence: kvonpressentin@sun.ac.za
[1]Division of Family Medicine and Primary Care, Faculty of Medicine and Health Sciences, Stellenbosch University, PO Box 241, Cape Town 8000, South Africa

from their LMIC (low and middle income country) counterparts [12].

Defining the roles of the family physician (or general practitioner) with postgraduate training has been a complex undertaking since the origins of academic family medicine in the 1960's [13–16]. The golden thread remains the commitment to the individual within the context of their family and community. The roles of the FP are based on values and principles that are shared almost universally [11, 17]. However the roles and scope of practice are also contextually defined by factors such as whether the FP is the first contact person, whether the FP also provides hospital based care and the skills-mix in the PHC team [11, 18].

In the African LMIC region, healthcare is characterised by a significant imbalance between the high burden of disease and the scarcity of healthcare workers to address this burden, especially doctors, nurses and midwives [19–21]. Family medicine only obtained recognition in the past two decades, with South Africa obtaining family medicine "specialty status" in 2007 [22]. The 2009 WONCA (World Organisation of Family Doctors) Africa regional conference reached a consensus statement on family medicine in Africa, describing the role of the FP as "a clinical leader and consultant in the primary health care team, ensuring primary, continuing, comprehensive, holistic and personalized care of high quality to individuals, families and communities." This consensus document forms the core understanding and basis for further development of family medicine in Africa [23].

In South Africa, a recent national position paper summarised the local consensus on the roles and competencies required of FPs [22]. This paper represents the viewpoint of the South African Academy of Family Physicians (SAAFP) and the College of Family Physicians of South Africa (CFPSA), and articulates the potential contribution of FPs to district health services within the national policy framework. Key elements of this policy framework include the National Development Plan, policy on Human Resources for Health and draft legislation on health system re-engineering towards establishing universal health coverage and national health insurance [24–26]. Six key roles for the FP were described (Fig. 1) [22], which link closely with regional and international trends:

- Care provider: a competent clinician, able to deal with the majority of the health problems in the community that he or she serves, within the district hospital or primary care setting, and competent in relational skills (including patient centeredness, communication skills and bio-psychosocial approach).
- Consultant: as part of a well-functioning healthcare team, he or she provides support to other practitioners (e.g. clinical nurse practitioners and medical officers) by seeing referred patients in primary care facilities or district hospitals.
- Capacity builder: as a senior clinician, he or she is responsible for the mentoring and training of less qualified clinicians within the primary health care or district hospital teams.
- Clinical trainer: he or she may need to function as the clinical supervisor in the workplace for medical students, clinical associate trainees, interns or registrars.
- Clinical governance leader: responsible for improving the quality of clinical services within the sub-district and facility where he or she is appointed.
- Champion of community-orientated primary care (COPC): supports the development of a COPC approach to the district health system, particularly the development and integration of ward-based outreach teams (a team of community health workers responsible for a geographically defined group of households).

In South Africa policymakers and managers of the health services continue to hold diverse views on the value of FPs and provinces have significant autonomy when deciding whether to employ FPs at scale [22, 27]. Although the entry of FPs into the healthcare system is relatively recent, evidence of their impact would contribute to decision making. Prior to 2007 FPs were trained in a variety of part-time programmes, whereas after 2007 FPs were trained in full-time registrar posts to a set of national learning outcomes and started entering the health system from 2011. Within the African region evidence of their impact would also be of value to countries that are contemplating the training of FPs or

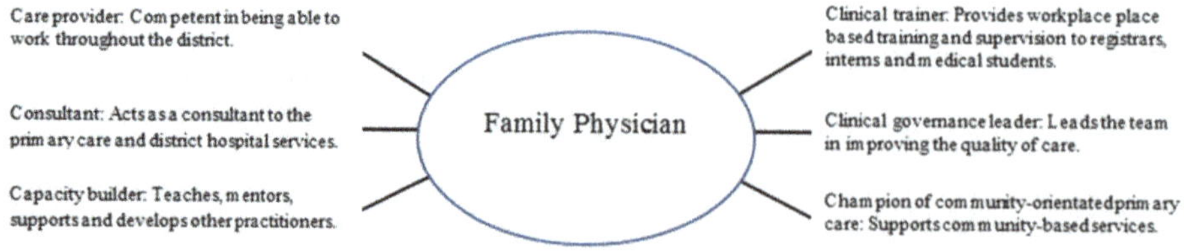

Fig. 1 The six key roles of the South African family physician [22]

deciding on whether to scale up training [28]. The African continent remains the only continent that has not widely embraced the training of FPs [12].

In order to collect evidence of the early impact of FPs in South Africa a national research project utilised four different methods – a quasi-experimental study, a survey of FPs using a validated 360-degree impact assessment tool, correlation of FP supply with routine district health indicators and interviews with district managers. This article presents the findings from the survey and the other studies will be reported elsewhere. Using a validated 360-degree impact assessment tool [29], this study aimed to evaluate the impact of FPs within the district health services of South Africa from the perspective of those working around them at district hospitals or primary care facilities. The study also intended to compare their perceived impact with that of medical officers who had not received postgraduate training. Secondary outcomes include comparing the perceived impact of FPs between rural and metropolitan (urban) contexts, by facility type (district hospitals and community health centres), and training programme model (graduation before and after 2011).

Methods

Study design

A cross-sectional survey of the perceived impact of FPs was conducted using a validated 360-degree FP impact assessment tool [29]. The STROBE (Strengthening the Reporting of Observational Studies in Epidemiology) checklist for cross-sectional studies was used to guide this report [30].

Setting

The study was conducted in public sector district health services (DHS) within seven out of the nine provinces of South Africa, as determined by the provincial footprint of the six participating universities.

FPs in the public sector are primarily employed within the DHS, and are typically based at a district hospital (DH), community health centre (CHC) or sub-district and provide support to the sub-district's PHC services. Some FPs are also based at the regional hospital (within a family medicine, emergency medicine or out-patient department) or at the level of the district, either as a district FP with a general clinical governance role or a more specific role for maternal and child health care as a member of a District Clinical Specialist Team (DCST) [22].

Characteristics and selection of participants

All FPs working in the DHS (public sector) of these seven provinces were invited to participate (via the collaborating academic family medicine departments, who consulted their departmental databases of all the DHS-employed FPs). FPs working at regional or tertiary hospitals, those working only at the district level (DCST or district office) or those working in the private sector, were excluded as their scope of practice did not encompass that of the six agreed FP roles as described in the national position paper [22].

After accepting the invitation, providing their written informed consent and receiving a briefing on the data collection procedure, each FP generated a list of 25–30 potential respondents from within their work environment (this list included the co-workers' job titles and contact information). This list of potential respondents was converted by the lead researcher into an Excel document and sorted into three categories: people who the FP reports to (e.g. managers), people who work alongside the FP (e.g. senior medical officers, pharmacists) and people who report to the FP (e.g. junior medical officers, nurses). For each participating FP, five respondents were randomly selected from each of these categories. The final list of participants contained the study codes of the FP (self-assessment) and his/her 15 selected co-workers (sixteen respondents in total).

Data collection tool

This study made use of a Family Physician Impact Assessment Tool, which was developed, validated and piloted previously in the Western Cape Province of South Africa [29]. The tool comprises of a section that provides information on use of the tool, a section that gathers information about the respondents and a section that asks about six domains representing each of the six previously described FP roles (Fig. 1).

Each domain consisted of a number of positively-phrased statements as items, with six response options in a Likert scale format: not performed by the FP (0), strongly disagree (1), disagree (2), agree (3) and strongly agree (4). Respondents could also state that they were not able to answer that question.

One additional item was added for each domain as a whole, asking the respondents to compare the impact of the FP to that of the medical officers at the same facility. This additional item had seven Likert scale options: does not perform this role (0), significantly less impact (1); less impact (2); same impact (3); more impact; (4), significantly more impact (5); and unable to answer.

Respondents were asked to complete the tool either on a hard copy (printed booklet) or online via a secure webpage (Stellenbosch University: Checkbox® survey software version 6) [31].

Data collection process

The research team included local co-ordinators from each of the academic family medicine departments and a total number of 16 fieldworkers were trained. A fieldwork protocol ensured a uniform approach to conducting the fieldwork. The fieldwork team contacted the FP and each respondent (in person, via email or phone call) and invited them to complete the paper or online version of the tool. The completed paper tools were collected in a secure box in a neutral space within the facility or collected in person by the fieldwork team. Data were collected between March 2015 and February 2016. Data collected on paper were captured with EpiData version 3.1 [32] via a double-entry method and using checks to minimize data entry errors. Answers to the individual statements were substituted for numbers according to the Likert scale. The data captured online were exported to Excel as a SPSS compatible file. The data from the two versions were combined into a single database. This database was checked for any errors and protected.

Data analysis

Data analysis was performed using IBM SPSS version 23 [33] and a data analysis protocol. Descriptive analysis was performed to describe the FPs in terms of the number of respondents, provincial distribution, location (metropolitan vs. rural), DHS facility type (district hospital vs. community health centre) and training model (qualification as FP before 2011 and ≥ 2011).

Data analysis of the perceived impact for each domain or role was conducted at the level of the FP (the unit of analysis), which required aggregating the respondent-level data into domain mean values. The data analysis protocol specified that no score per domain at individual respondent level will be calculated into the total mean score at the level of the FP, should more than 50% of the items (questions) in a domain not be answered.

A weighted mean score for each FP role was calculated based on the Likert scale from 0 to 4. The mean score was weighted according to the number of respondents per FP as the assessment would be more valid with more respondents. The weighted mean score could then be interpreted as:

- Score < 1.5: No impact in this area
- Score ≥ 1.5 but < 2.5: Little impact in this area
- Score ≥ 2.5 but < 3: Moderate impact in this area
- Score ≥ 3: High impact in this area

A comparison was made between the various roles to assess if the perceived impact of the FPs differed between the roles. A repeated measures analysis of variance (ANOVA) was used to obtain an overall p-value (Wilks' Lambda test statistic) for the differences between the six roles. Subsequently, paired samples t-test analyses were performed to compare the six individual roles against each other (15 pairs in total were compared). Using the Bonferroni correction, the level of α (critical p-value) was divided by the number of tests [34]. The new α for comparing the weighted means between the individual domains was calculated by dividing 0.05 with 15, which resulted in a new critical p-value of 0.0033 for the between-role comparisons.

The FP's perceived impact in each role was compared to the medical officers. The score for the comparative evaluation between FPs and the other medical officers (Likert scale from 0 to 5) was interpreted as follows:

- Score < 2.5: In favour of the medical officers for a particular role
- Score ≥ 2.5 but < 3.5: No perceived difference between medical officers and the FP for a particular role
- Score ≥ 3.5: In favour of the FP for a particular role

The independent samples test (t-test for equality of means) was used to assess the relationship between the mean scores for each domain and the secondary outcomes (metropolitan vs. rural, district health facility type, qualification before and after 2011).

Ethical considerations

This study was approved by the Health Research Ethics Committee, Stellenbosch University (reference S15/01/003), as well as the relevant institutions and provincial authorities in the study setting (the full list is available as an Additional file 1). All respondents gave their written informed consent and study codes were used to enter the information into the anonymised database.

Results

A total number of 52 FPs enrolled for the survey with a total number of 542 respondents. The average response rate of the eligible, invited FPs was 56.5% (see Table 1) and the mean number of respondents per FP was 10.4 (SD = 3.9; minimum 1 and maximum 18), which indicated a response rate of 63.9% (542/848) for the invited respondents.

The distribution of enrolled FPs by rural vs. metropolitan location, facility type and training programme was fairly equal (Table 2). The enrolment by province was unequally distributed. Table 3 outlines the four different groups of respondents who evaluated the enrolled FPs. Only 30 of the 52 enrolled FPs (57.7%) completed the tool as a self-assessment. An additional 14 FPs participated as respondents for other FPs, which meant that of all the respondents, 44 (8.1%) were FPs.

Table 4 presents the weighted and unweighted mean values for each domain and demonstrates a close correlation. The FP was seen to have a high impact in all six roles apart from that of capacity builder, which was rated

Table 1 Family physician and respondent enrolment per province

Province	Family physicians employed in DHS at facility level		Total number of respondents per province	
	Invited and eligible	Enrolled	Invited	Enrolled
Free State	4	3	48	48
Gauteng	28	12	192	107
KwaZulu-Natal	8	6	96	76
Mpumalanga	12	5	80	53
North West	5	5	80	71
Northern Cape	2	2	32	24
Western Cape	33	19	304	163
Total	92	52	848	542

as a moderate impact. The perceived impact for the role of capacity builder was significantly ($p < 0.001$) lower compared to the other roles. The remaining between role-comparisons were not significantly different. The mean values for each role are visually represented in the radar graph (Fig. 2). FPs were also perceived to have a greater impact than the medical officers across all six roles with a mean score above 3.5 (Table 5). No significant differences were found when comparing the weighted means according to rural vs. metropolitan location, facility type (DH vs. CHC), and the training model (Table 6).

Discussion

Summary

The impact made by family physicians in DHS facilities across seven South African provinces was perceived by co-workers as high for five of the six agreed roles: care provider, consultant, clinical trainer, leader of clinical governance and champion of community-orientated primary care. Their impact in the role of capacity builder was significantly less than the other roles although still seen as a moderate impact. Furthermore, co-workers rated their FP's impact across these six roles as higher than the other doctors at the same facility. The perceived beneficial impact was experienced equally across the whole study setting, as no significant differences were found when comparing location, facility type or training model.

Table 2 Distribution of enrolled FPs by DHS facility type, rural/metropolitan location and training programme type

Rural/Metropolitan			FP training programme		Total
			New	Previous	
Rural	Facility type	CHC	5	6	11
		DH	9	9	18
	Total		14	15	29
Metro	Facility type	CHC	3	11	14
		DH	6	3	9
	Total		9	14	23
Total	Facility type	CHC	8	17	25
		DH	15	12	27
	Total		23	29	52

CHC community health centres, *DH* district hospitals

Comparison with existing literature

Overall perceived impact for the different roles

The role of the FP in COPC was perceived to be much higher in the national study compared to the initial pilot study. This may be due to the greater involvement of family medicine departments in the implementation of COPC in provinces such as Gauteng and the limited commitment of the Western Cape, where the pilot study was conducted, to implement COPC as part of PHC re-engineering.

Conversely, the role of the FP in building the capacity of the healthcare team was rated much lower in the national study compared to the pilot study. This might be due to the emphasis on implementing clinical governance in the districts included in the pilot study [35]. In other provinces the DCSTs may have taken more of a lead in capacity building around maternal and child health [36]. FPs in the Western Cape may also have had

Table 3 Profile of respondents ($N = 542$)

Respondent Category	n (%)
Managers (including district, facility and operational managers)	111 (20.5)
Colleagues (including other family physicians, senior medical officers, allied health workers and pharmacists)	169 (31.2)
Junior colleagues (including family medicine registrars and junior doctors) and colleagues who consult the family physician (including nurses and community health workers)	164 (30.3)
Family physician self-evaluations	30 (5.5)
Undefined role (including missing data for this variable)	68 (12.5)
Total	542 (100.0)

Table 4 Mean values per domain (family physician role)

Domain	Unweighted means		Weighted means	
	N	mean (SD)	N	mean (SD)
Care provider	52	3.31 (0.36)	52	3.33 (1.26)
Consultant	52	3.23 (0.36)	52	3.24 (1.25)
Capacity builder	52	2.93 (0.36)	52	2.95 (1.16)
Clinical trainer	52	3.21 (0.37)	52	3.24 (1.30)
Clinical governance leader	51	3.13 (0.63)	51	3.11 (1.29)
Champion of community-orientated primary care	52	3.25 (0.36)	52	3.26 (1.30)

Table 5 Perceived impact in each role compared to the other doctors at the facility

Additional question for each domain	Unweighted means	Weighted means
	Mean (SD)	Mean (SD)
Care provider	3.91 (0.65)	3.87 (1.54)
Consultant	3.92 (0.63)	3.87 (1.55)
Capacity builder	3.63 (0.60)	3.61 (1.47)
Clinical trainer	3.89 (0.72)	3.86 (1.59)
Clinical governance leader	3.91 (0.87)	3.82 (1.62)
Champion of community-orientated primary care	3.99 (0.58)	3.94 (1.54)

*A mean value greater than 3.5 is in favour of the family physician making a greater impact than the other doctors at the facility for this role (Likert scale 0–5)

a greater emphasis on educational skills in their training programme [37].

A new postgraduate training programme was introduced post-2007 aimed at equipping the new graduates with the competencies needed for their six roles. This study, however, did not demonstrate a significant difference in perceived impact between FPs graduating from the old and new programmes. This may be attributed to the many years of vocational experience of FPs trained previously that ensured they developed the competencies required for their roles [22]. In addition, newly qualified FPs may require some time to grow into all six roles, especially the leadership roles, which require a degree of seniority and maturity [22].

Comparison of their impact relative to the medical officers

An ongoing concern voiced by managers in the health system revolves around the perceived benefit of employing a FP with postgraduate training vs. a MO with a lower salary package [22, 38, 39]. This study found that FP co-workers (including the facility managers who function closer to the FP's circle of control and influence) rated their perceived impact higher compared to the other doctors within the facility for all six roles.

Relationship between their impact in these roles and other indicators of health system performance and clinical processes

The study was not designed to demonstrate a causative link or correlation between the six FP roles and health outcomes. Nevertheless the six roles are incorporated by the DOH into the job description of FPs as these roles are important to strengthening the DHS and national health priorities [24, 26]. If policy makers agree on the potential value embodied by these six roles, further investment in the training and employment of FPs within the DHS should be promoted.

The link between FP supply and health system indicators has been explored and an ecological study did not show a demonstrable correlation from the macro-perspective of the district, as the FP supply was still too low [40]. A cross-sectional study, however, demonstrated

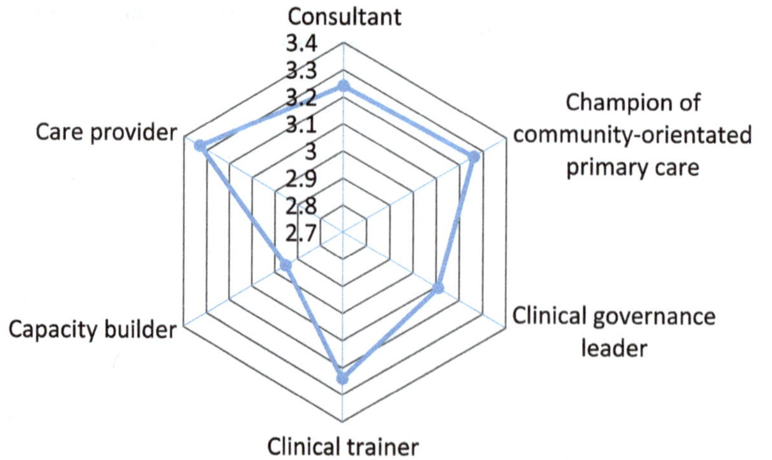

Fig. 2 The overall perceived impact of the participating family physicians across the seven provinces (weighted means)

Table 6 Comparison of weighted means for secondary outcomes

Domain		N	Mean (SD)	t	*p*-value
Rural vs. metropolitan location					
Care provider	rural	29	3.39 (1.13)	0.441	0.661
	metro	23	3.24 (1.42)		
Consultant	rural	29	3.31 (1.16)	0.468	0.642
	metro	23	3.15 (1.38)		
Capacity builder	rural	29	2.99 (1.12)	0.286	0.776
	metro	23	2.90 (1.23)		
Clinical trainer	rural	29	3.27 (1.19)	0.183	0.856
	metro	23	3.20 (1.46)		
Clinical governance leader	rural	28	3.17 (1.30)	0.365	0.717
	metro	23	3.04 (1.29)		
Champion of community-orientated primary care	rural	29	3.31 (1.18)	0.289	0.774
	metro	23	3.21 (1.45)		
DHS facility type					
Care provider	CHC	25	3.27 (1.14)	− 0.285	0.777
	DH	27	3.37 (1.38)		
Consultant	CHC	25	3.22 (1.12)	− 0.129	0.898
	DH	27	3.26 (1.38)		
Capacity builder	CHC	25	2.97 (1.04)	0.096	0.924
	DH	27	2.94 (1.28)		
Clinical trainer	CHC	25	3.26 (1.15)	0.109	0.914
	DH	27	3.22 (1.45)		
Clinical governance leader	CHC	24	3.26 (1.18)	0.776	0.441
	DH	27	2.98 (1.38)		
Champion of community-orientated primary care	CHC	25	3.27 (1.15)	0.043	0.965
	DH	27	3.26 (1.44)		
New vs. previous training model					
Care provider	new	23	3.27 (1.23)	− 0.284	0.778
	previous	29	3.37 (1.30)		
Consultant	new	23	3.11 (1.22)	− 0.650	0.519
	previous	29	3.34 (1.29)		
Capacity builder	new	23	2.74 (1.10)	−1.208	0.233
	previous	29	3.13 (1.19)		
Clinical trainer	new	23	3.07 (1.27)	− 0.842	0.404
	previous	29	3.37 (1.33)		
Clinical governance leader	new	22	2.77 (1.17)	− 1.664	0.102
	previous	29	3.37 (1.33)		
Champion of community-orientated primary care	new	23	3.08 (1.24)	− 0.914	0.365
	previous	29	3.41 (1.34)		

*significant at $p < 0.05$

how FPs add value to in-hospital clinical care (especially in terms of paediatric care) [41]. Qualitative studies have also explored this question from the perspective of the district managers and suggested that family physicians have had a positive impact on the quality of clinical processes across the quadruple burden of diseases, and some impact on health services performance (in terms of improved access to care, better coordination, and the provision of a more comprehensive and efficient service) [22, 38, 42].

Implications for research and practice

Given the alignment of these six roles with national priorities for strengthening the DHS and the perceived impact of FPs demonstrated in this study, there is a need to employ FPs at scale and to strengthen the training programmes (including number of registrar posts) as described in the national position paper [22].

The finding of a lower perceived impact in the capacity building role may require more research to understand the factors involved, such as the implementation of clinical governance in districts or training provided to registrars for this role.

The Family Physician Impact Assessment tool could be used to evaluate the perceived impact of FPs in other African or LMIC health systems, providing that the FPs are similarly positioned within the PHC teams and share the same roles. This will require adaptation and validation of the instrument for the new context, but may produce useful data for between country-comparisons.

This study should be repeated after 5-years in order to evaluate changing perceptions of the impact of FPs as more FPs are employed and the health system undergoes further transformation.

Limitations

This study was conducted congruent to the methods described in the pilot study, by conducting the analysis at the level of the FP (and not at the level of the individual respondent) [29]. The weighting of means to control for the variation in respondent numbers per FP resulted in larger standard deviations, which decreased the likelihood of finding statistically significant findings when comparing sub-groups. The weighting was applied in the direction of FPs with more respondents, as this increased the number of observations per FP which should result in a more valid 360-degree appraisal [43].

The potential bias of asking the FPs to nominate respondents was addressed in the pilot study's article [29]. The researchers implemented the pilot study's recommendation of selecting respondents randomly from the total pool of eligible people in each category [29]. Further bias may be introduced by only considering responses from FPs (and their co-workers) who chose to enrol for this study (this enrolment bias may have excluded better and/or worse performing FPs). The enrolment procedure included several strategies to help convince eligible FPs of the social and scientific value of the study, and inform them of the measures employed to ensure anonymity. Fortunately, Table 2 demonstrates the equal distribution of enrolled FPs by location, facility type and training model. As the tool included responses from the FPs themselves a sub-analysis was performed to see if excluding the self-assessments would alter the results. This sub-analysis demonstrated that the same results were obtained for the six domains as well as for the comparison of the FP's perceived impact to that of the other medical officers. The unequal distribution by province was predetermined by the differences in employment of eligible FPs [39]. The exclusion of two South African provinces (Eastern Cape and Limpopo) was predetermined by the provincial footprint of the academic family medicine departments. The number of eligible FPs in these excluded provinces was small and their omission from the survey is unlikely to have a substantial effect on the findings.

Conclusions

FPs working within the DHS have a high perceived impact in their roles as care providers, consultants, clinical trainers, leaders of clinical governance and champions of community-orientated primary care, and a moderate perceived impact as capacity builders. Their impact was perceived to be greater than the medical officers at the same facilities across all six roles. The impact was the same regardless of location, facility type or training model. The findings support the need to increase the deployment of family physicians in the DHS and to increase the number being trained as per the national position paper.

Abbreviations

ANOVA: Analysis of variance; CFP(SA): The College of Family Physicians of South Africa; CHC: Community health centre; COPC: Community-orientated primary care; DCST: District clinical specialist team; DH: District hospital; DHS: District health system; FP: Family physician; LMIC: Low and middle income country; MO: Medical officer; PHC: Primary health care; SAAFP: South African Academy of Family Physicians; SD: Standard deviation; STROBE: Strengthening the Reporting of Observational Studies in Epidemiology; WHO: World Health Organization; WONCA: World Organisation of Family Doctors

Acknowledgements

The authors wish to thank the family physicians and their co-workers for welcoming the fieldwork teams into their facilities. The authors would also like to acknowledge Dr. K Pasio for sharing his experience on using the 360-degree Family Physician Impact Assessment Tool. The authors also wish to thank the 16 members of the research teams for their help in collecting and capturing the data: Sr D Cairncross, Mr. L Chinhoyi, Mr. A Geiger, Sr J Mokaya and Mr. D September (Stellenbosch University); Mr. D Greeves and Mr. B Mashaba (Sefako Makgatho Health Sciences University); Ms. Z Gumede and Sr S Mkhize (University of KwaZulu-Natal); Sr G Mathebula and Dr. P van Niekerk (University of Pretoria); Mr. J Botes, Mr. T Mokhobo and Sr M Els (University of the Free State); and, Ms. T Rwafa and Dr. O Femi (University of the Witwatersrand). In addition, the authors would also like to thank Ms. S Munshi (University of the Witwatersrand) for her help during the initial planning phase of the study, as well as Dr. L Campbell (University of Kwa-Zulu Natal) for coordinating the data collection in the Kwa-Zulu Natal province.

Funding
This study was conducted with the financial assistance of the European Union. The contents of this document are the sole responsibility of the authors and can under no circumstances be regarded as reflecting the position of the European Union. Additional funding was received from the Discovery Foundation (South Africa) and the Faculty of Medicine and Health Sciences, Stellenbosch University, South Africa. The funders of this study had no part in the design of the study and collection, analysis and interpretation of data, nor in writing the manuscript.

Authors' contributions
KBvP and RJM conceptualised the study. LBR, RPGB, IG, WJS and TME provided critical input during the design and data collection phases of the study (such as checking the list of FPs who qualified for the study, helping to recruit suitable members to the fieldwork team, and assisting KBvP during the training of the fieldwork team and coordinating the data collection). KBvP prepared the database and conducted the data analysis with TME under the supervision of RJM. KBvP drafted the manuscript under the supervision of RJM. All authors reviewed the manuscript, gave critical input and approved the final manuscript.

Authors' information
At the time of conducting the study, KBvP and RJM were both located at the Division of Family Medicine and Primary Care, Stellenbosch University, in South Africa and co-ordinating a national project entitled "Strengthening primary health care through primary care doctors and family physicians" that was funded by the European Union. Subsequent to completing the study, KBvP started working as a family physician within the Eden district health system, Western Cape Department of Health, where he supervises postgraduate family medicine trainees. RJM is KBvP's PhD supervisor and head of the Division of Family Medicine and Primary Care, Stellenbosch University. LBR, RPGB, IG and WJS are academic family physicians based at the family medicine departments (respectively at the University of Witwatersrand, the University of Pretoria, the Sefako Makgatho Health Sciences University and the University of the Free State), which participated in the national, European Union-funded project. TME is a consultant biostatistician in the Biostatistics Unit, Faculty of Medicine and Health Sciences, Stellenbosch University.

Consent for publication
Not applicable.

Competing interests
The authors declare that they have no competing interests.

Author details
[1]Division of Family Medicine and Primary Care, Faculty of Medicine and Health Sciences, Stellenbosch University, PO Box 241, Cape Town 8000, South Africa. [2]Department of Family Medicine, School of Clinical Medicine, University of the Witwatersrand, Johannesburg, South Africa. [3]Department of Family Medicine, University of Pretoria, Pretoria, South Africa. [4]Family Medicine, Sefako Makgatho Health Sciences University, Pretoria, South Africa. [5]Family Medicine, University of the Free State, Bloemfontein, South Africa. [6]Biostatistics Unit, Centre for Evidence based Health Care, Department of Global Health, Stellenbosch University, Cape Town, South Africa.

References
1. World Health Organization. The World Health Report 2008: Primary Health Care Now More Than Ever. World Health Organization [Internet]. 2008 [cited 2017 July 15]. Available from: http://www.who.int/whr/2008/en/. Accessed 15 July 2017.
2. Shi L. The impact of primary care: a focused review. Sci. 2012;2012:1–22.
3. De Maeseneer J. Primary health care in Africa: now more than ever! Afr J Prim Health Care Fam Med. 2009;1(1):1–3.
4. Howe AC, Mash RJ, Hugo JF. Developing generalism in the south African context. S Afr Med J. 2013;103(12):899–900.
5. World Health Organization. Primary Health care, including health system strengthening. Sixty-second World Health Assembly Resolution. WHA62.12. 2009 May 22 [cited 2017 July 15]. Available from: http://www.who.int/hrh/resources/A62_12_EN.pdf. Accessed 15 July 2017.
6. Van Weel C, De Maeseneer J. Now more than ever: world health assembly revisits primary health care. Prim Health Care Res Dev. 2010;11(1):1.
7. Chan M. The rising importance of family medicine. Keynote address presented at: World Organization of Family Doctors (WONCA) 20th World Conference; June 25, 2013 [cited 2017 July 15]; Prague, Czech Republic. Available from: http://www.who.int/dg/speeches/2013/family_medicine_20130626/en/. Accessed 15 July 2017.
8. Howe A. What's special about medical generalism? The RCGP's response to the independent commission on Generalism. Br J Gen Pract. 2012;62(600):342–3.
9. Bindman AB, Grumbach K, Osmond D, Komaromy M, Vranizan K, Lurie N, Billings J, Stewart A. Preventable hospitalizations and access to health care. J Am Med Assoc. 1995;274(4):305–11.
10. Forrest CB, Starfield B. The effect of first-contact care with primary care clinicians on ambulatory health care expenditures. Fam Pract. 1996;43(1):40–9.
11. Kidd M, ed. The Contribution of Family Medicine to Improving Health Systems: A Guidebook from the World Organization of Family Doctors. 2nd ed. London: Radcliffe Publishing Ltd; 2013.
12. Mash R. The contribution of family medicine to African health systems. Afr J Prim Health Care Fam Med. 2016;8(1):1–2.
13. Stange KC, Miller WL, McWhinney I. Developing the knowledge base of family practice. Fam Med. 2001;33(4):286–97.
14. Future of Family Medicine Project Leadership Committee. The future of family medicine: a collaborative project of the family medicine community. Ann Fam Med. 2004;2(suppl 1):S3–2.
15. McWhinney IR. William pickles lecture 1996. The importance of being different. Br J Gen Pract. 1996;46(408):433–6.
16. Stephens GG. The intellectual basis of family practice. Fam Pract. 1975;2(6):423–8.
17. Bentzen BG, Bridges-Webb C, Carmichael L, Ceitlin J, Feinbloom R, Metcalf D, McWhinney I, Rajakumar MK. The role of the general practitioner/family physician in health care systems: a statement from WONCA. Bangkok: WONCA; 1991 [cited 2017 July 15]. Available from: https://medfamcom.files.wordpress.com/2009/10/wonca-statement-1991.pdf. Accessed 15 July 2017.
18. Gibson C, Arya N, Ponka D, Rouleau K, Woollard R. Approaching a global definition of family medicine the Besrour papers: a series on the state of family medicine in the world. Can Fam Physician. 2016;62(11):891–6.
19. Fulton BD, Scheffler RM, Sparkes SP, Auh EY, Vujicic M, Soucat A. Health workforce skill mix and task shifting in low income countries: a review of recent evidence. Hum Resour Health. 2011;9(1):1.
20. Mayosi BM, Lawn JE, Van Niekerk A, Bradshaw D, Karim SS, Coovadia HM. Lancet South Africa team. Health in South Africa: changes and challenges since 2009. Lancet. 2012;380(9858):2029–43.
21. Kinfu Y, Dal Poz MR, Mercer H, Evans DB. The health worker shortage in Africa: are enough physicians and nurses being trained? Bull World Health Organ. 2009;87(3):225–30.
22. Mash R, Ogunbanjo G, Naidoo SS, Hellenberg D. The contribution of family physicians to district health services: a national position paper for South Africa. S Afr Fam Pract. 2015;57(3):54–61.
23. Mash R, Reid S. Statement of consensus on family medicine in Africa: conference report. Afr J Prim Health Care Fam Med. 2010;2(1):1–4.
24. National Planning Commission. National Development Plan 2030: our future – make it work. Pretoria: Presidency of South Africa; 2012.
25. National Department of Health. Human resources for health for South Africa: strategy for the health sector 2012/13–2016/17. Pretoria: National Department of Health; 2011.
26. National Health Insurance in South Africa. Policy (white) paper. Government notice no. 1230, government gazette no. 39506. Pretoria: National Department of Health; 2015.
27. Moosa S, Mash B, Derese A, Peersman W. The views of key leaders in South Africa on implementation of family medicine: critical role in the district health system. BMC Fam Pract. 2014;15(1):125.
28. De Maeseneer J. Scaling up family medicine and primary health care in Africa: statement of the Primafamed network, Victoria Falls, Zimbabwe. Afr J Prim Health Care Fam Med. 2013;5(1):61–3.

29. Pasio KS, Mash R, Naledi T. Development of a family physician impact assessment tool in the district health system of the western Cape Province, South Africa. BMC Fam Pract. 2014;15(1):204.
30. Kelley K, Clark B, Brown V, Sitzia J. Good practice in the conduct and reporting of survey research. Int J Qual Health Care. 2003;15(3):261–6.
31. Checkbox Survey Solutions. Checkbox Survey, Inc. 2017 [cited 2017 July 15]. Available from: https://www.checkbox.com/. Accessed 15 July 2017.
32. Christiansen TB and Lauritsen JM. (Ed.) EpiData - Comprehensive Data Management and Basic Statistical Analysis System. Odense Denmark, EpiData Association, 2010 [cited 2017 July 15]. Available from: http://www.epidata.dk. Accessed 15 July 2017.
33. IBM Corp. Released 2015. IBM SPSS Statistics for Windows, Version 23.0. Armonk: IBM Corp; 2015.
34. Armstrong RA. When to use the Bonferroni correction. Ophthalmic Physiol Opt. 2014;34(5):502–8.
35. Gunst C, Mash RJ, Phillips LC. A reflection on the practical implementation of the clinical governance framework in the Cape Winelands District of the western cape. S Afr Fam Pract. 2016;58(6):236–41.
36. National Department of Health. Handbook for district clinical specialist teams. Pretoria: National Department of Health; 2014.
37. De Villiers MR, Cilliers FJ, Coetzee F, Herman N, Van Heusden M, Von Pressentin KB. Equipping family physician trainees as teachers: a qualitative evaluation of a twelve-week module on teaching and learning. BMC Med Educ. 2014;14(1):228.
38. Swanepoel M, Mash B, Naledi T. Assessment of the impact of family physicians in the district health system of the western cape, South Africa. Afr J Prim Health Care Fam Med. 2014;6(1):1–8.
39. Mash R, Von Pressentin K. Family medicine in South Africa: exploring future scenarios. South African Family Practice [Internet]. 2017[cited 2017 July 15]: 1–4. Available from: http://www.tandfonline.com/doi/full/10.1080/20786190.2016.1272231. Accessed 15 July 2017.
40. Von Pressentin KB, Mash RJ, Esterhuizen TM. Examining the influence of family physician supply on district health system performance in South Africa: an ecological analysis of key health indicators. Afr J Prim Health Care Fam Med. 2017;9(1):1–10.
41. Von Pressentin KB, Mash RJ, Baldwin-Ragaven L, Botha RPG, Govender I, Steinberg WJ, Esterhuizen TM. Measuring the influence of family physicians within the South African district health system: a cross-sectional observational study. The Annals of Family Medicine. Forthcoming 2018; 16(1):28–36.
42. Von Pressentin KB, Mash RJ, Baldwin-Ragaven L, Botha RP, Govender I, Steinberg WJ. The bird's-eye perspective: how do district health managers experience the impact of family physicians within the South African district health system? A qualitative study. South African Family Practice. 2018;60(1):13–20.
43. Donnon T, Al Ansari A, Al Alawi S, Violato C. The reliability, validity, and feasibility of multisource feedback physician assessment: a systematic review. Acad Med. 2014;89(3):511–6.

13

Irish general practitioners' view of perinatal mental health in general practice

Maria Noonan[1*], Owen Doody[2], Andrew O'Regan[3], Julie Jomeen[4] and Rose Galvin[5]

Abstract

Background: Identification of perinatal mental health problems and effective care for women who experience them are important considering the potentially serious impact that they may have on the wellbeing of the woman, her baby, family and wider society. General practitioners (GPs) play a central role in identifying and supporting women and this study aimed to explore GPs' experiences of caring for women with perinatal mental health problems in primary care. The results of this study may provide guidance to inform policy, practice, research and development of curriculum and continuous professional development resources.

Method: In-depth semi-structured interviews were undertaken between March and June 2017 with GPs ($n = 10$) affiliated with a University training programme for general practice in Ireland. Thematic data analysis was guided by Braun and Clarkes (2013) framework.

Results: Data were categorised into three themes with related subthemes: identification of perinatal mental health problems, decision making around perinatal mental health and preparation for a role in perinatal mental health. GPs described the multifaceted nature of their role in supporting women experiencing perinatal mental health issues and responding to complex psychological needs. Inbuilt tools on existing software programmes prompted GPs to ask questions relating to perinatal mental health. Limited access to referral options impacts on assessment and care of women. GPs desire further continuous professional development opportunities delivered in an online format and through monthly meetings and conference sessions.

Conclusions: GPs require access to culturally sensitive; community based perinatal mental health services, translation services and evidence based perinatal psychological interventions. A standardised curriculum on perinatal mental health for trainee GPs needs to be established to ensure consistency across primary care and GP education should incorporate rotations in community and psychiatry placements.

Keywords: General practice, General practitioners, Qualitative research, Primary healthcare, Training, Perinatal mental health

Background

The perinatal phase, encompassing pregnancy through to the first year after birth, is recognised as a risk period for the development, relapse or recurrence of mental health problems [1, 2]. Women can experience an array of mental health difficulties in this period ranging from depression and anxiety to more serious disorders such as severe depression and psychosis, which are encompassed under the term perinatal mental health problems (PMHPs) [2]. In the UK, population prevalence rates of mental health disorders in early pregnancy has been reported as 27% (95% CI 22–32%), equating to one in four women [3]. Depression and anxiety are the two most common PMHPs that women will experience with prevalence rates in Ireland for antenatal depression at 15.8% [4] and rates for postnatal depression (PND) are reported as 13.2% at six weeks and 9.8% at twelve weeks [5]. Furthermore, perinatal depression and anxiety are

* Correspondence: Maria.noonan@ul.ie
[1]Department of Nursing and Midwifery, Faculty of Education & Health Sciences, Health Sciences Building, University of Limerick, Limerick, Ireland

frequent co-morbidities [6]. Identification of PMHPs and effective care for women who experience them is important considering the potentially serious impact that they may have on the wellbeing of the woman, her family and wider society [7, 8].

For the majority of women in Ireland, GPs are the first point of contact in the perinatal period and women attend their GP for an initial examination before 12 weeks and thereafter for a set number of antenatal visits [9]. Women will be in contact with a midwife for the booking visit where midwives enquire about emotional issues [9] however, screening for current symptoms of PMHPs using assessment tools is not routinely completed [10]. Postnatal care is primarily provided by Public Health Nurses who screen for PND and anxiety using the Whooley questions and Edinburgh Postnatal Depression Scale and refer to the GP for diagnosis and treatment interventions [9]. Women are entitled to attend their GP for a two week and six-week postnatal check [9] which may be the last routine appointment opportunity for GPs to focus on the mothers' perinatal wellbeing [11] and offers a safety net to identify poor PMH [12]. Once a PMHP is identified, GPs are usually the first point of contact for women and healthcare professionals (HCPs) and can play a central role in the woman's recovery through referral to other specialist services, management by monitoring of the woman's condition or prescribing medication [11].

Current policy and guidance largely overlook the role of GPs in PMH [13]. Few researchers have explored GPs' views and experiences of recognising and differentiating PMHPs and treatment and caring strategies offered by GPs to women [1, 13] with studies generally employing quantitative methods [1]. Furthermore, calls have been made for further research to explore the management of anxiety disorders and to gain an understanding of barriers to disclosure and recognition of PMHPs in practice [1, 14]. Therefore, this study sets out to explore GPs' experiences of caring for women with PMHPs and their views on how best to prepare future GPs for a role in the provision of effective PMH care. To our knowledge, this is the first study to explore GPs role in PMH in the Irish context and is timely in light of the current review of Ireland's National Mental Health Policy 'A Vision for Change' and the publication of 'Specialist Perinatal Mental Health Services, Model of Care for Ireland' [15, 16]. The findings of this study may provide guidance to commissioners of PMH services on the support needs of GPs providing care to women who experience PMHPs and their families. The findings also serve to guide development of education and training resources for GPs. The reporting of this study was informed by COREQ criteria [17].

Methods

An exploratory qualitative design, was employed as its emphasis on context, meaning and experience was considered appropriate to answer the research questions [18, 19]: What are GPs' views, experiences, educational and training needs in supporting women with PMHPs. The University of Limericks, research ethics committee approved the study. All GP tutors affiliated with the Graduate Entry Medical School of that university were contacted by email, provided with information about the study and invited to participate ($N = 72$). Tutors facilitate an early patient contact programme for students and their practices are broadly representative of the national sample of GP tutors. The inclusion criteria were that participants must be registered with the Medical Council of Ireland and have a caseload that includes pregnant and postnatal women.

GPs were purposefully sampled and fifteen GPs responded to the invitation to participate. Recruitment and data collection were undertaken from March 2017 to June 2017 and ceased after ten interviews were conducted as no new information was emerging and data saturation was reached. Within the sample variants were sought relating to GP experience, gender, urban/rural setting, single/group practice and cultural diversity care provision. Characteristics of GPs interviewed ($n = 10$) are provided in Table 1.

Interviews were conducted using a pilot tested interview schedule which consisted of open-ended questions derived from the literature [1, 13, 14] and through discussion among the research team which included a practising GP (Table 2). GPs were asked to recall their experiences of providing care to women with PMHPs to ensure that data was representative of their practice. Interviews took place in the university ($n = 3$), GP practice ($n = 3$) and by phone ($n = 4$) and at a time convenient to the GP. Before interviews commenced participants had an opportunity to ask questions about the study and reflect on participation prior to giving written (face-to-face) or verbal (phone) consent. All interviews were audio recorded with consent, lasted 30–70 mins and were conducted by MN who was unknown to the participants. In addition, after each interview the researcher recorded field notes, reflected on data collection, summarised findings identified emerging codes as data collection and analysis proceeded simultaneously.

Interviews were transcribed verbatim, anonymised and verified for accuracy by reading transcriptions and

Table 1 Participant demographic details

Years of experience	Practice Type	Gender
< 5 years ($n = 1$)	Urban ($n = 7$)	Female ($n = 5$)
5–10 years ($n = 5$)	Rural ($n = 3$)	Male ($n = 5$)
> 25 years ($n = 4$)		

Table 2 Interview schedule

1. Tell me about your experience of caring for women who experience PMHPs[a] in primary care?
2. What facilitates you to identify women who may be experiencing psychological distress?
3. What facilitates you to care for women who experience PMHPs[a]?
4. What referral options are available to you in your practice?
5. Based on your experiences how best can a training programme prepare future GPs[b] for their role in PMH[c]?

[a] *PMHPs* perinatal mental health problems, [b] *GP* general practitioner, [c] *PMH* perinatal mental health

listening to recordings concurrently. Braun and Clarkes [19] framework guided thematic data analysis. Codes and themes were discussed, refined and agreed by authors who met regularly to discuss and compare summaries and where interpretation differed, they returned to original transcripts for clarification to reach a consensus about the meaning. Disconfirming evidence was sought and presented in the final analysis. Processes for ensuring data trustworthiness met criteria outlined by COREQ [17]. Methodological rigour was ensured by involvement of three researchers in coding and confirmation of themes, methodological coherence and sampling sufficiency. Furthermore, reflective sessions amongst the research team were undertaken at all stages of the process.

Results

The data were categorised into three main themes: Identification of PMHPs, decision making around PMH and preparation for a role in PMH (Table 3).

Theme 1: Identification of PMHPs

Within the interviews, there was a clear focus on GPs role and support for women experiencing PMHPs. GPs recalled encounters with women who experience PMHPs, identified factors they considered preconditions for disclosure and described their approaches to screening and assessment.

Table 3 Overview of themes and subthemes

Identification of PMHPs[a]	• Encountering emotional complexity in general practice • Preconditions for disclosure • Approaches to screening and assessment
Decision making around PMH[b]	• Contrasting referral options • It's out of my comfort zone
Preparation for a role in PMH[b]	• Luck of the draw GP[c] training • Continuous professional development opportunities

[a] *PMHPs* perinatal mental health problems, [b]*PMH* Perinatal Mental Health, [c] *GP* general practitioner;

Encountering emotional complexity in general practice

PMH was identified as a core component of antenatal and postnatal care offered by GPs who primarily encountered perinatal depression and anxiety in general practice. PND was conceptualised as different to depression that occurs outside of the perinatal period.

> *'In a way it has to be looked at separately, women are more vulnerable, they respond differently to medication, things can fluctuate more rapidly, pregnancy itself can bring on a crisis, the delivery itself can bring on a crisis so there are a number of stages and a number of flash point's' (P6).*

Risk factors were construed by GPs as adverse or vulnerability factors that put women at increased risk of PMHPs. A psychosocial aetiology appeared to be the dominant framework held by GPs when conceptualising anxiety.

> *'Pressure in society, a lot of women are working full time they might have a few kids at home, they have big mortgages, their husband is working a lot of the time and lot of it is maybe triggered by exhaustion or they are just juggling a lot' (P4).*

Some participants perceived that postnatal anxiety presentation for some women was associated with higher child consultations.

> *'I feel it's all about a lot of anxiety but it's packaged up as the child's problem and it's hard to disentangle that' (P2).*

GPs spoke about the difficulties of separating depression and anxiety and the interlink between them.

> *'Two sides of the one kind so when I talk of PND some of that would be more anxiety weighted than depressive symptoms'* (P1).

Severe PMHPs were considered by participants to be rare in general practice and when encountered, the consultation and circumstances left a long- lasting impression with participants *'She will stick in my head forever' (P6).* Participants had limited encounters with women who were suicidal antenatally and when they did were struck by the fact that pregnancy would not have affected her decision.

> *'The fact that she was pregnant didn't seem to be anything of a deterrent in relation to possibly killing herself which is surprising, I think it was because she was as depressed as she was the world was a bad*

place and bringing a baby into a bad place was no achievement' (P9).

However, they reported encounters with women postnatally with suicidal ideation.

'Certainly, they would be a lot of fleeting suicidal thoughts and even a bit of suicidal ideation but I don't think I have had anyone that had a formal plan' (P9).

GPs were conscious of a family approach to care and considered that opportunities for engaging men in conversations about their PMH were desired but limited as men rarely accompanied their partners on GP visits. Personal experiences through family, friends and self, increased GP awareness of PMHPs.

'It's more with time and personal experience of friends and self and what pregnancy means and what having children means I guess that you become more aware of it' (P2).

Preconditions for disclosure

Participants identified a number of preconditions that supported disclosure of psychological distress such as women's openness in relation to PMH issues and suggested that some women were reluctant to disclose their psychological distress particularly women from different ethnic and cultural backgrounds.

'There are certain expectations of them within their ethnic group not to have a psychological issue' (P7).

Participants felt that a lack of insight and persistence of stigma were key influencing factors on a woman's reluctance to disclose her feelings and what was important was being approachable:

'It's a place where they can discuss these things and without necessarily being labelled or admitted or put on medication' (P1).

Participants identified the importance of making time to listen to the woman however, participants also acknowledged that this is dependent on a number of factors:

'The art of practice is having that gap or space or vacuum in the consultation where you leave silence ... and if you are in listening mode...however it depends on how you say it...it depends on the day, depends on how you are feeling yourself, depends on how the practice is going' (P5).

Time was referred to by all participants as a barrier to engaging in effective PMH conversations.

'There is so much emotion around pregnancy and just having time to explore it can be difficult. Hugely time consuming and you can't really afford as a working-class GP' (P5).

GPs were conscious that responding to women experiencing psychological distress may result in longer consultations and this may impact on the time available for other patients presenting with various complexities waiting to see their GP. However, participants also acknowledged that they would make this time for the woman if required.

Building a personal connection was seen as an essential step in developing mutual trust and facilitating women to open up about their psychological distress as was having a good relationship and rapport with the woman. Participants reported that at times there can be a hesitancy to engage in PMH conversations.

'Can I be honest with you sometimes I wonder if you really want to open this can of worms and it's so much easier just to jolly along and check the BP, check the urine, check this and that and have them out the door and see the next patient' (P5).

'There are sometimes and I wouldn't lie that I would be absolutely hoping that the answer was going to be no problem' (P7).

These feelings for hoping the answer would be 'no' were driven by past experiences of dealing with mental health problems, lack of time, resources and referral options to support women.

Approaches to screening and assessment

A variety of approaches to assessment and screening for PMH issues were described by participants. Some participants would ask about the woman's PMH if they felt it might be an issue.

'If it's obvious or if there is a history you would, if it's volunteered you would and I will be perfectly honest now would you routinely ask about it, theoretically yes in practice maybe, maybe not' (P5).

Participants acknowledged that psychological distress in the antenatal period is poorly recognised:

'Antenatal care is very protocol driven therefore...it is very easy to ignore the psychological aspect' (P5).

In contrast, participants asked women about their PMH routinely as part of the two and six-week postnatal checks:

'We would be quite good in fact in asking and it's probably because of that little reminder on the screen' (P4).

However, GPs also acknowledged that the baby can become the focus of the postnatal visits.

'I would be guilty of focusing a lot on the child, that's the big excitement in the room' (P2).

Within the assessment process participants primarily referred to:

'A broad set of questions, you are not just looking at the person but you are looking at the complexities around their family, their environment, and their supports' (P4).

Participants referred to *'picking up on non-verbal cues'* (P6) and factors they considered to prompt them to engage and assess more:

'Your antenna would be raised by people coming clean with you that there is something going on...a history... the usual kind of joy isn't there, they're, quiet' (P5).

Participants also recalled encounters where women concealed their psychological distress.

'Anytime I met her she was pleasant and cheerful as she always was but obviously she could put it on for five or 10 minutes' (P9).

GPs described difficulties trying to understand the experience of psychological distress from the perspective of women from ethnic and culturally diverse backgrounds and expressed concerns that they may not be identifying those women's needs.

'Very long consultations and just trying to understand where they are coming from culturally can be difficult' (P1).

This left participant's questioning whether they were seeing the true extent of PMHPs:

'Are we *only seeing them when it reached boiling point because we [GPs] couldn't get on top of the problem before that' (P6).*

In addition, participants identified personal traits or characteristics such as perfectionism as aspects that create greater concern for the woman. Participants referred to using their clinical judgement to identify women experiencing psychological distress and suicide assessment involved a combination of clinical judgement, specific questions and assessment protocols. Within the assessment process participants were guided by information from a variety of sources particularly partners: *'It was he who actually told the story' (P9).* However, participants also commented that partners may interfere with the woman being able to discuss openly her mental health issues.

'I think they were actually stifled in being able to speak and talk and get it out because their partner was always sitting beside her' (P6).

Participants acknowledged that they did not formally screen for PMHPs and when screening tools were used it was primarily to confirm a diagnosis, differentiate between anxiety and depression, the co-existence of both and to aid referral decisions. Participants were aware of barriers to assessing PMH such as time, language barriers, fear of *'making the patient or yourself feel uncomfortable' (P3)* which led participants to wonder how often they missed psychological distress in general practice.

Theme 2: Decision making around PMH

This theme encompassed the contrasting referral options available to participants which affected assessment, treatment and referral decisions and GPs comfort with pharmacological decisions.

Contrasting referral options

Participants described making treatment decisions based on the individual needs of the woman and recommended lifestyle, social and self-management strategies for some women experiencing psychological distress and offered follow up appointments where appropriate. Participants spoke about the complexity of negotiating referrals and while counselling was identified as the main treatment option available to GPs in primary care, public generic counselling services have long waiting times and were considered difficult to access for both the woman and GP:

'We have to send the form; the patient has to ring to say did you get the form and I am now confirming that I am going to go and then they get an appointment, for someone who is very distressed and you are asking them to jump through hoops' (P9).

Thereby participants' considered counselling as 'hit and miss' and recommended private counselling to women who had financial capacity to access this option.

Three participants identified Cognitive Behavioural Therapy (CBT) as a treatment option however, mother infant mental health interventions and access to psychologists were not available to the majority of participants.

'CBT is often indicated as first line treatment but really it's not an option for a lot of women. They don't have the means to access it, they don't have the motivation to access online CBT so it really rules it out as an option' (P3).

Participants reported variable access to the multi-disciplinary team including psychiatrists, psychologists and occupational therapists. When participants had access to specialist PMH teams they felt this supported them in their treatment and referral decisions and to provide effective PMH care:

"We are lucky to have a good support' (P4).

The majority of participants relied on the community mental health services however, they did not see such services as the best option for women:

'Someone with PMH issues really does not belong in the general psychiatric outpatient clinic.' (P9).

A disjoint existed between services where women with severe PMHPs had received care in maternity services and then discharged to community mental health services where all contact with the maternity services ceased.

'There should have been a link across the divide...it's kind of now you're in the hospital, now you're out of hospital, now look after yourself and get back to where you were, it wasn't as cold as that and it wasn't intended like that, it's just the way it happened' (P9).

Participants identified supports required to enable them to undertake effective decision making in PMH including having access to referral and advise from specialist PMH teams with hospitalisation in a mother and baby unit reserved for severe cases with easy access to interpreter services, free accessible psychological services and preferably *'not a drug driven pathway' (P5).*

It's out of my comfort zone

Participants identified the antenatal period as a particular time when guidance from the psychiatrist was required particularly when considering pharmacological interventions:

'Dealing with psychotropic medications and pregnancy is out of my comfort zone' (P10).

One of the main concerns in relation to antenatal pharmacology was teratogenesis and women's reluctance to take medications. Medication was reserved for women who were not responding to psychological therapies:

'If they are not coming through with time as they might want to and sometimes doing all the right things and still there is this dead feeling' (P8).

Treatment for women experiencing anxiety focused on providing reassurance, acknowledging the woman's feelings and in some cases included pharmacological interventions. Participants were explicitly committed to working consensually with women and identified the importance of including women in treatment decisions:

'Any decision that would be made around medicine, any kind of management would be made in conjunction with the patient' (P10).

Other factors that impacted on participants decision to prescribe medications included their own personal preferences, lack of referral options and women's reluctance to take medication particularly when breastfeeding. Participants also described the challenges associated with the decision not to prescribe pharmacological interventions:

'A challenge sometimes in consultations of any kind where you are not prescribing and you are trying to explain that you are still giving them a good service' (P1).

Theme 3: Preparation for a role in PMH

This theme comprised aspects relating to the luck of the draw within participants GP training and their engagement in continuous professional development (CPD) opportunities.

Luck of the draw GP training

Participants recalled limited information related to PMH as the focus of their specialist training was on obstetric and medical topics and in terms of practical experience:

'It can be luck of the draw what you do get exposed to' (P1).

As a result of limited training on PMH in GP training schemes participants were unprepared for their role:

'It's not something I came into medicine having a formula to talk about.'(P2).

Across interviews participants identified components of what they perceived would be effective training:

'Beyond just ticking boxes and try and provide holistic care for women which would include psychological assessment' (P5).

Participants also identified the need to prepare trainee GPs for their role in responding to women and their families experiencing psychological distress across cultures in the community setting. Based on their experiences, participants felt that an obstetrics, gynaecology and psychiatric rotation should be compulsory for all trainee GPs which includes a community mental health placement. In addition to support practice and training, participants highlighted that if PMH guidelines were to be developed then it would be *best to distil them into one or two pages (P5)* with *take home messages that are easily remembered (P2)* because appointments are short and GPs need timely access to information. Strategies for facilitating PMH education included input from service users and specialist PMH psychiatrists in GP training programmes.

Continuous professional development opportunities

Participants acknowledged that the difficulty for GPs is that they offer a generalist service making it difficult for them to have expertise in all areas including PMH:

'You are kind of jack-of-all-trades, you are master of none' (P5).

Participants reported having limited access to CPD opportunities specific to PMH with pharmacology being identified as a particular *'education niche' (P10)* other suggestions for CPD opportunities included PMH across cultures and paternal PMH. In addition to CPD related to PMH participants also noted a need for further educational opportunities for trainee GPs on looking after their own mental wellbeing:

'Those of us in the medical or allied professions can find it harder to admit that we are vulnerable at times' (P8).

Participants suggested that CPD could be delivered in the format of an e-learning module on PMH and sessions on PMH at monthly meetings and in the annual GP conference.

Discussion

Summary

GPs described the multifaceted nature of their role in supporting women with PMHPs and responding to complex psychological needs. However, meeting the needs of women was challenged at a personal and service level where women are conscious of the social context and expectation placed on them as mothers, while services and referral options available to GPs were limited, under resourced, fragmented and uncoordinated.

Strengths and limitations

This study used robust and transparent methods to conduct and report the study findings. Participants were from a range of urban and rural population practices, with experience ranging from four to thirty years leading to a varied sample of GPs. An in-depth description of methods, settings and results facilitates judgement of transferability. However, findings should be interpreted in the context of study limitations where the sample was affiliated to one country and participants were from a highly selective group of GPs who might be expected to have a better than average knowledge, especially as they agreed to take part in the study.

Comparison with existing literature

Participants primarily encountered depression and anxiety in practice, which consistent with previous work, were conceptualised in psychosocial rather than biomedical terms [13]. Participants' perceived that women with anxiety had higher presentations for child concerns and found it difficult to address this when consultations were infant related. This issue is acknowledged in the literature where women with postpartum anxiety were noted to have greater healthcare usage [20] and further research is required to explore the feasibility and process of enquiring about a woman's PMH at routine and opportunistic child consultations to improve outcomes for women [20].

GPs identified stigma as a barrier to help seeking which is consistent with the literature where women remain silent rather than confront the potential stigma of admitting psychological distress [21]. The taboo around mental health affects HCPs and women alike and may lead to a reluctance in discussing PMH [22]. Button et al. [21] calls for research to identify methods of assessment that elicit women's confidence in disclosing their feelings combined with increasing HCPs ability to detect psychological distress even when women are avoiding disclosure. Of note in this study was that the integration of PMH questions within GP computer databases reminded participants to enquire about the woman's mental health and this may be a strategy for implementing routine PMH assessment.

GPs identified cultural and linguistic barriers in their interpersonal encounters with women seeking PMH support. Women from ethnic minority groups may be less likely to consult GPs with PMH concerns and may be particularly disadvantaged in their access to appropriate PMH services because of lack of understanding of the woman's cultural differences and nuances around PMH [23, 24]. Therefore, in order to improve PMH outcomes for women from ethnic and culturally diverse backgrounds, GPs require access to; translation, interpreting and advocacy services, culturally specific validated assessment tools and education implemented within a system of culturally sensitive and PMH specific referral and support mechanisms [23, 24].

National and international guidance suggests that women with severe PMHPs need to be cared for by services with specialised knowledge and skills [16, 25] and participants in this study reported varied access to specialist and community PMH services. The analysis found that where GPs had limited access to care pathways and referral options including specialist PMH services that this impacted on assessment and treatment decisions. Access to specialist community PMH services has been identified as a key issue for GPs [13]. However, such services are often reserved for women with severe and complex PMH presentations while women with common PMHPs are primarily treated in primary care [26]. Furthermore, women known to services or those with a severe condition are more likely to receive appropriate treatment in comparison to women presenting for the first time with mild to moderate PMHPs [27].

Currently women who seek treatment for PMHPs have limited choice of care pathways and GPs have limited access to proven psychological therapies such as CBT [1, 25] with counselling identified as the main psychological therapy. This is similar to the international context where GPs consider PMHPs in the context of women's lives and are frustrated at the lack of psychological therapies [1, 13]. Furthermore, GPs described long waiting times for counselling services and this creates a socio-economic divide where women with resources are referred for private counselling whereas those less off have to wait for generic services with long waiting lists. Delays in accessing psychological therapies has been identified as a barrier to help seeking and support [21] and can exacerbate the woman's psychological distress and direct the GP to pharmacological treatment.

The findings of this study suggest that generally, GPs used pharmacology in the minority of cases and reported a preference for psychological therapies which is in keeping with women's preferences [21]. However, participants acknowledged that pharmacological interventions were the most appropriate strategy for some women which is congruent with the view that GPs should be more proactive about initiating treatment during the vulnerable perinatal period where severe PMHPs may impact on the child's emotional and behavioural development [13]. GPs were cognisant of the importance of actively involving women in decisions concerning medication and this acts to enhance the GP service user relationship [28].

Currently no national PMH guidance is available in Ireland and guidelines can offer a resource to enhance GPs' competence and support a consistent approach to education and PMH care provision including pharmacological interventions [29]. Furthermore, implementation of guidelines in practice can prevent against unconscious biases in consultations where GPs selectively collect and interpret evidence from their interactions with women which may lead to an incorrect diagnosis [13]. Guidance may be particularly important for GPs commencing their career in primary care who may lack the breadth of experience to provide effective PMH care [22].

Consistent with the literature, GPs felt that a greater emphasis on PMH in GP training programmes is required [12] and recommended that it would be compulsory for trainee GPs to undertake a psychiatric rotation. Research has found that GPs who had undertaken a psychiatric rotation were significantly more likely to report a higher confidence in their ability to recognise and manage psychiatric presentations in primary care (4.04 vs. 3.70, $F = 1.515$, $t = 2.794$, $p < 0.01$) [30]. Furthermore, extending rotation options to alternative community based mental health settings has been recommended [31].

Insights gained through education is identified as a key intervention to avoid distorted decision-making processes [13]. Furthermore, PMH training programmes promote consistency in the implementation of evidence-based practices which may result in greater equity in access to PMH services for women and their families [9, 32]. In line with international recommendations education should incorporate resilience training for GPs [31] with further research required to identify strategies to support the mental wellbeing of GPs [33].

Participants suggested that PMH CPD opportunities could be facilitated through e-learning modalities which can be easily completed in the context of current workloads. However, others have argued for CPD to be provided by local PMH specialist teams which would encourage dialogue across professions and shared decision-making [16]. A variety of PMH education strategies have been found to enhance HCPs confidence, knowledge, and practice regardless of education modality [29].

Implications for research and/or practice

To provide effective PMH care, GPs require timely access to national integrated guidance, culturally sensitive, community based PMH services, translation services, evidence- based perinatal specific psychological interventions and PMH support groups. The integration of validated PMH screening questions to detect a variety of moods within GPs computer data bases may facilitate PMH conversations and assessment. In addition, the coverage of PMH training in a curriculum for trainee GPs needs to be established to ensure consistency across primary care and incorporate rotations in community and psychiatry placements. Research using validated outcome assessment measures is required to examine the effects of such training on GPs practice.

Conclusion

GPs have an important role to play in supporting women with PMHPs however, they require further support to provide effective PMH care including access to CPD opportunities, specialist PMH and psychological services to meet the needs of increasingly diverse populations. The data and analysis emphasise the context of PMH care provision where GP who have access to specialist PMH services and psychological therapies felt well supported to provide effective care in comparison to GPs who have to negotiate complex referrals with limited access to services.

Abbreviations

CPD: Continuous Professional Development; GPs: General Practitioners; HCPs: Healthcare Professionals; PMH: Perinatal Mental Health; PMHPs: Perinatal Mental Health Problems

Acknowledgements

The authors gratefully acknowledge the participants who gave their time and shared their experiences for this research.

Funding

No funding.

Authors' contributions

Study design: MN, OD, RG, JJ, AOR; data collection: MN; data analysis: MN, OD, AOR, RG and manuscript preparation: MN, RG, OD, JJ, AOR. All authors have read and approved the final manuscript.

Consent for publication

Not applicable.

Competing interests

The authors declare that they have no competing interests.

Author details

[1]Department of Nursing and Midwifery, Faculty of Education & Health Sciences, Health Sciences Building, University of Limerick, Limerick, Ireland. [2]Department of Nursing and Midwifery, Faculty of Education & Health Sciences, Health Sciences Building, University of Limerick, Limerick, Ireland. [3]Graduate Entry Medical School, Faculty of Education & Health Sciences, University of Limerick, Limerick, Ireland. [4]Faculty of Health and Social Care, University of Hull, Hull, UK. [5]School of Allied Health, Faculty of Education & Health Sciences, Health Sciences Building, University of Limerick, Limerick, Ireland.

References

1. Ford E, Shakespeare J, Elias F, Ayers S. Recognition and management of perinatal depression and anxiety by general practitioners: a systematic review. Fam Pract. 2017;34(1):11–9. https://doi.org/10.1093/fampra/cmw101.
2. Noonan M, Doody O, Jomeen J, Galvin R. Midwives' perceptions and experiences of caring for women who experience perinatal mental health problems: an integrative review. Midwifery. 2017;45:56–71. https://doi.org/10.1016/j.midw.2016.12.010.
3. Howard LM, Ryan EG, Trevillion K, Anderson F, et al. Accuracy of the Whooley questions and the Edinburgh postnatal depression scale in identifying depression and other mental disorders in early pregnancy. Br J Psychiatry. 2018;212:50–6.
4. Jairaj C, Fitzsimons CM, McAuliffe FM, et al. A population survey of prevalence rates of antenatal depression in the Irish obstetric services using the Edinburgh postnatal depression scale (epds). Archives of Women's Health. https://doi.org/10.1007/s00737-018-0893-3.
5. Leahy-Warren P, McCarthy G, Corcoran P. Postnatal depression in first-time mothers: prevalence and relationships between functional and structural social support at 6 and 12 weeks postpartum. Arch Psychiatr Nurs. 2011;25(3):174–84.
6. Falah-Hassani K, Shiri R, Dennis C-L. The prevalence of antenatal and postnatal co-morbid anxiety and depression: a meta-analysis. Psychol Med. 2017;47(12):2041–53.
7. Bauer A, Parsonage M, Knapp M, Lemmi V, Adelaja B. The costs of perinatal mental health problems. London: Personal Social Services Research Unit. Centre for Mental Health and London School of Economics; 2014.
8. Stein A, Pearson RM, Goodman SH, Rapa E, Rahman A, McCallum M, Howard L, Pariante CM. Perinatal mental health 3 effects of perinatal mental disorders on the fetus and child. Lancet. 2014;384:1800–19. https://doi.org/10.1016/S0140-6736(14)61277-0.
9. Department of Health. Creating a better future together National Maternity Strategy. Dublin, Ireland: Department of Health; 2016.
10. Noonan M, Jomeen J, Galvin R, Doody O. Survey of midwives' perinatal mental health knowledge, confidence, attitudes and learning needs. Women and Birth. 2018. https://doi.org/10.1016/j.wombi.2018.02.002.
11. The National Child Birth Trust. The Hidden Half Bringing postnatal mental illness out of hiding. 2017, The National Childbirth Trust, London. https://www.nct.org.uk/sites/default/files/related_documents/NCT%20The%20Hidden%20Half_0.pdf
12. Khan L. Falling through the gaps: perinatal mental health and general practice. UK: Centre for Mental Health; 2015.
13. Ford E, Lee S, Shakespeare J, Ayers S. Diagnosis and management of perinatal depression and anxiety in general practice: a meta-synthesis of qualitative studies. Br J Gen Pract. 2017;67(661):e538–46. https://doi.org/10.3399/bjgp17X691889.
14. Noonan M, Doody O, O'Regan A, Jomeen J, Galvin R. Family physicians perceived role in perinatal mental health: an integrative review. BMC Family Practice. 2018, 19(154), available, https://doi.org/10.1186/s12875-018-0843-1.
15. Department of Health (Ireland). 'A Vision for Change': report of the Expert Group on Mental Health Policy. Dublin: Stationary office, 2006.
16. Health Service Executive. Specialists Perinatal Mental Health Services Model of Care for Ireland. Dublin: National Mental Health Division, Health Service Executive; 2017. https://www.hse.ie/eng/services/list/4/mental-health-services/specialist-perinatal-mental-health/specialist-perinatal-mental-health-services-model-of-care-2017.pdf.
17. Tong A, Sainsbury P, Craig J. Consolidated criteria for reporting qualitative research (COREQ): a 32-item checklist for interviews and focus groups. Int J Qual Health Care. 2007;19(4):349–57.
18. Green J, Thorogood N. Qualitative methods for Health Research. 3rd ed. London: Sage; 2014.
19. Braun V, Clarke V. Successful qualitative research a practical guide for beginners. London: Sage; 2013.
20. Ashford MT, Ayers S, Olander EK. Supporting women with postpartum anxiety: exploring views and experiences of specialist community public health nurses in the UK. Health and Social Care in the Community. 2017; 25(3):1257–64.
21. Button S, Lee S, Shakespeare J, Ayers S. Seeking help for perinatal psychological distress: a meta-synthesis of women's experiences. Br J Gen Pract. 2017. https://doi.org/10.3399/bjgp17X692549.
22. Bambridge GA, Shaw EJ, Ishak M, Clarke SD, Baker C. Perinatal mental health: how to ask and how to help. Obstet Gynaecol. 2017;19:147–53. https://doi.org/10.1111/tog.12376.

23. Prady SL, Pickett KE, Petherick ES, Gilbody S, Croudace T, Mason D, et al. Evaluation of ethnic disparities in detection of depression and anxiety in primary care during the maternal period: combined analysis of routine and cohort data. Br J Psychiatry. 2016;208(5):453–61. https://doi.org/10.1192/bjp.bp.114.158832.
24. Watt K, Abbott P, Reath J. Developing cultural competence in general practitioners: an integrative review of the literature. BMC Fam Pract. 2016;17:158. https://doi.org/10.1186/s12875-016-0560-6.
25. National Institute for Health and Clinical Excellence. Antenatal and postnatal mental health: Clinical management and service guidance. NICE clinical guideline. 2014;45 guidandce.nice.org.uk/cg192.
26. Khalifeh H, Brauer R, Toulmin H, Howard LM. Perinatal mental health: what every neonatologist should know. Early Hum Dev. 2015;91:649–53. https://doi.org/10.1016/j.earlhumdev.2015.08.010.
27. The Regulation and Quality Improvement Authority. Review of Perinatal Mental Health Services in Northern Ireland. 2017. Available to access at: https://www.rqia.org.uk/RQIA/files/28/28f4ee85-a5e9-4004-b922-525bc41ae56d.pdf.
28. Megnin-Viggars O, Symington I, Howard LM, Pilling S. Experience of care for mental health problems in the antenatal or postnatal period for women in the UK: a systematic review and meta-synthesis of qualitative research. Arch Womens Ment Health. 2015;18:745–59.
29. Legere LE, Wallace K, Bowen A, McQueen K, Montgomery P, Evans M. Approaches to health-care provider education and professional development in perinatal depression: a systematic review. BMC Pregnancy and Childbirth. 2017;17:239. https://doi.org/10.1186/s12884-017-1431-4.
30. Agyapong VIO, Jabbar F, Conway C. Shared care between specialised psychiatric services and primary care: the experiences and expectations of general practitioners in Ireland. Int J Psychiatry Clin Pract. 2012;16:293–9. https://doi.org/10.3109/13651501.2012.667115.
31. MIND. Better equipped, better care improving mental health training for GPs and practice nurses. London: MIND; 2016.
32. Morrell JC, Cubison J, Ricketts T, Williams AS, Hall P. Training Health-Care Professionals for the Assessment and Management of Perinatal depression and Anxiety. In: Milgrom GAW, editor. Identifying Perinatal Depression and Anxiety Evidence-Based Practice in Screening, Psychosocial Assessment, and Management. Oxford: Wiley Blackwell; 2015. p. 210–27.
33. Murray M, Murray L, Donnelly M. Systematic review of interventions to improve the psychological well-being of general practitioners. BMC Fam Pract. 2016;17:36. https://doi.org/10.1186/s12875-016-0431-1.

14

Diagnostic behaviour of general practitioners when suspecting Lyme disease: a database study from 2010-2015

Esmée Botman[1], C. Wim Ang[2], Johanna H. K. Joosten[3], Pauline Slottje[1,3], Johannes C. van der Wouden[1] and Otto R. Maarsingh[1*]

Abstract

Background: Due to the raised public awareness of Lyme Borreliosis (LB), its increased incidence and the increased availability of serological tests, the demand for diagnostic testing on LB has increased. This may affect the diagnostic behaviour of general practitioners (GPs). Aim of our study was to describe GPs' diagnostic behaviour when suspecting LB.

Methods: In this descriptive study from January 2010 to June 2015, we used the anonymized electronic medical records of 56,996 patients registered in 12 general practices in Amsterdam, The Netherlands. The target population was identified by means of an extensive search strategy, based on International Classification of Primary Care (ICPC-1) codes, free text and diagnostic test codes. All contacts related to LB were included in the analysis.

Results: 2311 patients were included, accounting for 3861 LB contacts and 2619 LB episodes. The distribution of LB contacts showed annual peaks during spring and summer. Serological testing was performed in 36.4% of LB episodes and was mostly requested in patients presenting with general symptoms (71.4%). Unnecessary testing often occurred and only 5.9% of the tests turned out to be positive by immunoblot. From January 2010 to June 2015, no significant differences were found in the number of requested serological tests. The level of serological testing during LB episodes differed significantly between the general practices (19.2% to 75.8%).

Conclusions: Contrary to clinical guidelines, GPs regularly requested serology even when there was a low suspicion of LB. The development of an easy-to-use diagnostic algorithm may decrease overuse of diagnostic tests and thereby reduce overtreatment of LB.

Keywords: Lyme disease, Diagnosis, General practice, Primary health care

Background

Lyme Borreliosis (LB) is the most common tick-borne disease in the world [1–4] caused by *Borrelia burgdorferi* sensu lato-spirochetes, of which *Borrelia afzellii* and *Borrelia garinii* are most prevalent in Europe [1, 5]. Over the past decades, the incidence of LB in Europe has increased to approximately 65,500 patients per year [6–9]. Raised public awareness of LB, its various clinical manifestations, its treatable character, the fear of disease among patients and the increased availability of serological tests have driven a rising demand for diagnostic testing [8, 10, 11]. Current European guidelines, although not tailored to primary care, clearly state that serological tests must only be done when there is a high suspicion of LB. This high a priori probability is mainly based on LB-specific symptoms (like symptoms suggesting Lyme arthritis or neuroborreliosis) [12, 13]. Requesting non-indicated tests may lead to false-positive results, since - depending on the assay - 3-9% of healthy controls is seropositive for Borrelia antibodies [14]. This is because serological tests do not differentiate between an active LB and an (asymptomatic) infection from the past [11]. Other reasons for a false-positive test result are infections with other related pathogens (e.g. syphilis), autoimmune disorders, or cross-reactivity between spirochetes. [15] In

* Correspondence: o.maarsingh@vumc.nl
[1]Department of General Practice & Elderly Care Medicine and Amsterdam Public Health research institute, VU University Medical Center, Van der Boechorststraat 7, 1081, BT, Amsterdam, The Netherlands

general, according to Bayes' theorem, the usefulness of a serological test for LB depends on the pre-test probability and the subsequent predictive values in the setting where the test is being used [2, 16, 17]. However, even in a tertiary, multidisciplinary setting it is challenging to either rule out or demonstrate an association with Borrelia burgdorferi sensu lato. [18] The seropositivity rates for LB vary throughout Europe, from 3.4% in the general population in Italy to 15.2% in France [14, 19, 20]. When testing high-risk populations, these seropositive rates will be even higher. In Poland, healthy forestry workers reach a seropositivity rate of 45% [19, 21]. Because positive test results are often interpreted as Borrelia being the causal agent of the symptoms, overtreatment is common in cases of false-positive test results. Previous studies in general practices have only focused on tick bites and erythema migrans (EM). In Belgium 50% of the patients presenting with a typical EM got serologically tested by the GP [9], contrary to national/international guidelines (i.e. patients presenting with EM should always receive antibiotic treatment, so serological testing has no additional value; moreover, a false negative test result may occur, which can be misleading [12, 13].

The aim of the present study was to describe GPs' diagnostic behaviour with respect to LB. Our study is the first to describe seasonal trends in LB contacts, to link symptoms to serology requests, and to investigate if GPs' diagnostic behaviour on LB has changed over the years 2010-2015.

Methods

An observational study was carried out with anonymized data extracted from the database of the Academic Network of General Practice of VU University Medical Center (ANH VUmc), Amsterdam. The database contains pseudonimized primary health care data. We used the anonymized data of 56,996 patients registered in 12 general practices (with more than 60 GPs) in Amsterdam, from January 2010 to June 2015. In the Netherlands, almost all non-institutionalised citizens are registered to a general practice and the GP acts as gatekeeper. We developed an extensive search and selection strategy, based on the International Classification of Primary Care (ICPC-1) codes, free text and diagnostic test codes, to identify contacts related to LB (see Fig. 1 for the flow chart, Appendix 1 for the search strategy, and Appendix 2 for the origin of the identified patients, divided by search strategy). Annotations of the GPs from all identified contacts (consultations, telephone, home visits, e-mails) were reviewed by one of the investigators (EB). Contacts not related to LB or tick bites were excluded (e.g. other insect bites). A random selection of 5% of the identified contacts was reviewed by a second, independent reviewer to check the reliability of the data extraction. Disagreements were resolved during a consensus meeting between investigator and independent reviewer.

The following data were extracted from the selected medical records (analytical sample): basic characteristics of the patients (i.e. sex, age at the time of the first LB contact), characteristics of the LB contact and episode (i.e. date of contact, type of contact, number of contacts), ICPC-1 code, symptoms registered, findings during physical examination, diagnosis and management (i.e. Lyme serology or referral). Contacts belonging to the same episode were merged for the analysis of presenting symptoms and diagnostic testing. In the analysis, a distinction was made between individual contacts and

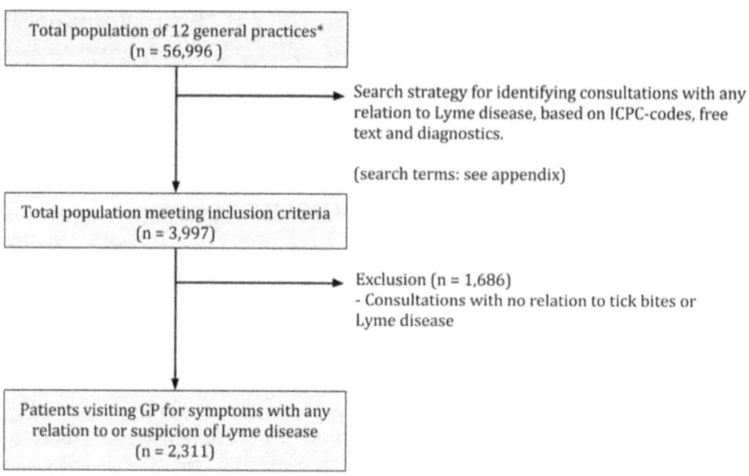

Fig. 1 Flowchart of the identification of general practice contacts related to Lyme Borreliosis. * Based on registered patients in 2014. GP: General Practitioner; ICPC-1 = International Classification of Primary Care

Table 1 Characteristics of patients and general practice contacts related to Lyme Borreliosis

Variables	Number	Percent
Patients ($N = 2311$)		
Gender, female	1371	59.3
Age, mean (95% CI)[a]	39.65 (38.85-40.52)	
≤ 18	389	16.8
19-64	1639	70.9
≥ 65	283	12.2
Contacts ($N = 3681$)		
Type of contact		
Consultations	2796	76.0
Telephone	869	23.6
Home visits	12	0.3
E-mail	4	0.1
Year of contact		
2010	635	17.3
2011	715	19.4
2012	548	14.9
2013	694	18.9
2014	740	20.1
2015[b]	349	9.5

CI Confidence Interval
[a]Age at time of the first contact of an episode
[b]Only first six months available

episodes that include all contacts concerning the same complaint. Also, a distinction was made between a definite tick bite and a possible tick bite; the latter was called 'insect sting' in the analysis.

The data contained different Lyme serology tests from different laboratories and it was not possible to identify the exact assay that was used for each patient. Based on the quantitative value and the cut-off level we could infer that the majority of the samples were screened with the Immunetics C6 ELISA kit (Immunetics Inc., Boston, USA). We used the available laboratory interpretation of the screening test. This included the requirement that all equivocal or positive screening test results had to be confirmed by an immunoblot. Laboratories classified immunoblot outcomes as 'negative', 'inconclusive' or 'positive'.

Descriptive analysis was performed using SPSS 23.0. Chi-square tests for trend (linear-by-linear) were used for comparing differences between years regarding contacts, episodes and serological tests.

The ANH database is run according to Dutch privacy legislation and contains pseudonymized general practice care data from all patients of the participating general practices, excluding those patients who object to this. Observational studies based on anonymized data from the ANH VUmc database are exempted from informed consent of patients.

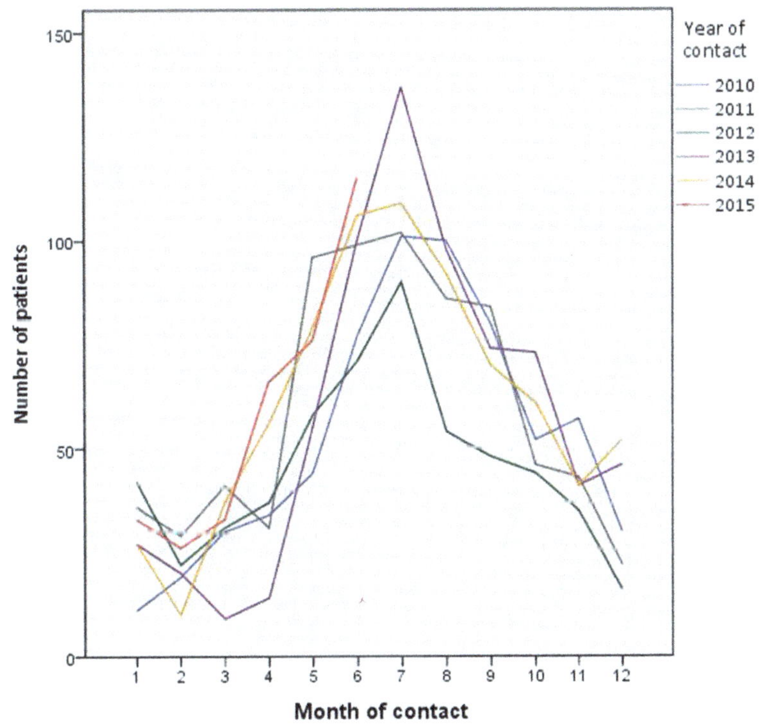

Fig. 2 Distribution of general practice contacts related to Lyme Borreliosis throughout the year*
* Contacts include consultations, visits, calls and e-mails. Data of 2015 were available until June

Table 2 Reasons for encounter registered in electronic medical record for episodes related to Lyme Borreliosis ($N = 2619$ episodes)

Registered reasons for encounter (during $N = 2619$ episodes)			Serological Testing		Positive immunoblot test result	
	N	%[c]	*N*	%[c]	*N*	%[c]
I. General symptoms						
Fatigue	458	17.5	357		20	
Malaise	162	6.2	89		4	
Gastro-intestinal	74	2.8	59		5	
Respiratory	39	1.5	34		3	
Other	233	8.9	151		12	
Total	966	36.9	690	71.4	44	6.4
II. Neurological symptoms						
Headache	105	4.0	72		6	
Dizziness	64	2.4	51		4	
Pain with radiation	50	1.9	34		6	
Numbness	41	1.6	26		4	
Paresthesia	47	1.8	26		2	
Other	96	3.7	70		5	
Total	403	15.4	207	51.4	27	13.0
III. Musculoskeletal symptoms						
Arthralgia	240	9.2	120		15	
Myalgia	92	3.5	61		4	
Total	332	12.7	181	54.5	19	10.5
IV. Diagnostic and therapeutic request[d]						
Serology request	196	7.5	154		18	
Referral request	31	1.2	15		5	
Antibiotics request	60	2.3	10		1	
Total	287	11.0	179	62.4	24	13.4
V. Psychological						
Fear of Lyme	434	16.6	146		14	
Other	27	1.0	23		1	
Total	461	17.6	169	36.7	15	8.9
VI. Skin abnormality						
Possible erythema migrans	120	4.6	34		6	
Local irritation tick bite	327	12.5	33		2	
Erythema migrans	136	5.2	25		7	
Sting bite	194	7.4	12		0	
Eczema	35	1.3	8		2	
Dermatomycosis	65	2.5	7		0	
Other	203	7.8	33		5	
Total	1080	41.2	152	14.1	22	14.5

Table 2 Reasons for encounter registered in electronic medical record for episodes related to Lyme Borreliosis (*N* = 2619 episodes) *(Continued)*

Registered reasons for encounter (during *N* = 2619 episodes)			Serological Testing		Positive immunoblot test result	
	N	%[c]	*N*	%[c]	*N*	%[c]
VII. Recent insect sting[a]						
Tick bite	914	34.9	121		5	
Insect bite	248	9.5	36		3	
Total	1162	44.4	157	13.5	8	5.1
Total[b]	4691	179.1				

[a]Recent is defined as a sting within 3 months prior to contact
[b]Adds up to more than 100%, because general practitioners may register more than one reason for encounter per episode
[c]Row percentages
[d]Request directly made by the patient

Results

Figure 1 provides a flowchart of the study. Twelve general practices were included (*N* = 56,996 patients), resulting in 2311 patients who visited the GP because of complaints or concerns related to LB in the period January 2010 to June 2015 (see Appendix 3 for practice characteristics). The reliability of the data extraction was acceptable: from a random selection of 5% of identified LB contacts, 6 out of 350 contacts (1.7%) had been classified incorrectly.

The basic characteristics of patients and their LB contacts are shown in Table 1.

The overall incidence of episodes related to LB was 8.8 per 1000 person years within the dataset of 56,996 patients. The incidence of LB episodes across the years 2010-2014 did not show a significant change ($p = 0.932$). Since data for 2015 were only partially available, 2015 was not included in this analysis. Each year, LB related contacts showed a peak during spring and summer (May until September; Fig. 2). The majority of patients (78.2%) contacted their GP only once within an LB episode. For LB episodes with 2 or more contacts, the mean interval between first and last contact was 45 days. Most patients (88%) experienced only one LB episode over the period January 2010 to June 2015.

Table 2 provides an overview of reasons for encounter during episodes related to LB (*N* = 2619 episodes). Also, the table illustrates per reason for encounter how often serological testing was ordered and how often this resulted in a positive immunoblot test result.

Symptoms most frequently registered by GPs in LB episodes were recent insect sting, defined as 'recent' when stung within three months prior to contact (*N* = 1162, 44.4% of episodes), skin abnormalities (*N* = 1080, 41.2%) and general symptoms like fatigue and malaise (*N* = 966, 36.9%; Table 2).

Lyme serology was requested during 953 out of 2619 episodes (36.4%). GPs mostly requested serology for episodes in which patients presented with general symptoms (*N* = 690, 71.4%). The percentage of positive test results was highest for the episodes in which patients presented with skin abnormalities (14.5%) and for episodes in which patients requested for a test themselves (13.4%; Table 2). GPs requested serology for 18.4% (*N* = 25 out of 136) of the episodes in which patients presented with typical EM, for 10.1% (*N* = 33 out of 327) of the episodes in which patients presented with a locally irritated tick bite, and for 13.2% (*N* = 121 out of 914) of the episodes in which patients presented with an asymptomatic tick bite.

From January 2010 to June 2015, the number of requested serological tests did not change significantly ($p = 0.190$). Of the 953 serological tests, 19.3% was screened positively. Only 5.9% of these were confirmed by the immunoblot. Referral to a specialist occurred in 7.6% of all LB episodes, mostly to neurologists (24.2%) or internists (21.7%; Table 3).

The general practices showed considerable differences with respect to serological testing during LB episodes, ranging from 19.2% to 75.8% of the LB episodes. There was a tendency for practices with lower serological testing rates to have higher positive tests rates (Fig. 3).

Discussion

Summary of main findings

This study was performed to describe GPs' diagnostic behaviour with respect to LB. As expected, LB contacts showed annual peaks during spring and summer. Of all episodes, 36.4% were followed by a serological test for LB. Tests were mainly performed for episodes in which patients presented with nonspecific complaints like fatigue and headache. Contrary to clinical guidelines, a serological test was performed in 18.4% of the episodes with a typical EM, 10.1% of the episodes with a locally irritated tick bite, and 13.2% of the episodes with an asymptomatic tick bite. Overall, only 5.9% of the serological tests turned out to be positive which is as high as the seropositivity rate of LB in the general population [14]. Also, considerable differences between the 12 general practices were found regarding the rates of serological requests. The number of LB contacts and requested serological tests did not change over the period January 2010 to June 2015.

Table 3 Referral to specialists for episodes related to Lyme Borreliosis ($N = 2619$ episodes)

Referral	Number	Percent
Non-referred	2421	92.4
Referred	198	7.6
Neurologist	48	24.2
Internist	43	21.7
Dermatologist	22	11.0
Lyme Centre[a]	16	8.1
Rheumatologist	12	6.1
Paediatrician	8	4.0
Other[b]	49	24.2
Total	2619	100.0

[a]Multidisciplinary centre specialized in Lyme Borreliosis
[b]E.g. cardiologist, rehabilitation specialist, and psychologist

Strengths and weaknesses

This study is the first to explore seasonal trends in LB contacts, to link symptoms with serology requests, and to investigate time trends in GPs diagnostic behaviour on LB over a period of four-and-a-half years. A strength of our study is the use of an extensive, combined search strategy (see Appendix 1). Such a search strategy is crucial, as single search strategies – based on either free text, ICPC-1 code, or diagnostic testing code – all would miss a significant proportion of the target population (see Appendix 2). For example, if one would not use the free text search, 610 patients (26.4% of all 2311 identified patients) and 1023 contacts (27.8% of all 3681 identified contacts) would have been missed. This would have led to an overestimation of the level of serological testing during LB related episodes. Some potential limitations need to be considered. Firstly, the quality of the data depends on the completeness and accuracy of registration by the GP and our selection and data extraction strategy. Relevant contacts may have been missed, which would then have resulted in an underestimation of the actual contact frequency for LB. However, we expect this to be unlikely, because we did not only rely on ICPC-1 codes but also included the free text annotations - which were mined on relevant search terms - and diagnostic testing codes. In addition, GPs affiliated to the ANH VUmc database receive regular training in EMR coding and registration. Secondly, episodes in which both patient and GP did not suspect nor mention LB were not included. Therefore, we were not able to measure underdiagnosis, i.e. not requesting a test although indicated. Finally, we studied data from general practices in an urban area, which may limit the generalizability to rural areas, or other (European) areas, given the reported increasing gradient from west to east (highest in central-eastern Europe), and decreasing gradient from south to north in Scandinavia and from north to south in Italy, Spain and Greece [20].

Comparison with existing literature

The seropositive prevalence of LB in the general Dutch population is 5-10% [11, 12, 14, 22]. Given the low percentage of seropositive patients (5.9%) in our study population, it is likely that GPs regularly requested serology when there only was a low suspicion on LB [23]. This is substantiated by the finding that GPs mostly requested serology for episodes in which patients presented with general/nonspecific symptoms. According to the current guidelines, EM and asymptomatic tick bites should not be followed by a serological test on LB [12, 13]. Nevertheless, the GPs in our sample performed serological testing in one fifth of all patients with EM. This may seem substantial, but other international studies present much higher percentages, i.e. 50% and 68% in Belgium and France, respectively [9, 24]. Also, 121 out of 914 (13.2%) asymptomatic tick bites were

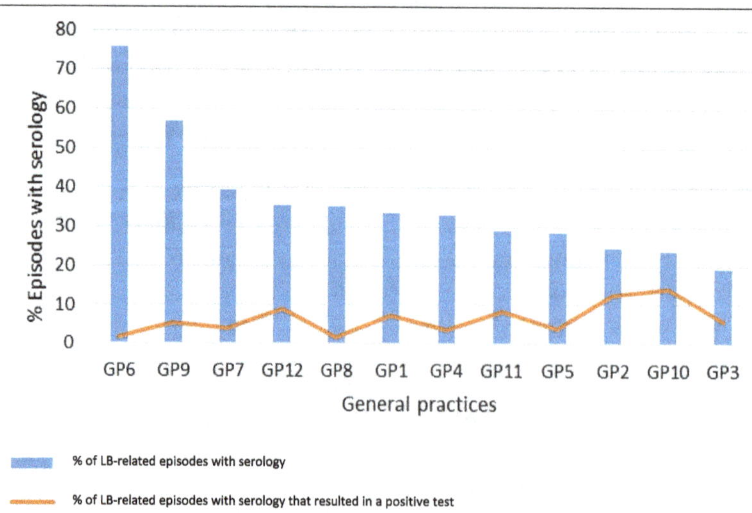

Fig. 3 Serology requests and positive test rate in LB-related episodes per general practice

serologically tested. In Belgium, 17.5% of the asymptomatic tick bites got serologically tested [9].

In our study, serology was mostly requested for episodes in which patients presented with nonspecific symptoms. Previous studies showed that unexplained symptoms, other than LB, more frequently lead to laboratory testing by the GP [25, 26]. Reasons for ordering tests for patients with unexplained symptoms may be a limited tolerance to diagnostic uncertainty or time pressure [25]. Once a laboratory test has been requested, the threshold for more testing is low and many GPs are unaware of the consequences (like false positive findings) [25, 26]. For example, an Australian study showed that 64.2% of patients presenting with fatigue to their GP received laboratory testing. In only 4% of the patients the tests led to a significant clinical diagnosis [26]. Improving GPs' knowledge on the subject, combined with an easy-to-use diagnostic algorithm may increase confidence and reduce the overuse of diagnostic tests.

The large differences in serological testing between general practices suggest that - despite multidisciplinary guidelines - there is no consensus how to apply these guidelines in daily general practice and when to perform serological testing on LB.

Implications for clinicians and research

Hopefully, our study will initiate the development of an easy-to-use diagnostic algorithm for LB that is (also) applicable in daily general practice. Although the current scientific evidence for such an algorithm is limited, some promising potential predictors have been reported, like tick engorgement and patient-estimated duration of tick attachment. [10, 27] Future research may focus on the needs and expectations of patients and GPs during LB consultations, for example by a focus group study or semi-structured interviews. This may reveal clues to arrive at optimal (diagnostic) healthcare decisions with respect to LB.

Conclusions

This descriptive GP database study, covering the period January 2010 to June 2015, was the first to investigate seasonal trends in LB contacts, to link symptoms to serology requests, and to investigate GPs' diagnostic behaviour over time. The distribution of LB contacts showed annual peaks during spring and summer. Episodes in which patients presented with general symptoms, like fatigue, were most frequently followed by serological testing. Serological testing was performed in 36.4% of LB episodes; only 5.9% of these tests turned out to be positive. The high number of LB consultations with nonspecific complaints together with the low frequency of positive serological tests, and the considerable inter-practice differences indicate a high number of inappropriate tests and underscores the need for an easy-to-use diagnostic algorithm that is (also) applicable in daily general practice.

Appendix 1

Table 4 Search strategy in electronic medical records

Search term or code	Explanation
I. Free text	
Teek	Tick
Teke[b]	Tick
Lyme	Lyme Borreliosis
Ery[b]Migr[b]	Erythema migrans
EM	Erythema migrans
E.M.	Erythema migrans
Bor[b]elia	Lyme Borreliosis
II. ICPC-1 code	
S12	Insect sting
S12.01	Tick bite
A78	Other infectious diseases
A78.05	Lyme Borreliosis
III. Diagnostic test code[a]	
125	Borrelia Burgdorferi antibodies IgA
126	Borrelia B. confirmation test
127	Borrelia Burgdorferi antibodies IgG
2889	Borrelia Burgdorferi antibodies IgG liquor
128	Borrelia Burgdorferi antibodies
2404	Borrelia Burgdorferi index per total antibodies IgG/IgM
129	Borrelia Burgdorferi IgM
3104	Borrelia Burgdorferi antibodies IgM (1e mnt,gprd)
3434	Borrelia Burgdorferi antibodies IgM (quantitative)
2891	Borrelia Burgdorferi antibodies IgM liquor
2167	Borrelia Burgdorferi C6 protein
3101	Borrelia Burgdorferi C6 protein (quantitative)
3102	Borrelia Burgdorferi C6 protein (1e mnt, gprd)
2890	Borrelia Burgdorferi C6 protein liquor
2226	Borrelia Burgdorferi antibodies IgG (Westernblot)
2227	Borrelia Burgdorferi antibodies IgM (Westernblot)

Our search strategy was based on selected International Classification Primary Care (ICPC-1) Codes, words in free text annotations, and requests for serological tests for Lyme disease as recorded in routine primary care in the electronical medical records

ICPC-1 International Classification of Primary Care

[a]Tests were included when requested 8 days before or after a contact

[b]Wild card code, to include any variation in typing following trunk

Appendix 2

Table 5 Origin of identified patients and general practice contacts, divided by search strategy

Identified patients (*N* = 2311)				
Search strategy			Number of patients	%
I. Free text	II. ICPC-1 code	III. Diagnostic test code		
X	–	–	610	26.4
–	X	–	62	2.7
–	–	X	331	14.3
X	X	–	801	34.7
–	X	X	4	0.2
X	–	X	325	14.1
X	X	X	178	7.7
Total			2311	100
Identified general practice contacts (*N* = 3681)				
Search strategy			Number of contacts	%
I. Free text	II. ICPC-1 code	III. Diagnostic test code		
X	–	–	1023	27.8
–	X	–	182	4.9
–	–	X	797	21.7
X	X	–	1093	29.7
–	X	X	40	1.1
X	–	X	427	11.6
X	X	X	119	3.2
Total			3681	100

ICPC-1 = International classification of Primary care
X: Used as search term to identify patient and contacts, respectively
-: Not used in search

Abbreviations
ANH VUmc: Academic Network of General Practice of VU University Medical Center; CI: Confidence Interval; EM: Erythema migrans; GP: General Practitioner; ICPC-1: International Classification of Primary Care; LB: Lyme Borreliosis

Acknowledgements
Special thanks to all GPs who participate in the Academic Network of General Practice of VU University medical center (ANH VUmc) for extracting the data.

Funding
This study was not funded.

Authors' contributions
EB, JCvdW and ORM were involved in the design of the study. EB performed the statistical analysis. EB wrote the original draft. All authors (EB, CWA, JHKJ, PS, JCvdW and ORM) made substantial contributions to interpretation of data, critically revised the draft for important intellectual content, and approved the final version of the manuscript.

Consent for publication
Not applicable.

Appendix 3

Table 6 Characteristics of the general practices (*N* = 12)

General practice	Type of practice[a]	Number of patients per practice (annual mean)		Number of GPs
		2010	*2015*	
1.	Group	4531	5562	4
2.	Solo	2684	2717	1
3.	Group	4432	4705	8
4.	Duo	2848	3351	2
5.	Duo	2663	2887	2
6.	Duo	1881	2094	2
7.	Group	3284	5808	5
8.	Duo	2777	2949	2
9.	Group	8812	8984	5
10.	Group	4852	4763	4
11.	Group	8075	7870	6
12.	Group	5499	6390	4

[a]: Solo (1 GP), duo (2 GPs), or group (> 2 GPs)

Competing interests
The authors declare that they have no competing interests.

Author details
[1]Department of General Practice & Elderly Care Medicine and Amsterdam Public Health research institute, VU University Medical Center, Van der Boechorststraat 7, 1081, BT, Amsterdam, The Netherlands. [2]Department of Medical Microbiology & Infection Control, VU University Medical Center, Amsterdam, The Netherlands. [3]Academic Network of General Practice, Department of General Practice & Elderly Care Medicine, VU University Medical Center (ANH VUmc), Amsterdam, The Netherlands.

References
1. Sykes RA, Makiello P. An estimate of Lyme borreliosis incidence in Western Europe. J Public Health (Oxf). 2017;39(1):74–81.
2. Stanek G, Fingerle V, Hunfeld KP, Jaulhac B, Kaiser R, Krause A, Kristoferitsch W, O'Connell S, Ornstein K, Strle F, et al. Lyme borreliosis: clinical case definitions for diagnosis and management in Europe. Clin Microbiol Infect. 2011;17(1):69–79.
3. Stanek G, Wormser GP, Gray J, Strle F. Lyme borreliosis. Lancet. 2012; 379(9814):461–73.
4. Steere AC, Strle F, Wormser GP, Hu LT, Branda JA, Hovius JW, Li X, Mead PS. Lyme borreliosis. Nat Rev Dis Primers. 2016;2:16090.
5. Rudenko N, Golovchenko M, Grubhoffer L, Oliver JH Jr. Updates on Borrelia burgdorferi sensu lato complex with respect to public health. Ticks Tick Borne Dis. 2011;2(3):123–8.
6. Brouwer ML, Rietmeijer-Mentink M, Sprong H, Van der Wouden JC, Bindels PJE. Tick bites: a dilemma in general practice. Huisarts Wet. 2013;56(7):5.
7. Hofhuis A, Harms M, Bennema S, van den Wijngaard CC, van Pelt W. Physician reported incidence of early and late Lyme borreliosis. Parasit Vectors. 2015;8:161.
8. Rizzoli A, Hauffe H, Carpi G, Vourc HG, Neteler M, Rosa R. Lyme borreliosis in Europe. Euro Surveill. 2011;16(27)
9. Vanthomme K, Bossuyt N, Boffin N, Van Casteren V. Incidence and management of presumption of Lyme borreliosis in Belgium: recent data from the sentinel network of general practitioners. Eur J Clin Microbiol Infect Dis. 2012;31(9):2385–90.
10. Ang W, Wolfs TFW. Diagnosis of Lyme borreliosis. Huisarts Wet. 2015;58(5):5.

11. Coumou J, Hovius JW, van Dam AP. Borrelia burgdorferi sensu lato serology in the Netherlands: guidelines versus daily practice. Eur J Clin Microbiol Infect Dis. 2014;33(10):1803–8.
12. Dutch Guideline Lyme Disease, July 2013. http://www.tekenbeetziekten.nl/wp-content/uploads/2014/08/CBO-richtlijn-Lymeziekte-versie-2013.pdf. Accessed on October 5th, 2017.
13. Belgian Guideline Lyme Borreliosis (Infection with Borrelia), 2016. Belgian Antibiotic Policy Coordination Committee (BAPCOC). http://overlegorganen.gezondheid.belgie.be/sites/default/files/documents/gids_lyme_borreliose_nl_march2017.pdf. Accessed on October 5th 2017.
14. Ang CW, Brandenburg AH, van Burgel ND, Bijlmer HA, Herremans T, Stelma F, Lunel FV, van Dam AP, Dutch Working Group on Diagnosis of Lyme B. A Dutch nationwide evaluation of serological assays for detection of Borrelia antibodies in clinically well-defined patients. Diagn Microbiol Infect Dis. 2015;83(3):222–8.
15. Lindsay LR, Bernat K, Dibernardo A. Laboratory diagnosis of Lyme disease. CCDR. 2014;40(11):9.
16. Leeflang MM, Ang CW, Berkhout J, Bijlmer HA, Van Bortel W, Brandenburg AH, Van Burgel ND, Van Dam AP, Dessau RB, Fingerle V, et al. The diagnostic accuracy of serological tests for Lyme borreliosis in Europe: a systematic review and meta-analysis. BMC Infect Dis. 2016;16:140.
17. Tugwell P, Dennis DT, Weinstein A, Wells G, Shea B, Nichol G, Hayward R, Lightfoot R, Baker P, Steere AC. Laboratory evaluation in the diagnosis of Lyme disease. Ann Intern Med. 1997;127(12):1109–23.
18. Coumou J, Herkes EA, Brouwer MC, van de Beek D, Tas SW, Casteelen G, van Vugt M, Starink MV, de Vries HJ, de Wever B, et al. Ticking the right boxes: classification of patients suspected of Lyme borreliosis at an academic referral center in the Netherlands. Clin Microbiol Infect. 2015;21(4):368. e311-320
19. Zakutna L, Dorko E, Mattova E, Rimarova K. Sero-epidemiological study of Lyme disease among high-risk population groups in eastern Slovakia. Ann Agric Environ Med. 2015;22(4):632–6.
20. Hubalek Z. Epidemiology of Lyme borreliosis. Curr Probl Dermatol. 2009;37:31–50.
21. Chmielewska-Badora J, Moniuszko A, Zukiewicz-Sobczak W, Zwolinski J, Piatek J, Pancewicz S. Serological survey in persons occupationally exposed to tick-borne pathogens in cases of co-infections with Borrelia burgdorferi, Anaplasma phagocytophilum, Bartonella spp. and Babesia microti. Ann Agric Environ Med. 2012;19(2):271–4.
22. Coumou J, van der Poll T, Speelman P, Hovius JW. Tired of Lyme borreliosis. Lyme borreliosis in the Netherlands. Neth J Med. 2011;69(3):101–11.
23. Lakos A, Igari Z, Solymosi N. Recent lesson from a clinical and seroepidemiological survey: low positive predictive value of Borrelia burgdorferi antibody testing in a high risk population. Adv Med Sci. 2012;57(2):356–63.
24. Letrilliart L, Ragon B, Hanslik T, Flahault A. Lyme disease in France: a primary care-based prospective study. Epidemiol Infect. 2005;133(5):935–42.
25. van der Weijden T, van Bokhoven MA, Dinant GJ, van Hasselt CM, Grol RP. Understanding laboratory testing in diagnostic uncertainty: a qualitative study in general practice. Br J Gen Pract. 2002;52(485):974–80.
26. Wilson J, Morgan S, Magin PJ, van Driel ML. Fatigue–a rational approach to investigation. Aust Fam Physician. 2014;43(7):457–61.
27. Hofhuis A, van de Kassteele J, Sprong H, van den Wijngaard CC, Harms MG, Fonville M, Docters van Leeuwen A, Simoes M, van Pelt W. Predicting the risk of Lyme borreliosis after a tick bite, using a structural equation model. PLoS One. 2017;12(7):e0181807.

15

Participation in medical activities beyond standard consultations by Swiss general practitioners

Julian Jakob[1,2,5*], Christine Cohidon[1,3], Jacques Cornuz[1] and Kevin Selby[1,4]

Abstract

Background: Few data exist to support the observation that general practitioners (GPs) occupy many important positions in our communities or to characterize which GPs devote more of their time to such activities. We sought to characterize community-based complementary medical activities performed by GPs in the canton Vaud, Switzerland.

Methods: All GPs in a region were invited to participate in a cross-sectional study ($n = 600$) examining engagement in complementary activities beyond standard ambulatory consultations. Categories included teaching, care giving in specific structures, roles as medical experts or company doctors, community care giving, and others completed by the GP. GPs were asked the number of hours devoted monthly to each activity and whether or not they are remunerated for this work.

Results: One hundred and sixty-eight GPs responded (28%), with 149 (92%) reporting that they were engaged in at least one activity beyond their in-office consultations, including 117 (72%) in community care-giving (ex: care for addictions or refugees). Altogether, GPs spend on average 5.8 h a week on these activities. One-hundred and twenty-three GPs (82%) were remunerated for at least one of their complementary engagements. Predictors of participation in a larger number of complementary activities were working in a rural area (IRR 1.29, 95% CI 1.05 to 1.57) and having a higher weekly workload (IRR 1.01 for each additional hour, 95% CI 1.01 to 1.02).

Conclusion: The vast majority of GPs engage in activities beyond their standard clinic tasks and they are typically reimbursed. GPs in rural areas and those who work more hours per week are more likely to engage in complementary activities.

Keywords: Primary care, Community medicine, Rural area, Complementary activities, Cross-sectional

Background

A shortage of general practitioners (GPs) has been predicted for the coming years [1], due to the rising demand of health care services, restrictions on incoming medical school students (*numerus clausus*) and not enough young physicians choosing primary care specialties [2]. Beyond its impact on basic medical care, this shortage could cause an inadequate supply of GPs for various community activities, and rural areas may be affected most [3]. We know anecdotally that besides the *standard* activities provided by every GP, defined as traditional in-office consultations with patients and associated administrative tasks, medical doctors often occupy additional, *complementary* functions. Acting as company doctors, providing care in nursing homes, or insuring the education of students and residents appear to be most common [4]. However, rising demand for complementary community activities could exacerbate the shortage of GPs available for standard consultations [5]. On the other hand, GPs may find complementary activities desirable because they provide variety, stable income, and predictable hours, thus increasing the

* Correspondence: julian.jakob@students.unibe.ch
[1]Department of Ambulatory Care and Community Medicine, Lausanne University, Rue du Bugnon 44, 1011 Lausanne, Switzerland
[2]Institute of Primary Health Care (BIHAM), University of Bern, Bern, Switzerland

desirability of being a GP and potentially attenuating the GP shortage [6].

Currently, there are few data focusing on complementary activities performed by GPs outside the exam room. Cohidon et al. described a clear increase in the proportion of Swiss physicians who perform paid complementary activities, such as teaching, being engaged in a nursing home or involved in private enterprises besides the standard in-office health care delivery, from 28% in 1993 to 66% in 2012 ($p < 0.001$) [7]. Thirty-nine percent of GPs in the US report being engaged in voluntary medical activities [8], while 90% of GPs consider public roles important [9]. Dimensions of community engagement to improve medical care delivery in variable settings have been proposed [10]. However, these studies used narrow definitions of complementary activities, did not specify participation rates and time spent on each type of activity, and did not specifically study associations between GP characteristics and practice location with engagement in these activities. This information could have important policy implications and be used to attract attention to the important role GPs play in our community.

The goal of this study was to characterize and quantify complementary medical activities performed by GPs in the canton Vaud, Switzerland.

Methods

Setting and design

We performed a cross-sectional study of GPs in the canton of Vaud, Switzerland during the summer of 2016, first using paper questionnaires during a continuing medical education course, and later an online form distributed by email. GPs were explicitly informed on the title page of the online form to fill it only if they had not previously participated in the study during a continuing medical education course. This questionnaire had been developed with consultation of authors who had published studies about similar primary care topics [7]. Primary care in Switzerland is formed by a combination of physicians licensed in General Internal Medicine and General Medicine, referred to jointly here as general practitioners (GPs). Vaud is the third largest Swiss canton, with over 750,000 inhabitants, mostly French-speaking. Members of *Médecins de famille Vaud*, a professional association representing nearly all GPs in the canton, were invited to participate ($n = 600$) between June and August 2016. Paediatricians were not included. We used paper questionnaires during continuing medical education courses including around 100 physicians in this time period, followed by a mass email to all members. A reminder was sent one month after the first email.

Survey instrument

We defined *standard* activities done by every GP as in-office consultations, completed by documentation of the visit and associated administrative tasks only. All medical activities that are not performed routinely by every physician and sometimes even require a special license, such as teaching (2 questions, pre- and post-graduate), care giving in specific structures (5 questions, i.e. schools and nursing homes), engagement as medical expert or company doctor (2 questions with 5 sub-items, i.e. insurance companies), community care giving (6 questions, i. e. supporting patients suffering from addictions, sporting events) and others as specified by the GP itself, were considered as *complementary* activities. In addition to Cohidon et al.'s definition of complementary paid activities, we included non-remunerated activities, but did not ask about office management and health care coordination engagements as these are part of a GP's daily routine [7]. For each complementary activity, the GPs were asked the mean number of hours monthly spent on it, averaged over a year. GPs were asked to answer whether they receive financial compensation, though the amount or nature of such a financial compensation was not of interest in this study. The end of the questionnaire included demographic questions such as physician gender, year of birth and graduation, office size and location, country in which GPs completed their medical education, whether they belong to a medical network and average hours spent on standard in-office consultations. The French-language questionnaire and the resulting dataset are available upon request.

Statistical methods

Descriptive statistics were presented using frequencies and means with standard deviations where appropriate. Activities left blank on otherwise complete questionnaires were considered as non-engagement in the complementary activity in question. A Poisson regression model was built on the primary outcome of the number of activities each GP is engaged in. Provider (gender, age, years since diploma, country of medical training, hours worked per week) and practice (urban vs rural location, solo vs group practice and participation in a network) characteristics were included, first in univariate analyses. Variables significant to a p-value less than 0.2 were retained for multivariate modelling using stepwise regression. Given the significant co-linearity between age and years since obtaining diploma, only years since obtaining diploma was retained for the multivariate model. Main predictors for engagement in complementary activities were presented through incident risk ratios (IRR), an IRR of 1.01 corresponding to 1% higher chance to be engaged in one additional complementary activity.

Table 1 Demographic distribution of GPs participating ($n = 162$)[a]

General characteristics	
Mean age – years (±SD)	54.3 (±9.2)
Female gender – N (%)	55 (32.7%)
Country of medical education Switzerland – N (%)	147 (87.5%)
Mean years since doctor's diploma – years (±SD)	28.2 (±9.8)
Specific characteristics	
In solo practice – N (%)	48 (30.2%)
Physician's office location rural - N [%]	48 (28.6%)
Mean number of hours worked per week - h (±SD)	42.7 (±13.3)
Median number of hours worked per week - h (IQR)	43 (31–50)
Physicians working full time[b] - N (%)	84 (51.8%)
Member of a medical network – N (%)	61 (36.3%)

[a]Six participants excluded because of missing demographic data
[b]In Switzerland, 50 h of activity weekly are considered a 100% workload

Statistical analyses were performed in STATA (Version 14.0, Stata Corp, College Station, USA).

Results

Of 600 GPs in Canton Vaud, 168 completed a survey (28%), 121 online and 47 using a paper form (see Table 1). Demographic characteristics concerning mean age, female gender proportion and mean hours worked per week were comparable to those published by the *Foederatio Medicorum Helveticorum* (FMH) yearly on physician's demographics in Switzerland (comparison not shown) [11]. Six questionnaires out of 168 (3.5%) had missing demographic data. Further, 20% of positive responses did not specify the number of hours per month, and 22% did not specify whether they receive remuneration.

Overall, 92% (149) of GPs were engaged in at least one activity in addition to their standard consultations, 85% of respondents of the paper form and 94% of online participants, with as many as 12 activities per GP (Fig. 1). Overall, GPs spent 5.8 h per week on these activities and 83% of physicians were paid for at least one of their engagements (see Table 2). GPs were most implicated in community care giving (72% of GPs), but those engaged in teaching or care giving in specific structures (e.g. nursing homes) dedicated the most time (median > 12 h / month). When dividing the time dedicated per month by working days, GPs spent a daily average of 19 min on teaching and 20 min in specific external structures (e.g. nursing homes). Frequent responses in the field 'other' were participating in research projects, organizing quality circles and being members of medical or non-medical foundations.

The primary predictors of engagement in a greater number of complementary activities were working in a rural area (incident rate ratio (IRR) of 1.29 for higher number of complementary activities, 95% CI 1.05–1.57) and a greater weekly workload of standard consultations (IRR 1.01 for higher number of complementary activities per hour spent in-office, 95% CI 1.01–1.02, or IRR 1.14 for 10 additional worked hours, 95% CI 1.06–1.24). Female gender, years since obtaining medical diploma and being member of coordinated network were not associated with engagement in complementary activities in our multivariate analysis (see Table 3).

Discussion

In this cross-sectional survey of GPs in Vaud, Switzerland, the vast majority of participants was engaged in one or more complementary activities and

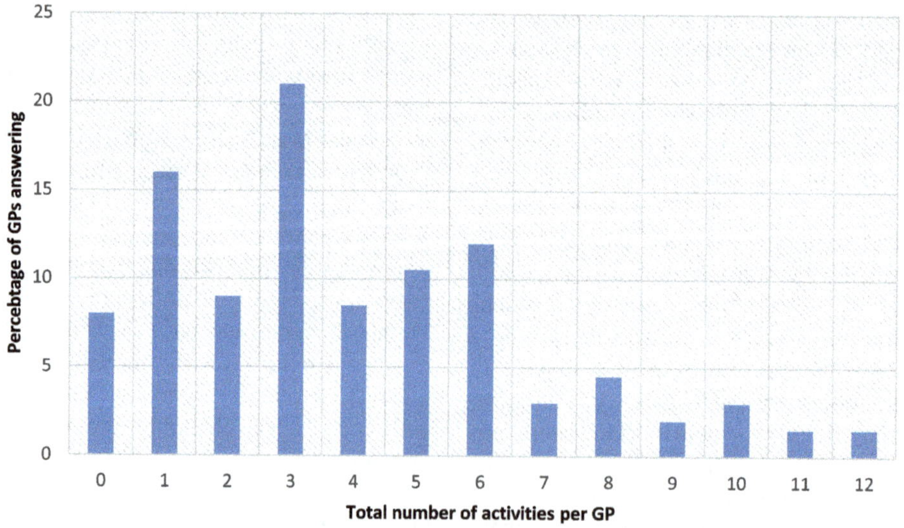

Fig. 1 Total number of activities performed by general practitioner (GP), ranging from 0 to 12 ($N = 162$).[a]Six participants excluded because of missing demographic data

Table 2 Number of, workload, remuneration and characteristic of participating GPs stratified by activity categories ($n = 162$)[a]

Category [question number]	Number of GPs (%)	Median hours per month spent on this activity	Number of GPs reporting at least one remunerated activity (% of GPs implicated)	Gender female	Mean age (±SD)	Practice in rural area
At least one activity [All questions: 1–17]	149 (92%)	23.4 h / mth	123 (83%)	47 (32%)	54.5 (±9.23)	45 (30%)
Teaching [1, 2]	83 (51%)	12.2 h / mth	74 (89%)	21 (38%)	55.2 (± 1.02)	27 (56%)
Care giving in specific structures [3–7]	90 (56%)	12.1 h / mth	74 (77%)	27 (49%)	55.1 (± 0.99)	32 (67%)
Medical expert or company doctor [8, 9]	66 (41%)	7.8 h / mth	52 (81%)	16 (29%)	55.0 (± 1.11)	24 (50%)
Community care giving [10–15]	117 (72%)	7.6 h / mth	73 (61%)	31 (58%)	54.6 (± 0.86)	38 (79%)
Other activities [16, 17]	41 (25%)	7.7 h / mth	29 (69%)	9 (16%)	57.1 (± 1.19)	12 (25%)

[a]Six participants excluded because of missing demographic data

spent a considerable amount of time on these tasks. The primary predictor of participating in complementary activities, beyond working more hours per week on standard consultations, was practicing in a rural area, where other health care providers may be hard to reach [12].

As the shortage of GPs in Switzerland is predicted to be greatest rural areas [3], not only do these areas face a drop in the provision of basic medical services, but also potentially in diverse fields of health care delivery such as in-office teaching, nursing home care and other community activities. One possibility is that rural physicians participate in more complementary activities in order to increase their income. However, a study in Germany, which has a similar health-care system as Switzerland, showed nearly equal incomes of rural and urban GPs through standard in-office care, measured on the number of private insured patients [13]. Thus, remuneration of the complementary activities seems unlikely to be a major motivator.

In the current study, GPs reported spending an average of 19 min daily on teaching and 20 min in specific external structures (e.g. nursing homes), each corresponding to an average in-office consultation in Switzerland [7]. This is more than Gottschalk et al. reported for the USA in 2005 (13 and 5 min respectively) [14] but similar to findings from Granja et al. for Portugal in 2015 (15 min spent on teaching on average per day) [15], indicating that these health care areas may be relying more on GPs engagement over time. An increase in time spent on complementary activities would support Cohidon et al., who compared a more limited number of activities between 1993 and 2012 using a nation-wide sample of Swiss GPs and observed an increase from 28 to 66% of GPs involved in paid activities beyond their standard functions [7]. As in general, GPs

Table 3 Poisson regression model of physician characteristics associated with increasing number of activities outside regular practice ($N = 162$)[a]

Characteristic (N = 162)	Univariate IRR (95% CI)	$p=$	Multivariate IRR (95% CI)	$p=$
Gender (female) ($N = 55$)	0.66 (0.51–0.86)	0.002	0.80 (0.60–1.05)	0.11
Age (years)[b]	1.01 (1.00–1.02)	0.042	–	–
Years since obtaining medical diploma (years)	1.01 (1.00–1.02)	0.024		–
Trained in Switzerland ($N = 147$)	0.99 (0.69–1.42)	0.95	–	–
Hours worked per week on in-office care giving	1.02 (1.01–1.02)	< 0.001	**1.01 (1.01–1.02)**	**< 0.001**
Practice in rural area ($N = 48$)	1.32 (1.05–1.65)	0.015	**1.29 (1.05–1.57)**	**0.01**
Solo practice (N = 48)	0.94 (0.72–1.22)	0.63	–	–
Physician member of coordinated network (ie Delta network) ($N = 61$)	1.20 (0.96–1.49)	0.11	–	–

IRR Incident rate ratio. Statistically significant values in multivariate regression are shown in bold
[a]Six participants excluded because of missing demographic data
[b]Age not included in multivariate model despite being at $p < 0.05$ because of significant co-linearity with years since obtaining medical diploma

tend to spend only about half their time on direct in-office patient contact [5], it is clear that out-of-practice medical services are taking an important role in their working days [16].

Given the number and variety of community roles filled by GPs, the new generation of medical professionals who value an equilibrated work-life balance and lighter weekly workload [17] may not be able to cover all needs. On the other hand, as complementary activities seem to strengthen the attractiveness of primary care [18, 19], GPs may favour complementary activities at the expense of in-office consultations. Regardless, the augmenting implication of GPs in these complementary activities can be explained either by an augmented need for GPs in out-of-practice medical care delivery or by the wish of primary physicians for a broader spectrum of work tasks.

Women appear to participate in fewer activities in univariate analyses (IRR 0.66 (95% CI 0.51–0.86)), however this result is no longer statistically significant when accounting for other physician and practice characteristics. This may be due to the observation that women in our study were younger than participating men, as age was significantly associated with more involvement in complementary activities. In the USA, spending more hours per week on standard consultations and working in a rural area were both independently associated with higher rates of participating in volunteer activities [8].

Strengths and limitations

We had a relatively small sample size with a low response rate. As the study is based on self-reported data, possible declaration bias including recall bias cannot be excluded. Declaration bias including recall bias could result in GPs over- or underestimating their complementary engagement. As we are investigating the association between physician variables and engagement in complementary activities, differential recall bias seems unlikely to explain our primary results of an association between greater involvement and working in rural areas. Given our broad definition of complementary activities, it may not be surprising that most GPs are involved in at least one activity. Enabling participation through paper form during continuing medical education courses in addition to an online survey allowed us to achieve a more diverse sample, as GPs who filled out the paper form reported fewer complementary activities than GPs answering online. Further, while we asked about remuneration, GPs did not specify the exact amount. Important discrepancies between financial incentives perceived in the different categories could not be detected through this study. Our study shows interesting trends, but is from only one sample and should be confirmed using similar definitions in other settings.

Conclusions

GPs provide not only excellent primary care in Switzerland [20], but as this study shows, play an important role in a multitude of educational, professional, and community activities. These findings support the importance of ensuring a steady supply of GPs. There are few existing studies that attempt to quantify these relevant aspects of complementary health care delivery, despite widespread reports of GP shortages. Presenting the broad spectrum of activities incorporated in primary care in the medical curriculum could help motivate young physicians to become GPs.

Abbreviations

CI : Confidence interval; FMH : Foederatio Medicorum Helveticorum (Swiss Physician's Association); GPs : General practitioners; IRR : Incident risk ratio; SD : Standard Deviation; US : United States (of America)

Acknowledgements

The authors would like to thank Sébastien Jotterand, Michael Klay, Jean Perdrix, Céline Braconnier and Stefanie Hostettler for their important contributions to this study.

Funding

This study has been funded through the Policlinique Médicale Universitaire, University of Lausanne fund for research with no additional external support.

Authors' contributions

JJ and JC created the questionnaire, CC and KS analyzed the data and performed the statistical analyses, JJ and KS wrote the draft manuscript. All authors reviewed older versions of this manuscript and read and approved the final manuscript.

Competing interests

The authors declare that they have no competing interests.

Author details

Department of Ambulatory Care and Community Medicine, Lausanne University, Rue du Bugnon 44, 1011 Lausanne, Switzerland. [2]Institute of Primary Health Care (BIHAM), University of Bern, Bern, Switzerland. [3]Institute of Family Medicine, Department of ambulatory care and community medicine, University of Lausanne, Lausanne, Switzerland. [4]Kaiser Permanente Division of Research, 2000 Broadway, Oakland, USA. [5]Policlinique Médicale Universitaire, Rue du Bugnon 44, CH-1011 Lausanne, Switzerland.

References

1. Pécoud A. De la pléthore à la pénurie de médecins : tentative de comprendre. Rev Med Suisse. 2016;89
2. Waeber G, Pécoud A, Cornuz J, Gaspoz JM, Perrier A. Relève en médecine interne générale: enjeux et perspectives. Rev Med Suisse. 2009;188
3. Weigel AM, Ullrich F, Shane DM, Mueller KJ. Variation in primary care service patterns by rural-urban location. J Rur Health. 2016;32:196–203.
4. Monnier M. Médecins de premier recours en Suisse romande: Qui sont-ils? Que font-ils? Prim Care. 2004;41
5. Gilchrist V, McCord G, Schrop SL, King BD, McCormick KF, Oprandi AM, et al. Physician activities during time out of the examination room. Ann Fam Med. 2005;3:494–9.

6. Jaccard Ruedin H, Weaver F. Ageing workforce in an ageing society - Combien de professionnels de santé seront nécessaires en Suisse d'ici 2030? Neuchâtel: Observatoire suisse de la santé (Obsan); 2009.
7. Cohidon C, Cornuz J, Senn N. Primary care in Switzerland: evolution of physicians' profile and activities in twenty years (1993-2012). BMC Fam Pract. 2015;16:107.
8. Grande D, Armstrong K. Community volunteerism of US physicians. J Gen Intern Med. 2008;23(12):1987–91.
9. Gruen RL, Campbell EG, Blumenthal D. Public roles of US physicians: community participation, political involvement, and collective advocacy. JAMA. 2006;296(20):2467–75.
10. Pathman DE, Steiner BD, Williams E, Riggins T. The four community dimensions of primary care practice. J Fam Pract. 1998;46:293–303.
11. Hostettler S, Kraft E. FMH Aerztestatistik 2015. http://www.fmh.ch/files/pdf17/SAEZ_12-13_Artikel_Aerztestatistik_2015_D.pdf. Accessed 27.09.2017.
12. Weinhold I, Gurtner S. Understanding shortages of sufficient health care in rural areas. Health Policy. 2014;118(2):201–14.
13. Steinhaeuser J, Joos S, Szecsenyi J, Miksch A. A comparison of the workload of rural and urban primary care physicians in Germany: analysis of a questionnaire survey. BMC Fam Pract. 2011;12:112.
14. Gottschalk A, Flocke SA. Time spent in face-to-face patient care and work outside the examination room. Ann Fam Med. 2005;3(6):488–93.
15. Granja M, Ponte C, Cavadas LF. What keeps family physicians busy in Portugal? A multicentre observational study of work other than direct patient contacts. BMJ Open. 2014;4(6):e005026.
16. Chen MA, Hollenberg JP, Michelen W, Peterson JC, Casalino LP. Patient care outside of office visits: a primary care physician time study. J Gen Intern Med. 2011;26(1):58–63.
17. Bickel MA, Brown AJ. Generation X: implications for faculty recruitment and development in academic health centers. Acad Med. 2005;80:205–10.
18. Le Floch B, Bastiaens H, Le reste YJ, Lingner H, Hoffman D, Czachowski S, et al. Which positive factors determine the GP satisfaction in clinical practice? A systematic literature review. BMC Fam Pract. 2016;17:133–41.
19. Bitterman H, Vinker S. Extending the boundaries of family medicine to perform manual procedures. Isr J Health Policy Res. 2014;3:35.
20. OECD Reviews of Health Systems, Switzerland, 2011. http://www.oecd.org/els/health-systems/oecdreviewsofhealthsystems-switzerland.htm. Accessed 27 Sept 2017.

16

How general practitioners understand and handle medically unexplained symptoms

Erik Børve Rasmussen[1*] and Karin Isaksson Rø[2]

Abstract

Background: Medically unexplained symptoms (MUS) are a common yet challenging encounter in primary care. The aim of this study was to explore how general practitioners (GPs) understand and handle MUS.

Methods: Three focus group interviews were conducted with a total of 23 GPs. Participants with varied clinical experience were purposively recruited. The data were analysed thematically, using the concept of framing as an analytical lens.

Results: The GPs alternated between a biomedical frame, centred on disease, and a biopsychosocial frame, centred on the sick person. Each frame shaped the GPs' understanding and handling of MUS. The biomedical frame emphasised the lack of objective evidence, problematized subjective patient testimony, and manifested feelings of uncertainty, doubt and powerlessness. This in turn complicated patient handling. In contrast, the biopsychosocial frame emphasised clinical experience, turned patient testimony into a valuable source of information, and manifested feelings of confidence and competence. This in turn made them feel empowered. The GPs with the least experience relied more on the biomedical frame, whereas their more seasoned seniors relied mostly on the biopsychosocial frame.

Conclusion: The biopsychosocial frame helps GPs to understand and handle MUS better than the biomedical frame does. Medical students should spend more time learning biopsychosocial medicine, and to integrate the clinical knowledge of their peers with their own.

Keywords: Medically unexplained symptoms, Primary care, Clinical knowledge and experience, Medical models, Framing

Background

Medically unexplained symptoms (MUS) is an umbrella term used to refer to various symptoms that 'have no identified organic basis' [1], and 'for which no adequate medical explanation can be found after a proper medical examination' [2]. As such, MUS force general practitioners (GPs) to base clinical judgements on something other than biomedical evidence [3]. Cases involving MUS are said to 'test the credibility of the doctor (...) for his or her inability to label the patient's complaint' [4], and it is well documented that MUS can be a challenge to both patient and doctor [5–7]. Those difficulties notwithstanding, MUS are among the largest categories of complaints in primary health care [8, 9]. In a recent Danish study, almost one in three patients belonged to this category [10]. Consequently, GPs need to understand and handle these patients' complaints. Yet, not enough is known about how GPs actually do this. In this article, we therefore explore GPs' approaches to understanding and handling MUS.

We use the concept of *frame* to explore GPs' approaches to MUS. Frames are shared ways of 'organising experience' [11, 12]. Each complaint can be interpreted under different framings, and each frame indicates different approaches to patient management. Studies suggest that whereas patients expect or demand that GPs employ a biomedical frame, GPs prefer a biopsychosocial frame [13–17]. This is perhaps not surprising, as the biopsychosocial model is at home in primary health care. Yet other studies suggest the opposite [18, 19];

* Correspondence: erik-borve.rasmussen@hioa.no
[1]Centre for the study of professions, OsloMet – Oslo Metropolitan University, P.O. Box. 4, St. Olavs plass, N-0130 Oslo, Norway

patients want support and compassion, but GPs provide somatic screening and intervention. Either way, the literature indicates a *tension* between a biomedical frame centred on disease and a biopsychosocial frame centred on the sick person [20]. This tension is heightened by health insurance policies and welfare bureaucracies that favour biomedicine [21, 22]. Little is known about how GPs negotiate those tensions, or how choice of frame affects patient management. This paper therefore explores how medical frames organise GPs' understanding of MUS, and how this enables (or disables) patient management. To that end, we conducted focus group interviews with GPs about MUS.

Methods

Design, setting and participants

Three focus group (FG) interviews were conducted in Norway in the first quarter of 2015. The number of groups was considered appropriate for an explorative study. Recruitment took advantage of established groups in the continuing medical education program (see Table 1 for group characteristics). In Norway, there is a five-year specialization program to become a specialist GP, which includes regular group supervision. The groups were informed about the study beforehand, and none refused to participate. We purposively sampled groups with varied experience [23], in terms of years and place of practice. FG1 mainly included non-specialists in training, most of whom work in suburbs around Oslo; FG2 was a mixture of doctors in training and experienced specialists in general practice, most of whom work in rural areas in the east of Norway; FG3 included experienced specialists, most of whom work in Oslo. The interviews were audio recorded and lasted for 90–120 min.

FGs are 'artificially set up situations' [24], 'created and managed by the researcher' [25], where participants and researchers *co-construct* [26] the data. It is therefore important to clarify researcher contributions to the data [27, 28]. EBR is a sociologist, KIR is a medical doctor trained in occupational medicine. EBR moderated the three interviews, KIR assisted. The semi-structured interview guide centred on experience with MUS and patient management (see Additional file 1). We asked about their experience with MUS, about what they considered typical features of patients with MUS, about what one should or should not do, and why. Moreover, we asked about the distinction between diseases and non-diseases, and about what diagnoses they used and why. We treated 'MUS' mainly as *placeholder* for conditions for which there are no biomedical evidence, meaning that apart from that criterion, we did not specify what conditions to discuss: we wanted them to decide. However, we did ask specific questions about sick listing, and in doing so, we implicitly excluded retired patients with MUS or patients with MUS who were already on permanent disability benefits.

FGs are good for producing concentrated amounts of data about issues for which it would be difficult to gather large sets of observations [25]. Additionally, by having groups of GPs engage each other in debate, FG methodology allowed us to use their experiences and perspectives as tools for exploration; they could give informed responses and rebuttals in ways we could not. Allowing participants' responses to each other to drive the interviews was also a fruitful way of exploring those aspects we did not know in advance to look for.

Table 1 Focus group composition and participant characteristics

	Experience (yrs.)			Specialist (yrs.)			Age (yrs.)			Gender	
	< 5	5–10	10 >	Not	< 5	5 >	< 40	40–50	50 >	F	M
FG1	7	1	1	8	–	1	6	3	–	4	5
FG2	1	3	5	2	2	5	1	3	5	4	5
FG3	–	3	2	–	3	2	–	5	–	4	1

Ethics, consent and permissions

The Norwegian Social Science Data Services approved the study (project number 41259). All participants gave written consent to participating, and for using the data in publications. Participants were also given the option to check the data used for publication.

Analysis

EBR transcribed in NVivo, drawing on Barbour's [29] annotation style. Italic font indicates emphasis; added information is in parentheses; brackets are used to describe events instead of representing them verbatim (typically non-lexical utterances, e.g. '[mhm]'); three stops indicate pauses in speaking ('...') or breaks in quotation ('(...)'). All quoted excerpts were translated by EBR.

Our disciplinary backgrounds allowed us to combine methodological skill with analytical sensitivity informed by clinical experience. Although sense making was an analytical interest from the outset, our interest specifically in clinical experience and medical frames grew out of interpretative engagement with the data and the literature. After initial analysis and coding done separately by EBR and KIR, we discussed and decided on a strategy for further analysis. EBR analysed the data thematically, broadly in line with Braun and Clarke [30], combining *descriptive* and in vivo coding styles [31]. The final analysis made sense of the various ways the GPs understood and handled MUS in our data. The two main themes are presented as medical frames in the following section.

Results

When discussing MUS, our participants alternated between 1) a biomedical frame, centred on disease, and 2) a biopsychosocial frame, centred on the sick person. Each frame accentuated different aspects of MUS. In the following, we describe how each frame organises GPs' understanding of MUS, and how this affects them, and their approach to handling patients.

MUS in the biomedical frame

The biomedical frame accentuated what is missing in MUS (objective signs of disease), and problems thought to flow from this absence. Consider excerpt A from FG1:

GP1

[T]here are rarely any specific issues with subjective *complaints*. That's definitely what I find the most difficult [mhm]. What the patient says and feels, that's what you have to deal with. And it's very difficult to assess, say, pain, objectively. Or to assess ... sadness, objectively [yes], anxiety, worries. So really, we're in a situation where we have to *listen* to the patient, and perhaps sick list based on that. And, when the law says that (...) we have the *opportunity* to sick list, even when we cannot *point* to anything *specific*. Then we have no choice but to trust the patient. And, of course, in principle, the patient decides what he or she wants to *say*. And then that can be entirely correct, or it could be entirely wrong [in-breath yes]. But often it's somewhere in between. Those are the difficult sick listing cases, definitely [mhm] ....

GP2

I think it's difficult too, with regards to the legislature. Because it clearly *states* that there should be a 'disease, injury or defect' (a legislative paraphrase) [mhm]. Usually, it's more of a borderline issue [mhm] (...).

GP3

And some of those sick notes are usually not the ones that last two- or three days. It's the ones that are a bit longer that are difficult, when it comes to unclear symptom constellations, or how to put it? I think *that's* where you're *dependent* on what the patient *says* (...).

GP2

There are many difficulties with the whole issue of fatigue. Examined, and yet we can't find anything, and then there are often a lot of burdens in their lives, which leads to the fatigue. And what are we to *do* about it [mhm]. Because, to sick list them ... I mean, there's no *disease* [mhm]. The way I see it.

GP3

Mhm. Tremendously difficult. (FG1).

The excerpt exhibits what was typical and related features of the biomedical framing of MUS. First, the focus throughout is on *the lack of objective evidence.* Thus, according to the GPs, 'there are rarely any specific issues' with MUS, GPs 'can't find anything', possibly because 'there's no disease' to be found (all from excerpt A). Some also pointed to the lack of scientific knowledge and explanation. For instance, one regretted not having 'an explanation for these conditions (MUS) in medical science' (FG2). When employing the biomedical frame, GPs thus understood and defined MUS negatively, in contrast with "normal" conditions for which evidence is obtainable and medical science has explanations on offer.

A second feature, and related to the former, is the strong emphasis on *subjective testimony as a problem.* Without objective evidence, GPs 'have no choice but to trust the patient' (GP1 excerpt A), i.e. they are '*dependent* on what the patient *says*' (GP3 excerpt A). Having to trust the patient was unpopular, as it involved the risk of being misinformed or even deceived. Patient testimony was thus framed as unreliable: it could be 'entirely correct, or it could be entirely wrong' (GP1 excerpt A). In other words, subjective testimony was considered a problematic source of knowledge about patients' conditions. Health insurance policy stipulates that impairment should have disease as its primary cause. Without evidence, the plausible presence of disease must be determined based on testimony. In the biomedical frame, sick listing thus becomes a problem of trust, and this is why some GPs felt it difficult to act responsibly as gatekeepers (see excerpt A).

Third, related to both lacking evidence and the low epistemic value attributed to testimony were frequent references to *negative feelings*, such as uncertainty and doubt. Some physicians were afraid that the patient might have a serious undetected problem, as expressed by a participant in FG2: 'Perhaps there's something else that I haven't seen?' Others emphasised how inability to obtain evidence spawned feelings of uncertainty, doubt and powerlessness. Consider excerpt B:

(...) we start to doubt how sick the patient is. Because we can't quite objectively *grab a hold* of these things. We can't do any blood tests, we can't scan them or anything. And then we begin to doubt a little. (FG2).

The GP explicitly ties his doubt to the inability to 'objectively grab a hold' of MUS. It is because he 'can't do any blood tests' or the likes that he begins 'to doubt how sick the patient is'. It is noteworthy that lack of evidence results in doubts in patients rather than doubt in medical knowledge. Some voiced suspicion of malingering. For instance, a participant in FG3 talked about two cases concerning young men with back pains. She 'couldn't find anything wrong' with their backs and concluded that they were unhappy with their jobs and wanted sick notes for their 'supposed back pains'. Some also complained about feeling powerless. Consider excerpt C:

I can urge, or give medical *counsel*, and I can *suggest* that we try and up the workload in accordance with what is considered medically appropriate. But, in the end, when she says 'No, I actually *cannot* work more (...) I have no choice but to *trust* the patient, and I really feel forced into doing what she wants [in-breath yes, mhm]. (FG1).

We emphasise that GPs *feel* powerless; their powers are no more restricted here than they are with biologically verifiable diseases like hyperthyroidism (legally, GPs cannot *make* patients do anything – they must counsel). But with MUS, GPs *feel* inhibited. Note also that the participant believes the patient to be healthier than the patient does. The GP's problem, then, is the lack of authoritative warrants. Without evidence to back him, he feels that he cannot (or should not) force or sway the patient.

The biomedical frame thus accentuated the lack of objective evidence, the problem of trust and subjective testimony, and various troubling emotions. For those reasons, the frame also brought up frequent references to how MUS made GPs' work difficult. Because the symptoms are 'difficult to assess', sick listing becomes difficult ('what are we to do about it?'), elevating the risk of going into what one GP called 'a stalemate', i.e. an unfruitful therapeutic situation (FG1).

MUS in the biopsychosocial frame

In contrast to the biomedical frame, the biopsychosocial frame accentuated what is present, and opportunities that flow from this presence. Thus, when talking about MUS in the biopsychosocial frame, the GPs emphasised understanding, confidence and competence. Consider excerpt D:

> A *nice* aspect of being a GP is getting to know people over time. And I'm thinking of my patient list a bit like my flock. I'm looking out for them, over time, to get the most out of it. They're going to be as comfortable as possible, so they can go to work, make money, pay taxes. And that means that you get to know people, and you can tell 'Will it pay off to invest in a small sick note? Be a little proactive about it [mhm]?' So that they'll return to work *quicker*? Almost like a preventive measure [mhm]. And I do have quite a few 'good girls' and a few 'good boys', who will at times stretch the rubber band a bit too far [M: mhm]. And then, some people need a little sick leave. So you've got to be watchful (...). (FG3).

Excerpt D exhibits several prominent accents of the biopsychosocial frame. First, the participant expresses an *understanding* of the condition of patients he characterises as 'good girls' and 'good boys' – Norwegian slang for dutiful persons who tend to exert themselves too far. He also explains the condition by way of metaphor, saying such patients 'will at times stretch the rubber band a bit too far' – i.e. the body's ability to recuperate (elasticity), is lost. In other words, he (feels that he) knows what is troubling his patient. Other patient types were suggested, such as 'the double-labouring woman', 'between 37 and 43 years old, with three kids (...) and a job in the care services', whose conditions were understandable to the participants: 'It's in the *entire* system, the *entire* body, and the burden becomes *too heavy*' (FG2). This was typical of the biopsychosocial frame: MUS were discussed in terms of patient types the participants understood and could accept.

Second, because the participant in excerpt D feels confident that he understands, he also seems *confident about how to handle* these patients. He 'can tell' when a brief sick leave 'will pay off', and so he is 'watchful'. In other words, he (believes that he) knows what to do. As a result, he does not seem worried about sick listing patients with MUS. In his experience with these patients, using sick notes for the present condition can work 'like a preventive measure' for a later longer, and possibly irreversible illness trajectory. Understanding MUS in terms of patient types thus seems clinically efficacious. The contrast with the biomedical framing of MUS in this regard is striking.

Third, the participant in excerpt D ties his understanding with his *clinical experience*: it is because he gets 'to know people over time' that he 'can tell' what is wrong. This, we suggest, is a seminal effect of the biopsychosocial frame: it invites GPs to draw on their clinical experience to make sense of MUS. It is not simply that GPs come to trust what their patients say. By drawing on their extensive clinical experience, GPs can acquire a holistic understanding of the sick person, enabling them to act with confidence. Note that 'understanding' does not imply veracity – the GP could have the wrong idea. What is implied is rather that the patient's complaint is rendered meaningful in a clinically helpful way. Moreover, because GPs get 'to know people over time', trust is not (as much of) an issue. The credibility of patients' suffering is not called into question. Consider excerpt E:

GP1

You have to *see* them over *time*, you have to get to *know* people, so you can *sense-*, or *form* a picture, over time. Is it *real*? Do they *have* these troubles, these impairments they claim to have? That you don't have instruments to measure. And I'm thinking *this* is where being a doctor is *exciting* [Yes]! This is where the art of medicine comes in! And where people knowledge comes in! Whereas with these other conditions, if a leg is *broken* or you've *seen* a heart attack on EKG. *Alright* then (inaudible, chuckles) that's technique. But its not much of an *art of medicine.* (...).

GP2

I think that when you *know* the patient, like (GP1) says, over a quite *extended* period of time, I think most of us would agree that ... the suffering is *there.* I think one *feels* that quite well, that there is no *doubt* that these patients suffer, and are *sick.* (FG2).

The emphasis on clinical experience ('people knowledge') and 'the art of medicine' was at times coupled with a distancing from scientific medicine and medical training, as in excerpt F:

> (...) I feel that, in the course of an ordinary day, I can see *rather* a *lot* of patients, without having to use what I learnt in medical school, like *academic* or *scientific* (training). It's more like ... 'yes, mhm, yes I understand, mhm' (pretending to answer a patient). I mean, *that's* what we spend our time doing. (FG1).

Thus, in the biopsychosocial frame, MUS concerns what they do know, instead of what they do not. Rather than worrying about the lack of objective signs of disease and evidence based treatment, talking about MUS in the biopsychosocial frame meant relying on clinical experience (with individual patients and patient types), informal explanatory models and interpretation. In the biopsychosocial frame, MUS thus become (more) tangible.

Differences between groups

The use of frames differed across the focus groups. The group with specialists in training (FG1) relied heavily (though not entirely) on the biomedical frame. In contrast, the group of experienced specialists (FG3) relied almost exclusively on the biopsychosocial frame for discussing MUS. FG2, the group with the most variation in clinical experience, slightly emphasised the biopsychosocial frame. Similarly, outspoken preference for biomarkers ('the more objective (...) the more we like it') was frequently expressed in FG1 (the juniors), less frequently in FG2 (mixed group), and not once in FG3 (the seniors). Moreover, expressions of insecurity and frustration regarding patient management was frequently expressed in FG1, in contrast to FG3, whose members seemed confident about themselves and their own judgement. When the seniors in FG3 and FG2 voiced their frustration, it typically concerned bureaucrats and consulting physicians who did not accept the GPs' clinical judgement and instead instigated 'the burden of evidence' on them.

Discussion

Our analysis has shown how two medical frames shaped GPs' understanding of MUS, and how this affected them and their approach to handling patients. Biomedical framing emphasised what is missing (objective evidence) , made what is present (patient testimony) problematic, and manifested feelings of uncertainty, doubt and powerlessness. By comparison, biopsychosocial framing seemed to lessen and even solve some of those problems. In particular, it made the conditions understandable and turned patient testimony into a valuable source of information, which in turn made GPs more comfortable and confident. A main reason for these differences, we suggest, is that whereas the biomedical frame invites GPs to draw on formal and scientific knowledge (of little use with MUS), the biopsychosocial frame invites GPs to draw on their clinical experience to make sense of their patients' problems. This enables them to make clinically efficacious distinctions between patients with MUS that give direction to clinical judgement.

In terms of patient handling, biomedical framing centred on what the patient has (disease or not). Since this is precisely what cannot be biomedically determined, handling (such as sick listing) became problematic. In contrast, biopsychosocial framing centred on how to improve the patient's condition. For instance, the GPs suggested that short-term sick listing can alleviate stress and prevent long-term absence from work, and that being compassionate and supportive can help patients cope with their situation. Paraphrasing Stone [32], the biomedical frame thus manifested "the botanist", bent on scientific classification, whereas the biopsychosocial frame manifested "the gardener", bent on nurturing and making things "grow". In terms of handling MUS, the latter mode currently seems more appropriate and effective.

Finally, the GPs with the most experience tended mostly to employ the biopsychosocial frame, whereas those with the least experience tended to rely more on the biomedical frame.

Choosing medical frames

The biopsychosocial model is at home in primary health care, and seems better suited for handling MUS. So why was biomedical framing a prominent feature in the FGs? In short, because framing is not simply a matter of personal choice. For one, GPs' framing practices are subject to external pressure: there is a strong institutional emphasis on the biomedical model of disease. Formally speaking, health related benefits are contingent on a biomedical account [21, 22]. When trying to secure disability pension for patients whom they consider sufficiently impaired, GPs therefore bear 'a burden of evidence', as one participant put it (FG2). Moreover, there is a strong cultural preference for clear-cut biomedical diseases and diagnoses in medicine [33–35]. As one participant put it, 'The more objective the findings, the more we like it, because that means we can verify it [mhm]. What we *don't* like are conditions where you have *zero* objective findings (...)' (FG1). GPs are thus part of a culture that values objective evidence and unambiguous disease (and this preference is not restricted to medicine [36]). There is thus an impetus towards a biomedical framing of MUS. As one participant said, 'we have to try to *create* this "cause effect" model that we should feel makes sense *ourselves*, that the patient should feel makes sense and that NAV (the national insurance bureaucracy) should feel makes sense' (FG2). For these reasons, framing is not simply a matter of choice.

Situating our findings

Our study is small, and the findings cannot be generalized to all GPs. However, although few studies have explored the effect of medical frames, our findings and their theoretical underpinnings are supported by – and shed light on tensions within – existing research literature.

First, regarding the negative effects of biomedical framing of MUS, studies typically report that GPs experience negative emotions when working with MUS, such as uncertainty, fear, frustration and powerlessness [2, 3, 37–41]. Yet few studies attempt to understand the cause of the negative emotions on a deeper level. We suggest viewing GPs' emotions as frame related, as expressions of whether or not a frame promotes action and understanding. On examining the data presented in these studies, this interpretation makes sense. For instance, a doctor in one study by Warner et al. said MUS are challenging because 'it doesn't fit the medical mould (...)' [38]. Our finding that GPs' biomedical framing makes subjective testimony problematic could also help explain why patients are reported to feel distrusted and misunderstood, and that they must struggle to be recognised as legitimate sufferers [1, 16, 42–45]. Although others have pointed to the lack of fit between biomedicine and MUS [46, 47], we have not found studies that show *how* biomedical framing makes MUS problematic. Our findings thus help tie frequently reported problems of MUS to the biomedical model of disease: it is against such a background that trust in patient testimony, and lacking objective evidence and scientific explanations, become problematic.

Second, our finding regarding the positive effects of biopsychosocial framing also finds support in the literature. Although rarely highlighted, several studies reporting negative emotions also show examples of GPs feeling confident about their ability to understand and handle MUS. And typically, this is when they depart from a biomedical frame. For instance, Wileman et al. [39] reports that despite the GPs' negative feelings, they 'felt that showing an empathy with the patient, and taking an interest in them (...), enabled the patient to gain personal trust in the doctor'. Moreover, the GPs 'felt they had the opportunity to 'know' such patients better (than other doctors), and build a relationship upon which successful management could be based' [39]. GPs are also typically reported to explain MUS by considering the sick person in his or her psychosocial context [2, 3, 37, 39, 40, 48–50]. While the link between this understanding and a form of biopsychosocial framing is rarely explicated, it is certainly indicated. Moreover, studies of sick listing MUS in primary care indicate the need to assess patients' complaints holistically, and emphasise the importance of trust and knowing the patient over time [49, 51, 52]. Finally, studies into occupational medicine support our claim that the epistemic valuation of patient testimony is frame related [12, 22]. In particular, Dodier's description of the "clinical frame" and the "solicitude frame" resemble our description of biomedical and biopsychosocial frames, respectively: in the latter, 'the patient's complaints have the status of an 'unconditional force' and their legitimacy is not therefore called into question' [12].

The work of Mik-Meyer [3, 49] approximates ours. She too finds that 'biomedical classification and diagnostic tools (...) were replaced with trust and confidence when doctors were working with patients with MUS' [3]. Yet Mik-Meyer claims that 'MUS create an important, new role for doctors', in which they 'are encouraged to make judgements on the basis on something other than purely objective medical findings (...)' [3]. We think that lacking objective evidence is an inherent part of clinical work. Instead of a new role, we suggest, what is required is the role belonging to what Jewson called "Bedside Medicine" [53], centred on the 'total psychosomatic disturbance' of the sick person. In other words, what is needed is a proper 'general physician' [54] (coupled, of course, with proper scientific research into the nature and causes of MUS).

Third, regarding our finding that the junior GPs relied the most on biomedical framing and expressed more insecurity and frustration than the seniors, the literature indicates that this is not coincidental. Studies suggest that understanding and handling MUS is more problematic for inexperienced GPs [41, 50, 55, 56]. Some indicate that 'physicians who are in practice longer experience less stress from uncertainty than those in practice for shorter periods of time' [57, 58]. Others report that junior GPs feel unsure of themselves specifically because of their lack of training and experience with MUS [41, 55], and are reported to be *less strict* gatekeepers than their experienced peers [59]. One possible reason for these findings is a selection mechanism, whereby those who are "biomedically minded" and insecure change job, whereas those who are biopsychosocially minded and comfortable stay. An alternative and likely complementary reason is that since biopsychosocial framing invites GPs to draw on their experience, there is a reciprocal relationship, wherein experience supports the frame, and the frame supports the use and generation of relevant experience. In other words, *biopsychosocial practice builds confidence.* More research is needed, and in that regard we note that experience is not limited to number of years – the type of experience (e.g. feeling that you succeed) likely matters most.

Conclusion

We suggest that biopsychosocial framing, combined with clinical experience, enables GPs to understand and handle MUS better than biomedical framing does. However, that does not necessarily imply that biopsychosocially minded GPs benefit patients and society. Although similarities between MUS have been found [54], it remains a differentiated patient group, and there are few widely acknowledged efficacy studies (even the cautious indications of PACE are now in question, see [60]). Studies indicate that many (but not all) patients want more support, compassion and understanding [18, 19], and for GPs to be attentive to their personal circumstance [61]. (Note that there is no contradiction between these wishes and believing that one's condition is rooted in an undetected somatic pathogen.) This supports the notion that biopsychosocial framing benefits patients as well as doctors. Moreover, fewer rounds of diagnostic screening and referral would save time and costs, which could benefit other patients. But there are also possible problems: biopsychosocial framing likely increases the tendency to medicalise ordinary troubles [62–64], and there is ample room for implicit bias [65, 66] in the clinical judgement of practitioners who are overly confident in their "people knowledge". Clearly, more research is needed.

Strengths and limitations

The strength of qualitative studies, such as focus-group interviews, is their ability to provide experience-based knowledge and insight, rather than a quantitative ranking of importance or the proportional distribution of opinions [25, 67]. Including doctors with different lengths of experience, specialists as well as physicians in training and doctors of both genders, ensures a diversity in experience, although we cannot draw robust conclusions. The inter-disciplinary collaboration between a sociologist (EBR) and a medical doctor (KIR) has potentiated critical reflection when interpreting the data. This can result in a more nuanced and balanced discussion, but in some cases also lead to less clear-cut conclusions than if only one perspective had prevailed. External validity or transferability can be assessed in relation to how the data are discussed [27]. As we show, our results are in line with previous research in this field. Moreover, we have presented our findings at medical and sociological conferences, and our conclusions were recognizable and credible to these different groups.

Implications

If biopsychosocial thinking and clinical experience are central to GPs' understanding and handling of MUS, than this should be reflected in research, teaching and practice. What is needed is an emphasis on the role of *clinical knowledge* [68, 69]. Clinical knowledge emerges in the course of practice, i.e. the daily chore of interpreting and interacting with patients, and applying general concepts to individual persons [68, 70, 71]. It is thus local, hermeneutic and experience based; its genesis bottom-up, contrasting top-down scientific and evidence-based knowledge. Such knowledge is the core of clinical reasoning and judgement [69, 71–73]. Yet not enough is known about its content and consequences [68, 74–76]. Thus, experienced-based ways of knowing must be studied further, so that they may be shared and scrutinised for the betterment of patients and practitioners [68]. In line with this, medical students should spend more time learning to think biopsychosocially, and to integrate the clinical knowledge of their peers and seniors with their own. There is no denying the success of the biomedical model, but its uses are limited: quality primary care is impossible without acknowledging that personality and circumstance are major constituents of patients' health [77, 78].

Abbreviations

FG: focus group; GP: general practitioner; MUS: medically unexplained symptoms

Acknowledgements

The authors would like to thank Berit Bringedal and Lars EF Johannessen for instructive comments, and the participants for their invaluable contributions.

Authors' contributions

Both authors contributed to the overall focus of the manuscript, based on discussion and preliminary analysis of the data. EBR is responsible for the research design, moderated the focus groups, transcribed and translated the data, performed the final analysis and wrote the majority of the manuscript. KIR assisted in the focus groups, and commented on the analysis and writing. Both authors read and approved the final manuscript.

Competing interests

The authors declare they have no competing interests.

Author details
[1]Centre for the study of professions, OsloMet – Oslo Metropolitan University, P.O. Box. 4, St. Olavs plass, N-0130 Oslo, Norway. [2]LEFO, Institute for studies of the medical profession, Oslo, Norway.

References

1. Nettleton S. 'I just want permission to be ill': towards a sociology of medically unexplained symptoms. Soc Sci Med. 2006 Mar;62(5):1167–78.
2. den Boeft M, Huisman D, van der Wouden JC, Numans ME, van der Horst HE, Lucassen PL, et al. Recognition of patients with medically unexplained physical symptoms by family physicians: results of a focus group study. BMC Fam Pract. 2016 May 12;17:55.
3. Mik-Meyer N. The social negotiation of illness: doctors' role as clinical or political in diagnosing patients with medically unexplained symptoms. Soc Theory Health. 2015 Feb;13(1):30–45.
4. Jutel A. Medically unexplained symptoms and the disease label. Soc Theory Health. 2010 Aug;8(3):229–45.
5. Czachowski S, Piszczek E, Sowinska A, Hartman TCO. Challenges in the management of patients with medically unexplained symptoms in Poland: a qualitative study. Fam Pract. 2012 Apr;29(2):228–34.
6. olde Hartman TC, Hassink-Franke LJ, Lucassen PL, van SKP, van WC. Explanation and relations. How do general practitioners deal with patients with persistent medically unexplained symptoms: a focus group study. BMC Fam Pract. 2009;10(1):68.
7. Shattock L, Williamson H, Caldwell K, Anderson K, Peters S. 'They've just got symptoms without science': medical trainees' acquisition of negative attitudes towards patients with medically unexplained symptoms. Patient Educ Couns. 2013;91(2):249–54.
8. Brown RJ. Introduction to the special issue on medically unexplained symptoms: background and future directions. Clin Psychol Rev. 2007 Oct; 27(7):769–80.
9. Burton C. Beyond somatisation: a review of the understanding and treatment of medically unexplained physical symptoms (MUPS). Br J Gen Pract. 2003 Mar;53(488):231–9.
10. Rosendal M, Carlsen AH, Rask MT. Symptoms as the main problem: a cross-sectional study of patient experience in primary care. BMC Fam Pract. 2016 Mar 10;17:29.
11. Goffman E. Frame analysis: an essay on the organization of experience. Vol. ix. Cambridge, MA, US: Harvard University Press; 1974. 586 p
12. Dodier N. Expert medical decisions in occupational medicine: a sociological analysis of medical judgment. Sociol Health Illn. 1994 Sep 1;16(4):489–514.
13. Allegretti A, Borkan J, Reis S, Griffiths F. Paired interviews of shared experiences around chronic low back pain: classic mismatch between patients and their doctors. Fam Pract. 2010 Dec;27(6):676–83.
14. Baker SC, Gallois C, Driedger SM, Santesso N. Communication accommodation and managing musculoskeletal disorders: doctors' and patients' perspectives. Health Commun. 2011 Jun 1;26(4):379–88.
15. May C, Allison G, Chapple A, Chew-Graham C, Dixon C, Gask L, et al. Framing the doctor-patient relationship in chronic illness: a comparative study of general practitioners' accounts. Sociol Health Illn. 2004 Mar;26(2): 135–58.
16. Peters S, Stanley I, Rose M, Salmon P. Patients with medically unexplained symptoms: sources of patients' authority and implications for demands on medical care. Soc Sci Med. 1998 Mar;46(4–5):559–65.
17. Toye F, Barker K. 'Could I be imagining this?' – the dialectic struggles of people with persistent unexplained back pain. Disabil Rehabil. 2010 Jan 1; 32(21):1722–32.
18. Salmon P, Ring A, Dowrick CF, Humphris GM. What do general practice patients want when they present medically unexplained symptoms, and why do their doctors feel pressurized? J Psychosom Res. 2005 Oct;59(4):255–60.
19. Salmon P, Dowrick CF, Ring A, Humphris GM. Voiced but unheard agendas: qualitative analysis of the psychosocial cues that patients with unexplained symptoms present to general practitioners. Br J Gen Pr. 2004 Mar 1;54(500):171–6.
20. Cassell E. The nature of suffering and the goals of medicine [internet]. New York NY: Oxford University Press; 1991.
21. Kalisch DW, Aman T, Buchele LA. Social and Health policies in OECD countries [internet]. Paris: organisation for economic co-operation and Development; 1998 Jul.
22. Meershoek A, Krumeich A, Vos R. Judging without criteria? Sickness certification in Dutch disability schemes. Sociol Health Illn. 2007 May 1;29(4):497–514.
23. Marshall MN. Sampling for qualitative research. Fam Pract. 1996 Jan 1;13(6):522–6.
24. Kitzinger J. The methodology of focus groups: the importance of interaction between research participants. Sociol Health Illn. 1994;16(1):103–21.
25. Morgan DL. Focus groups as qualitative research: SAGE Publications; 1996. 92 p
26. Wilkinson S. Focus groups in feminist research: power, interaction, and the co-construction of meaning. Womens Stud Int Forum. 1998 Jan;21(1):111–25.
27. Malterud K. Qualitative research: standards, challenges, and guidelines. Lancet. 2001 Aug 11;358(9280):483–8.
28. Tong A, Sainsbury P, Craig J. Consolidated criteria for reporting qualitative research (COREQ): a 32-item checklist for interviews and focus groups. Int J Qual Health Care. 2007 Dec 1;19(6):349–57.
29. Barbour RS. Analysing focus groups. In: Flick U, editor. The SAGE handbook of qualitative data analysis. London: SAGE; 2013. p. 313–26.
30. Braun V, Clarke V. Using thematic analysis in psychology. Qual Res Psychol. 2006 Jan 1;3(2):77–101.
31. Saldana J. The coding manual for qualitative researchers. SAGE; 2009. 369 p.
32. Stone L. Being a botanist and a gardener: using diagnostic frameworks in general practice patients with medically unexplained symptoms. Aust J Prim Health. 2013 May 27;19(2):90–7.
33. Album D, Johannessen LEF, Rasmussen EB. Stability and change in disease prestige: A comparative analysis of three surveys spanning a quarter of a century. Soc Sci Med. 2017 May 1;180(Supplement C):45–51.
34. Album D, Westin S. Do diseases have a prestige hierarchy? A survey among physicians and medical students. Soc Sci Med. 2008 Jan;66(1):182–8.
35. Rasmussen EB. Balancing medical accuracy and diagnostic consequences: diagnosing medically unexplained symptoms in primary care. Sociol Health Illn. 2017 Sep 1;39(7):1227–41.
36. Grue J, Johannessen LEF, Rasmussen EF. Prestige rankings of chronic diseases and disabilities. A survey among professionals in the disability field. Soc Sci Med. 2015 Jan;124:180–6.
37. Stone L. Making sense of medically unexplained symptoms in general practice: a grounded theory study. Ment Health Fam Med. 2013 Jun;10(2):101–11.
38. Warner A, Walters K, Lamahewa K, Buszewicz M. How do hospital doctors manage patients with medically unexplained symptoms: a qualitative study of physicians. J R Soc Med. 2017 Feb 1;110(2):65–72.
39. Wileman L, May C, Chew-Graham CA. Medically unexplained symptoms and the problem of power in the primary care consultation: a qualitative study. Fam Pract. 2002 Apr 1;19(2):178–82.
40. Woivalin T, Krantz G, Mäntyranta T, Ringsberg KC. Medically unexplained symptoms: perceptions of physicians in primary health care. Fam Pract. 2004 Apr 1;21(2):199–203.
41. Howman M, Walters K, Rosenthal J, Ajjawi R, Buszewicz M. "You kind of want to fix it don't you?" exploring general practice trainees' experiences of managing patients with medically unexplained symptoms. BMC Med Educ. 2016 Dec;16(1)
42. Aamland A, Malterud K, Werner EL. Patients with persistent medically unexplained physical symptoms: a descriptive study from Norwegian general practice. BMC Fam Pract. 2014 May 29;15(1):107.
43. Cooper L. Myalgic encephalomyelitis and the medical encounter. Sociol Health Illn. 1997 Mar;19(2):186–207.
44. Werner A, Isaksen LW, Malterud K. 'I am not the kind of woman who complains of everything': illness stories on self and shame in women with chronic pain. Soc Sci Med. 2004;59(5):1035–46.
45. Werner A, Malterud K. It is hard work behaving as a credible patient: encounters between women with chronic pain and their doctors. Soc Sci Med. 2003 Oct;57(8):1409–19.
46. Aronowitz RA. When do symptoms become a disease? Ann Intern Med. 2001 May 1;134(9_Part_2):803–8.
47. Chiong W. Diagnosing and defining disease. JAMA. 2001 Jan 3;285(1):89–90.
48. Horton-Salway M. Bio-psycho-social reasoning in GPs' case narratives: the discursive construction of ME patients' identities. Health (N Y). 2002 Oct 1;6(4):401–21.
49. Mik-Meyer N, Obling AR. The negotiation of the sick role: general practitioners' classification of patients with medically unexplained

symptoms. Sociol Health Illn. 2012 Sep;34(7):1025–38.
50. Stone L. Managing the consultation with patients with medically unexplained symptoms: a grounded theory study of supervisors and registrars in general practice. BMC Fam Pract. 2014;15:192.
51. Nilsen S, Werner EL, Maeland S, Eriksen HR, Magnussen LH. Considerations made by the general practitioner when dealing with sick-listing of patients suffering from subjective and composite health complaints. Scand J Prim Health Care. 2011 Mar 1;29(1):7–12.
52. Nilsen S, Malterud K, Werner EL, Maeland S, Magnussen LH. GPs' negotiation strategies regarding sick leave for subjective health complaints. Scand J Prim Health Care. 2015 Jan 2;33(1):40–6.
53. Jewson ND. The disappearance of the sick-man from medical cosmology, 1770-1870. Sociology. 1976 May 1;10(2):225–44.
54. Wessely S, Nimnuan C, Sharpe M. Functional somatic syndromes: one or many? Lancet. 1999 Sep 11;354(9182):936–9.
55. Yon K, Nettleton S, Walters K, Lamahewa K, Buszewicz M. Junior doctors' experiences of managing patients with medically unexplained symptoms: a qualitative study. BMJ Open. 2015 Dec 1;5(12):e009593.
56. Salmon P, Peters S, Clifford R, Iredale W, Gask L, Rogers A, et al. Why do general practitioners decline training to improve Management of Medically Unexplained Symptoms? J Gen Intern Med. 2007 May 1;22(5):565–71.
57. Gerrity MS, DeVellis RF, Earp JA. Physicians' reactions to uncertainty in patient care: a new measure and new insights. Med Care. 1990;28(8):724–36.
58. Gerrity MS, Earp JAL, DeVellis RF, Light DW. Uncertainty and professional work: perceptions of physicians in clinical practice. Am J Sociol. 1992 Jan 1; 97(4):1022–51.
59. Markussen S, Røed K, Røgeberg O. The changing of the guards. Can family doctors contain worker absenteeism? J Health Econ. 2013 Dec;32(6):1230–9.
60. Marks DF. Special issue on the PACE trial. J Health Psychol. 2017 Aug 1; 22(9):1103–5.
61. Houwen J, Lucassen PLBJ, Stappers HW, Assendelft PJJ, van Dulmen S, Hartman O, et al. Medically unexplained symptoms: the person, the symptoms and the dialogue. Fam Pract. 2017 Apr 1;34(2):245–51.
62. Illich I. Medicalization of life. J Med Ethics. 1975;1(2):73–7.
63. Conrad P. The medicalization of society: on the transformation of human conditions into treatable disorders. Baltimore MD: Johns Hopkins University Press; 2008. 224 p
64. Barker KK. The social construction of illness. Medicalization and contested illness. In: Bird CE, Conrad P, Fremont AM, Timmermans S, editors. Handbook of medical sociology. Nashville TN: Vanderbilt University press; 2010. p. 147–62.
65. Kahneman D. Thinking, Fast and slow. London: Penguin Books; 2011.
66. Groopman J. How doctors think. Houghton Mifflin: New York NY; 2007.
67. Malterud K. Shared understanding of the qualitative research process. Guidelines for the medical researcher. Fam Pract. 1993 Jul 1;10(2):201–6.
68. Malterud K. The art and science of clinical knowledge: evidence beyond measures and numbers. Lancet. 2001 Aug 4;358(9279):397–400.
69. Horton R. The interpretive turn. Lancet Lond. 1995;346(8966):3.
70. Malterud K. Clinical knowledge: facts or something more? Some epistemological points of view. Tidsskr Nor Laegeforen. 1993;113(26):3248–50.
71. Malterud K. Reflexivity and metapositions: strategies for appraisal of clinical evidence. J Eval Clin Pract. 2002 May 1;8(2):121–6.
72. Leder D. Clinical interpretation - the hermeneutics of medicine. Theor Med. 1990 Mar;11(1):9–24.
73. Montgomery K. How doctors think: clinical judgement and the practice of medicine. Oxford: Oxford University Press; 2006. VIII, 246 s
74. Malterud K. The legitimacy of clinical knowledge: towards a medical epistemology embracing the art of medicine. Theor Med. 1995 Jun 1; 16(2):183–98.
75. Malterud K. The social construction of clinical knowledge – the context of culture and discourse. Commentary on Tonelli (2006), integrating evidence into clinical practice: an alternative to evidence-based approaches. Journal of evaluation in clinical practice 12, 248–256. J Eval Clin Pract. 2006 Jun 1; 12(3):292–5.
76. Malterud K. Theory and interpretation in qualitative studies from general practice: why and how? Scand J Public Health. 2016 Mar 1;44(2):120–9.
77. Dixon DM, Sweeney KG, Gray DJ. The physician healer: ancient magic or modern science? Br J Gen Pr. 1999;49(441):309–12.
78. Olesen F, Dickinson J, Hjortdahl P. General practice—time for a new definition. BMJ. 2000 Feb 5;320(7231):354–7.

Use of diagnostic tests and the appropriateness of the treatment decision in patients with suspected urinary tract infection in primary care in Denmark

Gloria Córdoba[1*], Anne Holm[1], Tina Møller Sørensen[2], Volkert Siersma[1], Håkon Sandholdt[1], Marjukka Makela[3], Niels Frimodt-Møller[4] and Lars Bjerrum[1]

Abstract

Background: Inappropriate prescription of antibiotics is the leading driver of antimicrobial resistance (AMR). The majority of antibiotics are prescribed in primary care.

Understanding how general practitioners (GPs) use diagnostic tests and the effect on treatment decision under daily practice conditions is important to reduce inappropriate prescription of antibiotics. The aim of the study was to investigate the use of diagnostic tests in primary care patients with suspected urinary tract infection (UTI) and to assess the appropriateness of the treatment decision (TD) under daily practice conditions in Denmark.

Methods: Prospective observational study. Symptomatic adult patients consulting general practice with suspected UTI recruited over 12 months. The diagnostic workup was registered in a standardized form. The appropriateness of the TD was assessed based on the results of a culture performed at a reference microbiological laboratory. TD was considered appropriate if a patient had a positive culture and was prescribed antibiotics or had a negative culture and was not prescribed antibiotics. TD was considered inappropriate if a patient had a negative culture and was prescribed antibiotics (overtreatment) or had a positive culture and was not prescribed antibiotics (undertreatment).

Results: Four hundred and eighty-eight patients were included. Dipstick was used in 98% of the patients and urine culture was used in 89% of the patients; 317 had the culture performed in practice and 117 had the culture performed at the hospital. The appropriateness of the final TD was significantly ($p = 0.04$) lower in patients without culture (55%) than in patients with culture performed in practice (71%) or at hospital (69%).

Conclusion: In a context with wide availability of diagnostic tests, GPs use diagnostic tests for the decision-making process in all patients with suspected UTI. Urine culture is used in the majority of the patients and is associated with a higher proportion of appropriate treatment decisions. Performance of urine culture is therefore important in reducing inappropriate antibiotic prescribing in patients with suspected UTI seeking care in general practice in Denmark.

Keywords: Treatment decision, Point-of-care systems, Urinary tract infections, Anti- bacterial agents, Primary care, Diagnostic test

* Correspondence: gloriac@sund.ku.dk
[1]The Research Unit for General Practice and Section of General Practice, Department of Public Health, University of Copenhagen, Øster Farimagsgade 5, 1014 Copenhagen, Denmark
Full list of author information is available at the end of the article

Background

Optimizing the use of antimicrobials and increasing the investment in diagnostic tests are part of the key strategies of the World Health Organization (WHO) for counteracting the spread and development of antimicrobial resistance (AMR) [1].

Denmark has a low prescription rate of antimicrobials at primary health care level in comparison to other European countries [2]. Nonetheless, there is still a high use of antibiotics at primary health care level [3].

In Denmark, suspected Urinary tract infection (UTI) is a frequent cause for antibiotic prescribing [4] and use of point-of-care tests (POCTs) [5]. There are no national guidelines on the diagnostic procedures to be followed in patients with suspected UTI. It is up to the GPs as managers/owners of the practice to decide the type of urine tests that are available in their practice. Furthermore, it is up to the GPs as clinicians to decide whether a diagnostic test should be performed in a patient with suspected UTI.

There is wide availability of diagnostic tests, which can be used in patients with suspected UTI. The diagnostic workup may include 1) dipstick, 2) microscopy, 3) culture performed and interpreted in practice, and/or 4) culture sent to a hospital laboratory. All practices can send urine samples for culture at hospital and most practices have a small laboratory where they can perform simple testing. GPs receive a fee for performing tests in practice, and there is no economic restriction to the number of tests per individual patient.

The use of urine culture implies a two-step treatment decision: first a decision when the patient consults the GP (index consultation), and a second step after the result of the urine culture is available. For cultures performed in practice, the results can be seen 1 day after the index consultation, while it may take up to 3 or 4 days to receive the results from a hospital.

In busy primary care, diagnostic test results may not translate directly to treatment decisions [6, 7], as these decisions are affected by several contextual factors [8, 9]. Therefore, the impact of diagnostic workup on appropriate treatment should be assessed under daily practice conditions.

The aim of this study was to describe the use of diagnostic tests in patients with suspected UTI and to assess the impact of the diagnostic work-up on the treatment decision under daily practice conditions in Denmark.

Methods

Design and setting

The study protocol has been published previously [10]. An observational study of the management of patients with suspected UTI in general practice under daily practice conditions was carried out between December 2014 and December 2015. It was part of the context assessment of a quality improvement program aimed at reducing the inappropriate prescription of antibiotics in patients with suspected UTI.

Study population and data collection

A random sample of 500 practices from the capital region of Copenhagen was invited by letter to participate; 39 accepted the invitation. Each practice included up to 20 patients fulfilling four criteria: a) > 18 years of age, b) presence of dysuria and/or frequency, c) suspected UTI, d) not currently taking antibiotics. In a standardized form the GPs registered number of days with symptoms, types of symptoms, potential risk factors for UTI, diagnostic workup performed, and treatment decision.

Urine sample – Reference standard

All patients were requested to provide a mid-stream urine sample (approx. 20 ml) of which half could be used for diagnostic purposes in practice, and the other half (reference standard) was cultured at a reference laboratory (Statens Serum Institute, SSI). The sample analysed by SSI was preserved in boric acid and sent by certified post on the day of the consultation. Results from the reference standard analysis were not available for the participating GPs.

At SSI, cultures were analyzed by a microbiology technician who had no information about the clinical history of the patient. A positive culture was defined as growth of $\geq 10^3$ colony forming units per milliliter (CFU/ml) for *E. coli* and *S. saprophyticus*, $\geq 10^4$ CFU/mL for other typical uropathogens and $\geq 10^5$ CFU/ml for possible uropathogens according to the European Urinalysis Standards [11].

Definition of variables

As the main focus of analysis was the role of diagnostic tests in the decision-making process, treatment decision was selected as the primary outcome [10]. The appropriateness of the treatment decision was evaluated against the reference standard (i.e. culture at SSI). Treatment decision was considered as appropriate when a patient with a positive reference culture was prescribed antibiotics or a patient with a negative culture received no antibiotics. Treatment decision was considered as inappropriate for patients with a negative culture who received antibiotics (overtreatment) or patients with a positive culture who were not prescribed antibiotics (undertreatment).

UTI was defined as complicated if the patient was a man, a pregnant woman, a woman ≥65 years, had a relevant co-morbidity or was assessed by the nurse or GP to have complicated cystitis or pyelonephritis. An anamnestic score was calculated. It is the sum of positive findings recorded by the GP, in the standardized data collection form, during the anamnestic phase of the consultation (range 1–11).

The diagnostic pathways were categorized into three groups: a) no urine culture performed, b) urine culture performed in practice, and c) urine culture performed at the hospital.

Statistical analysis

The statistical analysis was performed in two steps. First, possible determinants for the use of the various diagnostic tests were investigated in logistic regression models. We tested the following predictor variables individually with practices as a random intercept. The predictors were: a) anamnestic information, b) availability of diagnostic tests and c) information from any diagnostic tests previously performed (See Additional file 1: Table S1).

Secondly, we used a permutation test to assess the impact of the diagnostic pathway variable on the treatment decision . The multinomial regression model was adjusted for the predictors that were significant in the first model and the differences in baseline characteristics of the diagnostic pathway groups. All analyses were performed in the R programming language and environment v3.3.2 "Sincere Pumpkin Patch" using the lme4 and nnet package [12].

Ethical aspects

The study was approved by the ethical committee of the Capital region (case number: H-4- 2014-097). Informed written consent was obtained from all patients participating in the study.

Results

Diagnostic workup

Four hundred and eighty-eight patients were recruited to the study. Dipstick was done in 480 (98%) patients and microscopy in 160 (32%) patients. 434 (89%) patients had a urine culture performed as part of the diagnostic work-up; done in practices in 317 (65%) and sent to hospital in 117 (24%) patients. The most common combination of diagnostic tests was dipstick and culture done in practice ($n = 240$, 49% of the patients) – Table 1.

Table 1 Distribution of the use of diagnostic tools and diagnostic pathways

	Total ($n = 488$)
Dipstick	480
Microscopy	160
Culture in practice	317
Culture sent to the hospital	117
Diagnostic pathways	
No urine culture ($n = 54$)	
Dipsticks	14
Microscopy	3
Dipsticks + microscopy	37
Urine culture in practice ($n = 317$)	
Dipsticks + urine culture in practice	240
Dipsticks + microscopy + urine culture in practice	76
Urine culture in practice	1
Urine culture sent to the hospital ($n = 117$)	
Dipsticks + urine culture in hospital	73
Microscopy + urine culture in hospital	4
Dipsticks + microscopy + urine culture in hospital	40

Dipstick results ($n = 480$) included reactions for nitrite and leucocytes. In 334 (69%) patients, the two reactions pointed in different directions: most frequently, the reaction for leucocytes was positive and for nitrite negative. 63 (13%) patients had negative reactions for both nitrite and leucocytes and 91 (18%) were positive for both.

Microscopy results ($n = 160$) included identification of ≥ 1 bacteria per High Power Field (HPF) in 106 (66%) patients; and identification of ≥ 1 white blood cell per HPF in 70 (43%) patients. Combination of ≥ 1 bacteria + ≥ 1 white blood cell per HPF in 30 (19%) patients.

The sensitivity of urine culture performed and interpreted in practice was 94% (95% CI 89%; 96%), specificity 51% (95%CI 43%; 59%), Positive Predictive Value – PPV 69% (95% CI 63%; 74%), Negative Predictive Value – NPV 88% (95% CI 79%;93%) – see Additional file 1: Table S2.

The sensitivity of urine culture performed at hospital was 90% (95% CI 80%; 95%), specificity 89% (95% CI 78%;94%), PPV 90% (95% CI 80%;95%), NPV 89% (95% CI 78%;94%) – see Additional file 1: Table S3.

Table 2 shows the distribution of baseline characteristics in patients without culture, those where culture was done in practices and patients whose culture was sent to hospital. The proportion of uncomplicated UTIs was higher (70%) in patients with no culture performed than in patients with practice culture (60%) or hospital culture (34%).

Identification of predictors for use of additional diagnostic testing is shown in Additional file 1: Table S1. Neither a suspected complicated UTI nor the results of dipstick or microscopy predicted the incorporation of urine culture within the diagnostic workup. The incorporation of a diagnostic test was predicted by the availability of diagnostic tests. For example, availability of a microscope in practice decreased the propensity of performing a culture in practice (OR 0.04, 95% CI 0.004; 0.5) and availability of culture in practice decreased the propensity of performing a culture at hospital (OR 0.01, 95% CI 0.001; 0.08).

The incorporation of a diagnostic test was predicted as well by anamnestic information. For example, a high anamnestic score decreased the likelihood of performing urine culture in practice OR 0.7 (95% CI 0.6; 0.9), but increased cultures at hospital OR 1.5 (95% CI 1.1; 1.9).

Offensive smell increased urine cultures at hospital OR 2.9 (95% CI 1.2; 7), but not in practice.

Table 2 Patients' baseline characteristics and diagnostic pathways

	No culture (n = 54)	Culture performed in practice (n = 317)	Culture performed at hospital (n = 117)
Prevalence confirmed UTI	29(54)	170(46)	62(52)
Uncomplicated UTI	38(70)	191(60)	41(34)
Women	51(94)	293(92)	110(94)
Younger patients (<=64 years)	41(76)	218(69)	88(75)
Number of days with symptoms (Median-IQR)	2(1;4)	2(1;5)	2(1;4)
Signs & Symptoms			
Dysuria	38(70)	214(67)	88(75)
Frequency	38(70)	211(66)	84(72)
Urgency	24(44)	152(48)	73(62)
Suprapubic pain	17(31)	85(27)	45(38)
Dysuria and frequency	25(46)	149(47)	62(52)
Dysuria and urgency	17(31)	106(33)	57(49)
Dysuria and suprapubic pain	11(20)	57(18)	32(27)
Flank pain	4(7)	53(17)	17(14)
Genital symptoms	4(7)	30(9)	16(13)
Reported Fever	1(2)	27(8)	9(7)
Offensive smell	6(11)	57(18)	26(22)
Macrohematuria	4(7)	31(10)	17(15)
UTI within 4 weeks	0	18(6)	14(12)
Other[a]	6(11)	27(8)	15(13)
Anamnestic score[b]	2(2;3)	3(2;4)	3(2;4)

Figures are n (%), if not marked otherwise [a] Signs and symptoms not listed in the questionnaire
[b]Median IQR (Interquartile range) of signs, symptoms and anamnesis of previous UTI (Score 1 to 11)

Diagnostic workup and treatment decisions

Table 3 shows the distribution of appropriate treatment decisions in the three diagnostic pathway groups. The distribution of the treatment decision was different between the three diagnostic pathways. For example, the day of the index consultation (i.e. first treatment decision), overtreatment was seen in 39% of patients without culture, 14% of those with culture in practice, and 27% of the patients with culture sent to hospital (*p*-value: 0.0001).

For the final treatment decision, an appropriate treatment decision was taken in: 55% of patients without culture, 71% of those with culture in practice, and 69% of the patients with cultures sent to hospital (*p*-value = 0.04).

Discussion

Summary of results

In a practice setting with wide availability of diagnostic tests, nearly all patients with suspected UTI are examined

Table 3 Appropriateness of the treatment decision and use of diagnostic tests

	First treatment decision (*p*-value = < 0.0001)[a]			Final treatment decision (*p*-value = 0.04)[b]		
	Appropriate	Overtreatment	Undertreatment	Appropriate	Overtreatment	Undertreatment
No culture[c] (n = 54)	30(55)	21(39)	3(6)	30(55)	21(39)	3(6)
Culture performed in practice (n = 317)	176(56)	46(14)	95(30)	227(71)	76(24)	14(5)
Culture performed at hospital (n = 117)	71(61)	32(27)	14(12)	81(69)	24(21)	12(10)

Appropriate = prescribing antibiotics when reference test is positive and not prescribing antibiotics when reference test is negative
Overtreatment = prescribing antibiotics when reference test is negative
Undertreatment = not prescribing antibiotics when reference test is positive
Permutation LR test to assess whether treatment decision at the day of the index consultation[a] or at the day of the final treatment decision[b] differs between groups: a) no culture, b) culture performed in practice, c) culture performed at hospital. Hierarchical model with practices as a random intercept and adjusted for: complicated versus uncomplicated UTI, offensive smell, anamnesis score, microscope and culture in practice availability
[c]When not performing culture, first treatment decision is the final treatment decision

with urine dipstick and for most, urine culture is part of the diagnostic workup. Neither a suspected complicated UTI nor the results of dipstick or microscopy predict the incorporation of urine culture within the diagnostic workup. Incorporation of urine culture within the decision-making process is associated with a higher proportion of appropriate treatment decisions.

Strengths and limitations

Although a randomized controlled trial might be considered the ideal design to assess the effect of diagnostic tests on treatment decisions, there is no consensus about the best study design to help understand the link between combination of diagnostic test, test interpretation and treatment decision [6, 13, 14]. Since our study aimed at describing the use of diagnostic tests and the appropriateness of the treatment decision under daily practice conditions, a prospective observational design was a sensible way of capturing the whole decision-making process from consultation to final treatment decision [15].

The observational study was carried out as part of the context assessment of a quality improvement program. It brings about some advantages and disadvantages.

On one hand, the external validity needs to be considered with caution. Only 39 practices out of 500 accepted to participate. Previous studies have shown that GPs that participate in research or quality improvement activities tend to prescribe fewer antibiotics and are possibly more interested in reducing inappropriate prescribing than their non-participating colleagues [16, 17]. Therefore, the differences shown in this study may be conservative.

On the other hand, observation bias was minimized by the fact that GPs were interested in obtaining an accurate recording of their decisions under daily practice conditions. This type of medical audit has been extensively used in Denmark for more than 25 years [18]. The cornerstone of the methodology is the bottom-up approach in which the GPs set their own improvement goals. Hence, there is no point to record data that do not reflect their everyday practice.

Finally, we cannot completely rule out residual confounding due to unmeasured variables. Nonetheless, the effect of clustering was considered in the assessment of predictors and differences between the diagnostic groups. The model to test the association between the diagnostic pathway groups and treatment decision was adjusted by the predictors for the combination of tests and differences in baseline characteristics between the diagnostic pathway groups.

Interpretation of the findings in relation to previous literature

This study shows the complexity of the decision-making process in a group perceived as "easy" patients in general practice [19].

International guidelines recommend the inclusion of urine culture as part of the diagnostic process only in suspected complicated UTI to target the right antibiotic choice [20, 21]. In our study, an uncomplicated versus complicated UTI did not predict the incorporation of urine culture within the diagnostic workup. It may be explained by the current debate on finding a new approach [22] to define the type of UTI based on burden of symptoms, risk factors, and availability of appropriate antimicrobial therapy. For example, in the no culture group the median anamnestic score was lower than in the other two groups. It means GPs possibly considered these patients as "uncomplicated cases". Furthermore, the higher the anamnestic score the higher the probability to send the urine culture to the hospital and the lower the probability to perform the urine culture in the practice.

Results from the tests performed previously did not predict incorporation of a test within the diagnostic work-up. It indicates a quality problem in the use of diagnostic tests. An obvious reason for the unsystematic use of diagnostic tests might be the payment scheme. Danish primary care system provides economic incentive for the GP to perform laboratory testing in practice, and this may have influenced the diagnostic workup.

Nonetheless, shortcomings of the dipstick and microscopy may lead to the incorporation of another test in order to gain certainty on the diagnosis. The use of dipsticks in primary care needs to take into consideration two important factors for the interpretation [11]. Firstly, a minimum bladder incubation time of 4 h, what is difficult if we take into consideration that one of the main motives of consultation is frequency. Secondly, common uropathogens such as Enterococcus spp. and Staphylococcus spp. do not reduce nitrites. Microscopy requires expertise and the sensitivity is low with colony counts $< 10^5$ [23]. Then, Danish GPs may rely more on the results of a urine culture.

Behavioural and medical reasons may explain the inclusion of urine culture in the diagnostic workup for most patients too.

Sackett et al. have long ago described four diagnostic approaches in clinical practice [24]. A mixture of the hypothetico-deductive strategy where the clinician gathers information to either confirm or refute his/her hypothesis and the complete history strategy could explain our results.

In a country with a strong antibiotic stewardship program, GPs are aware of the societal consequences of unnecessary use of antibiotics. They need to find a way to counteract the systematic error called "confirmation bias" [25]. This error arises from the tendency to seek and interpret evidence that predominantly confirms a pre-existing hypothesis. In our population, patients entered the study with a suspected UTI, thus for the GPs it may be difficult to withhold antibiotic prescribing. Not surprisingly, inappropriate use of antibiotics is mainly driven by overprescribing of antibiotics and only to a lesser extent by underprescribing.

Cardinal symptoms such as dysuria, frequency and urgency has a high negative predictive value [26]. It means, they are useful to rule out a UTI when absent. However, in our study population, one of the inclusion criteria was dysuria and/or frequency so the negative predictive value could not be used to rule out a UTI.

Urine culture performed in a laboratory is currently regarded as the best available test to rule in or out an infection [23]. Thus, GPs may see the use of urine culture as the best way to counteract "the confirmation bias".

The clinical history plays a role when GPs decide whether to perform a urine culture in the practice or send it to the hospital. This has an effect as well on treatment decision.

In patients whose urine culture was performed in practice, the expectation of obtaining a result the following day combined with low anamnestic scores encouraged both GPs and patients to withhold antibiotics. The day of the index consultation, only 14% of patients were over-treated. However, incorrect interpretation of the culture resulted in 24% overtreatment for the final treatment decision.

For patients with hospital culture, a few days' delay of culture result combined with a higher symptom score led to more antibiotic overprescribing at the day of the index consultation (27%). It is in line with a qualitative study on TDs in patients with suspected UTI, where GPs preferred to treat empirically due to the discomfort experienced by the patient [19].

Perspectives

Implementation of effective interventions to reduce inappropriate use of antibiotics requires thorough knowledge of the context in which the decision to prescribe antibiotics is taken [27]. For example, for the group of GPs that participated in this study, education on interpretation of urine culture in practice or improving communication with the microbiology department are interventions that might reduce the inappropriate prescribing of antibiotics.

This assessment should encourage the implementation of studies to assess the use of the available diagnostic tests to set-up improvement strategies that can reduce the unnecessary prescription of antibiotics within each context/country.

Finally, the results presented in this paper focus on the impact on treatment decision. Further research assessing the cost-effectiveness and impact on patients' outcomes should contribute with information to evaluate the multi-dimensional value of these diagnostic strategies.

Conclusion

In a context with wide availability of diagnostic tests, GPs use diagnostic tests in all the patients with suspected UTI. It may be explained by economic as well as medical/behavioural reasons. Inclusion of urine culture as part of the diagnostic workup leads to appropriate treatment decision in the majority of the patients. Performance of urine culture is important for reducing inappropriate prescribing in patients with suspected UTI seeking care in general practice in Denmark.

Abbreviations

AMR: Antimicrobial resistance; GP: General Practitioner; NPV: Negative predictive value; PPV: Positive predictive value; SSI: Statens Serum Institute; TD: Treatment decision; UTI: Urinary tract infection; WHO: World Health Organization

Acknowledgements

We would like to acknowledge the General Practitioners and patients that contributed with data for the study. We would like to thank as well Anette Hammerum, Frank Hansen and Nadia Xenia Olsen for their work in the processing of the urine culture at the Statens Serum Institute (SSI). Finally, our deep gratitude to the Audit Project Odense (APO) group for data management.

Funding

This study was fund by: a) 2016 fund (grant from the University of Copenhagen to promote interdisciplinary research), b) KAP-H (agency for quality in primary care at the capital region), c) læge Sofus Carl Emil Friis og Hustru Olga Doris Friis' legat.

Authors' contributions

GC AH TMS MM LB NF designed the study. VS HS supervised the statistical analysis and contributed with the interpretation. GC wrote the first draft and all authors critically revised the manuscript and approved the final version.

Competing interests

The authors declare that they have no competing interests.

Author details

[1]The Research Unit for General Practice and Section of General Practice, Department of Public Health, University of Copenhagen, Øster Farimagsgade 5, 1014 Copenhagen, Denmark. [2]Department of Veterinary Clinical Sciences, University of Copenhagen, Copenhagen, Denmark. [3]Finnish Office for Health Technology Assessment (FINOHTA) - National Institute for Health and Welfare, Helsinki, Finland. [4]Department of Clinical Microbiology, Rigshospitalet, Copenhagen, Denmark.

References

1. World Health Organization. Global action plan on antimicrobial resistance. 2015. http://www.who.int/antimicrobial-resistance/publications/global-action-plan/en/.
2. Adriaenssens S, Versporten A, Muller A, Minalu G, Faes C, Vankerckhoven V, et al. European surveillance of antimicrobial consumption (ESAC): outpatient antibiotic use in Europe (1997-2009). J Antimicrob Chemother. 2011;66 Suppl 6:vi3–12.
3. Statens Serum Institut. DANMAP 2015-use of antimicrobial agents and occurrence of antimicrobial resistance in bacteria from food animals, food and humans in Denmark. 2015. http://www.danmap.org/pdf.ashx?title=Reports&url=http%3A%2F%2Fwww.danmap.org%2FDownloads%2FReports.aspx%3Fpdf%3D1.
4. Aabenhus R, Hansen MP, Siersma V, Bjerrum L. Clinical indications for antibiotic use in Danish general practice: results from a nationwide electronic prescription database. Scand J Prim Health Care. 2017;35:162–9.
5. Haldrup S, Thomsen RW, Bro F, Skov R, Bjerrum L, Søgaard M. Microbiological point of care testing before antibiotic prescribing in primary care: considerable variations between practices. BMC Fam Pract. 2017;18:9.

6. Bossuyt PM, Lijmer JG, Mol BW. Randomised comparisons of medical tests: sometimes invalid, not always efficient. Lancet. 2000;356:1844–7.
7. Thompson M, Weigl B, Fitzpatrick A, Ide N. More than just accuracy: a novel method to incorporate multiple test attributes in evaluating diagnostic tests including point of care tests. IEEE J Transl Eng Heal Med. 2016;4:2800208.
8. Hulsher ME, Meer JW, Grol RP. Antibiotic use. how to improve it? Int JMed Microbiol. 2010;300:351–6.
9. Teixeira Rodrigues A, Roque F, Falcão A, Figueiras A, Herdeiro MT. Understanding physician antibiotic prescribing behaviour: a systematic review of qualitative studies. Int J Antimicrob Agents. 2013;41(3):203–12.
10. Cordoba G, Sorensen T, Holm A, Bjornvad C, Bjerrum L, Jessen L. Exploring the feasibility and synergistic value of the one health approach in clinical research: protocol for a prospective observational study of diagnostic pathways in human and canine patients with suspected urinary tract infection. Pilot Feasibility Stud. 2015;1:38.
11. European confederation of laboratory medicine. European urinalysis guidelines. Scand J Clin Lab Invest Suppl. 2000;231:1–86.
12. Bates D, Mächler M, Bolker B, Walker S. Fitting linear mixed-effects models using lme4. J Stat Soft. 2015;67:48.
13. Kennedy AG. Evaluating diagnostic tests. J Eval Clin Pract. 2016;22:575–9.
14. Trikalinos TA, Siebert U, Lau J. Decision-analytic modeling to evaluate benefits and harms of medical tests: uses and limitations. Med Decis Mak. 2009;29(5):E22–9.
15. Home P, Yang W, Zilov A, Soewondo P, Bech OM, Sekkal F, et al. How can observational trials inform and improve clinical practice? Observational studies: going beyond the boundaries of randomized controlled trials. Diabetes Res Clin Pract. 2010;88:S3–9.
16. Strandberg EL, Ovehed I, Troein M, Hakansson A. Influence of self-registration on audit participants and their non-participating colleagues. A retrospective study of medical records concerning prescription patterns. ScandJPrimHealth Care. 2005;23(1):42–6.
17. Akkerman AE, Kuyvenhoven MM, Verheij TJ, Van Dijk L. Antibiotics in Dutch general practice: nationwide electronic GP database and national reimbursement rates. Pharmacoepidemiol Drug Saf. 2008;17(4):378–83.
18. Munck AP, Hansen DG, Lindman A, Ovhed I, Forre S, Torsteinsson JB. A Nordic collaboration on medical audit. The APO method for quality development and continuous medical education (CME) in primary health care. Scand J Prim Heal Care. 1998;16:2–6.
19. Duane S, Domegan C, Callan A, Galvin S, Cormican M, Bennett K, et al. Using qualitative insights to change practice: exploring the culture of antibiotic prescribing and consumption for urinary tract infections. BMJ Open. 2016;6:e008894.
20. Scottish Intercollegiate Guidelines Network. Management of suspected bacterial urinary tract infection in adults: a national clinical guideline. 2015. http://www.sign.ac.uk/guidelines/fulltext/88/.
21. Gupta K, Hooton TM, Naber KG, Wullt B, Colgan R, Miller LG, et al. International clinical practice guidelines for the treatment of acute uncomplicated cystitis and pyelonephritis in women: a 2010 update by the Infectious Diseases Society of America and the European Society for Microbiology and Infectious Diseases. Clin Infect Dis. 2011;52(5):e103–20.
22. Johansen TE, Botto H, Cek M, Grabe M, Tenke P, Wagenlehner FM, et al. Critical review of current definitions of urinary tract infections and proposal of an EAU/ESIU classification system. Int J Antimicrob Agents. 2011;38:64–70
23. Schmiemann G, Kniehl E, Gebhardt K, Matejczyk MM, Hummers-Pradier E. The diagnosis of urinary tract infection: a systematic review. Dtsch Arztebl Int. 2010;107:361–7.
24. Sacket D, Haynes RB, Tugwell P, Guyatt G. In: 2nd, editor. Clinical epidemiology: a basic sciences for clinical medicine. New York: Little, Brown and Company; 1991.
25. Bornstein BH, Emler AC. Rationality in medical decision making: a review of the literature on doctors' decision-making biases. J Eval Clin Pract. 2001;7: 97–107.
26. Giesen LG, Cousins G, Dimitrov BD, van de Laar FA, Fahey T. Predicting acute uncomplicated urinary tract infection in women: a systematic review of the diagnostic accuracy of symptoms and signs. BMC Fam Pr. 2010;11:78.
27. Arnold SR. Straus SE. Cochrane Database Syst Rev: Interventions to improve antibiotic prescribing practices in ambulatory care; 2005. http://www.ncbi.nlm.nih.gov/pubmed/16235325

18

Multimorbidity: can general practitioners identify the health conditions most important to their patients?

Anouk Déruaz-Luyet[1], Alexandra A. N'Goran[1], Jérôme Pasquier[2], Bernard Burnand[2], Patrick Bodenmann[3], Stefan Zechmann[4], Stefan Neuner-Jehle[4], Nicolas Senn[1], Daniel Widmer[1], Sven Streit[5], Andreas Zeller[6], Dagmar M. Haller[7] and Lilli Herzig[1*]

Abstract

Background: Faced with patients suffering from more than one chronic condition, or multimorbidity, general practitioners (GPs) must establish diagnostic and treatment priorities. Patients also set their own priorities to handle the everyday burdens associated with their multimorbidity and these may be different from the priorities established by their GP. A shared patient–GP agenda, driven by knowledge of each other's priorities, would seem central to managing patients with multimorbidity. We evaluated GPs' ability to identify the health condition most important to their patients.

Methods: Data on 888 patients were collected as part of a cross-sectional Swiss study on multimorbidity in family medicine. For the main analyses on patients-GP agreement, data from 572 of these patients could be included. GPs were asked to identify the two conditions which their patient considered most important, and we tested whether either of them agreed with the condition mentioned as most important by the patient. In the main analysis, we studied the agreement rate between GPs and patients by grouping items medically-related into 46 groups of conditions. Socio-demographic and clinical variables were fitted into univariate and multivariate models.

Results: In 54.9% of cases, GPs were able to identify the health condition most important to the patient. In the multivariate model, the only variable significantly associated with patient–GP agreement was the number of chronic conditions: the higher the number of conditions, the less likely the agreement.

Conclusion: GPs were able to correctly identify the health condition most important to their patients in half of the cases. It therefore seems important that GPs learn how to better adapt treatment targets and priorities by taking patients' perspectives into account.

Keywords: Multimorbidity, Family medicine, Patient–provider agreement

* Correspondence: Lilli.herzig@hin.ch
[1]Institute of Family Medicine, University of Lausanne, 44 rue du Bugnon, 1011 Lausanne, Switzerland
Full list of author information is available at the end of the article

Background

Multimorbidity is defined as the co-occurrence of two (or three) or more chronic health conditions in one person without any condition being considered an index condition [1]. Faced with patients with multimorbidity, GPs must often set priorities between the different chronic conditions, as managing them all is often infeasible in everyday practice. Patients also set their own disease and treatment priorities to handle the everyday burdens associated with their multimorbidity and these may be different from the priorities established by their GP.

Evidence shows that good communication between patients and GPs leads to more agreement between them and a better care outcome [2]. However, studies examining the match between physicians' and patients' priority health conditions have produced contrasting results, and most of these studies were conducted in diabetic patients [3–5]. High levels of agreement on which conditions were considered important from patients' and GPs' perspectives have been reported previously, but levels of agreement were lower in patients reporting a poor health status [5]. A common patient–GP (or patient–provider) agenda is key to a successful therapeutic process, particularly in patients with multimorbidity, and this is generally dependent on good patient–GP communication and shared decision-making [2, 6, 7]. Our hypothesis was that more experienced GPs and GPs with a sub-specialization in psychosocial and psychosomatic medicine, based on the development of strong communication, would be positively associated with agreement between GPs and patients, as would a higher number of visits to the GP in the last 12 months and more years of follow-up by the same GP. In contrast, a high number of chronic conditions and a greater number of medical doctors involved in the patient's treatment could be a reflection of more complicated cases or sicker patients, for whom setting priorities would be more difficult. Lower health-literacy and less well-educated patients could also be factors complicating patient–GP communication and could be negatively associated with agreement rates between GPs and patients. The presumed direction of the association between the number of consultations handled by the GP each week was less clear-cut, however, as more consultations per week could mean either greater knowledge of each patient with multimorbidity or less time spent per consultation

Studies to date in primary care settings have reported low levels of agreement between patients and GPs on health and treatment priorities [8]. Qualitative studies have underlined that they do not seem to give the same level importance to the same conditions, and to some extent, GPs appear unaware of their patients' priorities [8–10]. Voigt et al. [8] showed that even if GPs were able to identify the number of health problems that their patients considered important, they did not give the same level of importance to the same conditions. Patients' ratings of health conditions have been shown to be related to their current experience of their condition, whereas GPs' ratings were more related to the condition's prognosis [9]. Thus, our aim was to evaluate whether GPs could identify the condition that their patients with multimorbidity considered most important. To the best of our knowledge, this is one of the first quantitative study addressing this topic.

Methods

We analyzed data from the Multimorbidity in Family Medicine study, a cross-sectional study in Switzerland. The study protocol and a detailed description of the database established have been published elsewhere [11, 12].

Setting and participants

Data collection took place in Switzerland between January and September 2015. A convenience sample of 100 GPs randomly enrolled patients during scheduled consultations at their private practices. Each GP was provided with a randomisation calendar specifying which patients to enrol on each half-day during the recruitment weeks. All multimorbid patients above 18 years old, followed by their GP for at least 6 months and suffering from at least three of the 75 chronic conditions on a predefined list based on the International Classification of Primary Care 2 (ICPC 2) were considered eligible [13, 14] and signed a written consent to participate to the study. GPs completed a paper-based questionnaire for each included patient and patients enrolled completed a telephone-based questionnaire. Only anonymous dates were transmitted to the research team. The study protocol (n° 314/15) was approved by the Human Research Ethics Committee of the Canton Vaud.

Variables

Outcome variable

We evaluated the agreement between what patients considered to be their most important health condition and what GPs thought patients considered to be their most important health condition. Conditions were considered to be "in agreement" if one of two conditions considered important by the GP belonged to the same group of conditions as the one considered most important by the patient; they were "in disagreement" otherwise. Agreement between GPs and patients was considered as a dichotomous variable.

Independent variables

The GP-related variables of interest were: sex, number of years of practice, number of consultations per week, practice location, and a sub-specialization in psychosocial and psychosomatic medicine, i.e., a postgraduate qualification to handle psychosomatic and psychosocial factors influencing the development and management of diseases. The patient-related variables were: age, sex, number of chronic conditions, level of education, number of medical doctors involved in the patient's treatment, number of visits to the GP in the last 12 months, and number of years with this GP.

Data sources

GP level

We asked the GPs to list the two health conditions they thought were most important to their patients.

Patient level

During a telephone interview, patients were asked, "If you had the power to heal one of your medical problems, which one would you choose first?" In the absence of a validated question on this topic, we designed this question during several internal consensus discussions. Although it did not precisely match the GPs' question, it could be answered by patients with lower levels of health literacy. In line with the study's protocol and its overall goals, interviewers were trained to conduct standardized telephone interviews. As a result, they did not to attempt to establish more precise patient answers when they might have been needed.

Measurement

Only answers that could be transferred into a corresponding ICPC-2 code were used. In the knowledge that patients and GPs may refer to the same conditions differently and with different levels of precision, we grouped related chronic conditions for agreement analyses. For the main analysis, we considered a classification involving 46 groups of diseases derived from the classification developed by van den Bussche et al. for elderly patients with multimorbidity and subsequently adapted specifically to our assessment by three members of the research team [15]. (Additional file 1: Table S1). We evaluated agreement between GPs' and patients' answers based on these 46 groups. To avoid over-interpretation, for both analyses, any responses that could not be unequivocally attributed to one group were considered as missing data. In a sensitivity analysis, we used fifteen chapters of the ICPC-2 classification to group items (General and unspecified; Blood/blood-forming organs and immune system; Digestive; Eye; Ear; Cardiovascular; Musculoskeletal; Neurological; Psychological; Respiratory; Skin; Endocrine/metabolic and nutritional; Urological; Female Genital; Male Genital). We excluded the two chapters on pregnancy and social aspects, which did not encompass chronic conditions per se [16]. We also considered answers in which more than one code was given, as follows. If all of the codes belonged to the same group or chapter, we attributed the condition to that group or chapter, respectively. If the codes did not belong to the same group or chapter, or if the group or chapter could not be clearly defined, the codes were considered as missing data.

Agreement was considered a binary outcome. Agreement occurred when the most important condition identified by the patient matched one of the two conditions given by the GP. The independent variables of number of years of practice, number of years of follow-up by the GP, the patient's age, and the number of visits to the GP in the last 12 months were considered as continuous variables. All other variables were considered as categorical variables. The different numbers of chronic conditions were stratified into three groups: "3", "4 or 5", and "6 or more" chronic conditions. This categorization was made according to the levels of multimorbidity defined by Kadam et al. [17]

Study size

In all, 888 patients were included in the cross-sectional study. After discarding patients with missing values for the matching variables, 841 patients remained. From these patients, we excluded those with ambiguous responses, i.e. responses that could not easily be assigned to one category. As a result, 579 and 593 were retained for the main and sensitivity analyses, respectively. We eliminated patients with incomplete data for any of the independent variables considered. Finally, 572 and 585 patients (64.4 and 65.9% of the original sample) were included in the main and sensitivity analyses, respectively. Patients discarded due to missing data were not different from the patients included in the main analysis in terms of sex (chi^2, 1 df, $p = 0.05$), number of chronic conditions (chi^2, 2 df, $p = 0.45$), level of education (chi^2, 6 df, $p = 0.25$), number of MDs involved in patient's treatment (chi^2, 3 df, $p = 0.24$), number of GP visits in last 12 months (t-test, $p = 0.86$). They were slightly older than patients included (mean age (SD): 74.3 (11.5) versus 72.2 (12.2), t-test $p < 0.05$).

Analyses

For both analyses, we examined whether one of the two conditions identified by the GP matched the most important condition identified by the patient. For the main analysis, agreement was evaluated with regards to 46 groups of conditions (Additional file 1: Table S1), whereas for the sensitivity analysis this was done with regards to 15 chapters of the ICPC-2 classification.

Statistical methods

We conducted bivariate and multivariate logistic regressions to evaluate the associations between GP-related and patient-related variables with the agreement variable and to evaluate any potential clustering effects around GPs' variables.

Results

Agreements between the most important health condition for patients and those perceived to be the most important to patients by GPs are reported in Table 1. In the main analysis, agreement occurred in 54.9% of cases ($N = 314$). For the sensitivity analysis, agreement occurred in 63.8% of the cases ($N = 373$) (Table 1). No clustering effects around GPs' variables were detected.

In the main model based on the classification of items in 46 groups, only the number of chronic conditions was significantly associated with the outcome both in univariate (Table 2) and multivariate analyses (Table 3).

More precisely, agreement between GPs and patients decreased as the number of chronic conditions increased. Compared to "3" chronic conditions, the odds ratios (95% confidence interval, CI) for agreement between when there were "4 or 5" and "6 or more" chronic conditions were 0.53 (95% CI, 0.31–0.89) and 0.59 (95% CI, 0.34–1), respectively. Thus, there was only a statistically significant difference in agreement when the "4 or 5" conditions group was compared to the "3" chronic conditions group. No cluster effects were observed around any of the GPs, and the rates of agreement were similar for all the GPs enrolled. Rates of agreement were 65.6, 50.8, and 55.1% for the "3", "4 or 5", and "6 or more" chronic conditions groups, respectively (Table 4).

The groups of conditions most frequently mentioned by patients as the most important conditions included Musculoskeletal conditions and pain and Spine conditions/back pain (groups 18, 19). For these two groups of conditions, rates of agreement between GPs and patients were 67.8 and 42.9%, respectively (Additional file 2: Table S2 a). Unfortunately for this analysis, the limited number of observations in some groups of conditions limited the interpretation of results.

The sensitivity analysis conducted on broader groups of conditions relating to chapters if the ICPC-2 showed similar results. Compared to "3" chronic conditions, the odds ratio for agreement between when there were "4 or 5" and "6 or more" chronic conditions were 0.6 (95% CI, 0.34–1.01) and 0.64 (95% CI, 0.36–1.09), respectively (Additional file 2: Table S2 b).

Discussion

When chronic conditions were classified into 46 categories, GPs were able to identify the condition most important to their patients in 54.9% of cases. The rate of agreement was higher (63.8%) when looking for agreement with items grouped in the chapters of the ICPC-2 classification. Differences between the perspectives of GPs and patients have previously been shown for such aspects of disease management as the cure or relief of symptoms [18], disease severity [19], and the level of suffering [20]. In the present study, back pain and musculoskeletal conditions, often symptomatic, were the conditions most often ranked first by patients. However, agreement with GPs on these conditions was contrasted, being higher than average for musculoskeletal conditions but lower for spine and back syndromes. Any interpretation of these analyses is limited by the reduced number of conditions per group. Nevertheless, these results seem to confirm that pain and symptomatic chronic conditions are patients' first priorities, whereas GPs' priorities may be more prognosis-based [7].

The only variable associated with a difference in the rates of agreement between GPs and patients was the number of chronic conditions. This was expected because the probability of patient–GP agreement is higher in patients with fewer health conditions [5, 6]. In the present study, however, the rate of agreement for patients suffering from 4 or 5 chronic conditions was lower than for patients with 3 chronic conditions, but the rate did not decrease further for patients suffering from 6 or more. This suggests that patient–GP agreement may depend somewhat on factors

Table 1 Patient–GP rates of agreement on the condition ranked as most important to the patient (data collection January–September 2015)

		46 groups of conditions ($N = 572$) N (%)		15 chapters of the ICPC-2 ($N = 585$) N (%)	
Agreement	The condition that the GP thinks is most important to the patient belongs to the same group/chapter as the condition considered most important by the patient.	217 (37.9)	314 (54.9)	260 (44.4)	373 (63.8)
	The condition that the GP thinks is the second most important to the patient belongs to the same group/chapter as the condition considered most important by the patient.	97 (17)		113 (19.3)	
Disagreement	The conditions that the GP thinks are most important to the patient do not belong to the same group/chapter as the condition considered most important by the patient.	258 (45.1)		212 (36.2)	

Table 2 Bivariate analyses of all the variables considered in the study (Data collection January–September 2015)

		46 groups of conditions ($N = 572$)			15 chapters of the ICPC-2 ($N = 585$)		
		No	Yes	*p*-value	No	Yes	*p*-value
Patient-related variables							
No. of chronic conditions+	3, N (%)	31 (12)	59 (18.8)	0.06	26 (12.3)	66 (17.7)	0.20
	4 or 5	121 (46.9)	125 (39.8)		98 (46.2)	154 (41.3)	
	6 or more	106 (41.1)	130 (41.4)		88 (41.5)	153 (41)	
Age++	Mean, years (SD)	73.1 (12.1)	71.5 (12.3)	0.11	73 (11.5)	71.9 (12.7)	0.28
Sex+	Male, N (%)	117 (45.3)	144 (45.9)	0.93	101 (47.6)	171 (45.8)	0.73
	Female	141 (54.7)	170 (54.1)		111 (52.4)	202 (54.2)	
Level of education+	Primary school/no diploma, N (%)	43 (16.7)	42 (13.4)	0.28	36 (17)	51 (13.7)	0.82
	Secondary school	20 (7.8)	24 (7.6)		16 (7.5)	28 (7.5)	
	Practical professional training	61 (23.6)	86 (27.4)		56 (26.4)	94 (25.2)	
	High school or equivalent	33 (12.8)	33 (10.5)		23 (10.8)	45 (12.1)	
	Vocational school or training	58 (22.5)	92 (29.3)		51 (24.1)	105 (28.2)	
	Non-university higher education	26 (10.1)	24 (7.6)		17 (8)	33 (8.8)	
	University	17 (6.6)	13 (4.1)		13 (6.1)	17 (4.6)	
No. of MDs involved in patient's treatment+	1, N (%)	73 (28.3)	81 (25.8)	0.81	58 (27.4)	98 (26.3)	0.75
	2	76 (29.5)	89 (28.3)		57 (26.9)	112 (30)	
	3	54 (20.9)	75 (23.9)		48 (22.6)	88 (23.6)	
	4 or more	55 (21.3)	69 (22)		49 (23.1)	75 (20.1)	
No. of GP visits in last 12 months++	Mean, N (SD)	12.9 (8.9)	13 (8.7)	0.87	13.2 (9.3)	13.2 (9.2)	0.95
No. of years followed by GP++	Mean, years (SD)	10.9 (7.9)	11.2 (8.5)	0.59	10.4 (7.9)	11.5 (8.4)	0.13
GP-related variables							
Sex+	Male, N (%)	196 (76)	220 (70.1)	0.13	152 (71.7)	271 (72.7)	0.85
	Female	62 (24)	94 (29.9)		60 (28.3)	102 (27.3)	
No. of years of practice++	Mean, years (SD)	17.3 (9.6)	18 (9.6)	0.42	16.5 (9.5)	18.2 (9.5)	0.03
No. of consultations per week+	≤ 30 N (%)	2 (0.8)	3 (1)	0.82	1 (0.5)	4 (1.1)	0.59
	]30–70]	72 (27.9)	84 (26.8)		60 (28.3)	96 (25.7)	
	]70–110]	117 (45.3)	148 (47.1)		100 (47.2)	176 (47.2)	
	]110–170]	59 (22.9)	64 (20.4)		46 (21.7)	79 (21.2)	
	> 170	8 (3.1)	15 (4.8)		5 (2.4)	18 (4.8)	
Practice location+	Urban, N (%)	109 (42.2)	136 (43.3)	0.97	92 (43.4)	157 (42.1)	0.86
	Suburban	108 (41.9)	129 (41.1)		85 (40.1)	158 (42.4)	
	Rural	41 (15.9)	49 (15.6)		35 (16.5)	58 (15.5)	
Sub-specialization in psychosocial & psychosomatic medicine	No, N (%)	236 (91.5)	294 (93.6)	0.34	198 (93.4)	347 (93)	1.00
	Yes	22 (8.5)	20 (6.4)		14 (6.6)	26 (7)	

Agreement is positive if one of the two conditions the GP considered as important to the patient belongs to the same category as the condition considered most important by the patient. Otherwise, it is negative. Difference between groups tested using: + Fisher test; ++ t-test; practice location was evaluated using zip codes and data obtained from the Swiss Federal Statistical Office

other than those evaluated in this study. Similarly to our results, a previous study showed that a GP's knowledge of a patient's health was not influenced by the patient's age, level of education, number of consultations in the previous 6 months or the duration of the patient–GP relationship [6]. Although the present study did not report the GP's sex, this did not seem to be associated with agreement on important health conditions [5].

Our study failed to show any positive associations between the rate of patient–GP agreement and a sub-specialization in psychosocial or psychosomatic medicine, a longer follow-up, or more frequent appointments. This was despite our anticipation that these factors would have given GPs greater knowledge of their patients. An alternative explanation could be that patients with more frequent appointments and longer follow-up

Table 3 - Multivariate analyses of all the variables considered in the study (Data collection January–September 2015)

		46 groups of conditions (N = 572)		15 chapters of ICPC-2 (N = 585)	
		Odds ratio (95% CI)	*p*-value	Odds ratio (95% CI)	*p*-value
Patient-related variables					
No. of chronic conditions	3 (reference)				
	4 or 5	0.53 (0.31;0.89)	0.02	0.6 (0.34;1.01)	0.06
	6 or more	0.59 (0.34;1)	0.05	0.64 (0.36;1.09)	0.11
Age	per year	0.99 (0.98;1.01)	0.22	0.99 (0.98;1.01)	0.32
Sex	Male (reference)				
	Female	0.98 (0.69;1.41)	0.92	1.11 (0.77;1.59)	0.59
Level of education	Primary school/ no diploma (reference)				
	Secondary school	1.17 (0.55;2.51)	0.68	1.18 (0.55;2.58)	0.68
	Practical professional training	1.53 (0.87;2.69)	0.14	1.16 (0.66;2.03)	0.60
	High school or equivalent	1.05 (0.54;2.05)	0.89	1.33 (0.68;2.65)	0.41
	Vocational school or training	1.66 (0.94;2.94)	0.08	1.45 (0.82;2.57)	0.20
	Non-university higher education	0.89 (0.42;1.89)	0.76	1.28 (0.59;2.8)	0.54
	University	0.79 (0.32;1.92)	0.60	0.91 (0.37;2.25)	0.84
No. of MDs involved in patient's treatment	1 (reference)				
	2	1.05 (0.66;1.67)	0.84	1.13 (0.7;1.82)	0.62
	3	1.22 (0.74;2.01)	0.44	1.07 (0.64;1.78)	0.80
	4 or more	1.11 (0.67;1.84)	0.69	0.87 (0.52;1.45)	0.59
No. of GP visits in last 12 months	per unit	0 (0;0)		0 (0;0)	
No. of years followed by GP	per year	1 (0.97;1.03)	0.92	1 (0.97;1.03)	0.95
GP-related variables					
Sex	Male (reference)				
	Female	1.49 (0.96;2.33)	0.08	0.99 (0.64;1.54)	0.96
No. of years of practice	per year	1.01 (0.99;1.04)	0.39	1.02 (0.99;1.05)	0.20
No. of consultations per week	≤ 30 (reference)				
	]30–70]	0.82 (0.1;5.49)	0.83	0.43 (0.02;3.26)	0.47
	]70–110]	1.01 (0.12;7.01)	0.99	0.43 (0.02;3.36)	0.48
	]110–170]	0.92 (0.11;6.56)	0.94	0.42 (0.02;3.38)	0.47
	> 170	1.36 (0.14;11.61)	0.78	0.78 (0.03;8.1)	0.85
Practice location	Urban (reference)				
	Suburban	0.92 (0.62;1.36)	0.68	1.08 (0.73;1.61)	0.70
	Rural	0.92 (0.54;1.59)	0.77	1 (0.58;1.73)	0.99
Sub-specialization in psychosocial & psychosomatic medicine	No (reference)				
	Yes	0.76 (0.38;1.49)	0.42	1.08 (0.53;2.26)	0.84

Table 4 Rates of agreement in relation to the number of chronic conditions, split into 46 groups and 15 chapters of the ICPC-2

Number of chronic conditions	Agreement on one of the 46 groups of conditions – main analysis (N = 572)				Agreement on one of the 15 chapters of the ICPC-2 classification – sensitivity analysis (N = 585)			
	No agreement		Agreement		No agreement		Agreement	
3	31	34.4%	59	65.6%	26	28.3%	66	71.7%
4 or 5	121	49.2%	125	50.8%	98	38.9%	154	61.1%
6 or more	106	44.9%	130	55.1%	88	36.5%	153	63.5%

suffer from more chronic conditions and are more complicated for GPs to handle.

Our study has some limitations. To identify the health conditions most important to patients, we asked them which of their chronic health problems they would like to heal first and second, given the opportunity. Although admittedly the question was not formally validated, both GPs and patients deemed the question appropriate during a pilot phase But, it slightly differed from the question asked to GPs. Using the term "healing" with patients might have encouraged them to list their most symptomatic conditions. But, as previous studies showed that in any case patients with multimorbidity generally prioritized the treatment of symptomatic diseases over asymptomatic diseases [5, 21, 22] we do not believe that this could have biased our study's outcome to a great extent. We also did not evaluate the importance of certain other factors previously identified as influencing patients' prioritization of health problems, such as emotional disorders interfering with day-to-day activities and perceived unfavorable diagnoses [9]. And we did not include detailed information about duration, severity, treatment side effects, or functional impairments linked to each condition. Finally, patients' priorities regarding multiple chronic conditions are likely to change over time in response to factors such as a worsening of one of the conditions [23], the negative effects of a treatment [24], or contact with health professionals [23, 24] and should be re-examined whenever the patient's clinical status changes [4].

An alternative explanation for the absence of positive associations between any of the patient or GP variables considered and the rate of patient-GP agreement could be related to a lack of patient-centered care. Indeed, patient-centered care could be a more holistic or better overall way of treating patients with multimorbidity; one more centered on general priorities such as staying alive, maintaining independence, reducing/eliminating pain, and reducing/eliminating symptoms rather than on treating specific health conditions or diseases. A study evaluating patients' prioritization of these outcomes reported that 76% ranked maintaining independence as the most important factor; this was followed by the relief of symptoms [25]. In another study of patients with multimorbidity, of those who ranked staying alive as their primary concern (11%), 66% ranked maintaining independence as their secondary concern [25].

Conclusion

The present national, cross-sectional study of multimorbidity in Switzerland is one of the first evaluations of GPs' ability to identify the chronic health condition that their patients consider most important. We showed that in more than half of the cases examined, GPs were able to identify this condition, as referenced in a classification of 46 groups of conditions. This rose to about two thirds of cases when the conditions were grouped by chapter in the ICPC-2 classification. In view of these results, it seems crucial that GPs evaluate, which conditions are most important to their patients and subsequently adapt treatment targets and priorities accordingly. Good communication and patient–provider agreement would seem to be essential in this regard. Further research is needed to understand the factors underlying rates of agreement between GPs and patients, as well as which aspects—specific health conditions and symptoms or a more comprehensive or alternately holistic treatment method—should be at the heart of the patient-centered care for patients with multimorbidity.

Abbreviation

GP: General practitioners

Acknowledgements

We would like to thank the 100 GPs who participated in this study for their valuable feedback, as well as all the participating patients.

Funding

The Swiss University Conference has granted financial support to reinforce teaching and research on primary care in Switzerland. Within this framework, the country's five institutes for Family Medicine (Basel, Bern, Geneva, Zürich, and Lausanne) collaborate as the Swiss Academy for Family Medicine (SAFMED). Part of the funding must be used for national research projects on family medicine.

Authors' contributions

ADL, AAN, NS, PB, BB, DW, RT, AZ, DMH, TR, and LH developed the protocol and defined the study's objectives. ADL, AAN, NS, PB, BB, DW, LH, RT, DMH, and AZ defined the list of variables to be collected. LH, SZ, SNJ constructed the item classifications. LH, AZ, DMH, and SS recruited the participating GPs. ADL, JP conducted the statistical analyses. All authors contributed to the development and revision of the manuscript and to the decision to submit it for publication. All authors read and approved the final manuscript.

Competing interests

The authors declare that they have no competing interests.

Author details

[1]Institute of Family Medicine, University of Lausanne, 44 rue du Bugnon, 1011 Lausanne, Switzerland. [2]Institute of Social and Preventive Medicine, Lausanne University Hospital, Lausanne, Switzerland. [3]Department of Ambulatory Care and Community Medicine, Lausanne University Hospital, Lausanne, Switzerland. [4]Institute of Primary Care, University of Zurich, Zurich, Switzerland. [5]Institute of Primary Health Care (BIHAM), University of Berne, Berne, Switzerland. [6]Centre for Primary Health Care, University of Basel, Basel, Switzerland. [7]Primary Care Unit, Faculty of Medicine, University of Geneva, Geneva, Switzerland.

References

1. Van den Akker MBF, Knottnerus JA. Comorbidity or multimorbidity: what's in a name? A review of literature. Eur J Gen Pract. 1996;2(2):65–70.
2. Starfield B, Wray C, Hess K, Gross R, Birk PS, D'Lugoff BC. The influence of patient-practitioner agreement on outcome of care. Am J Public Health. 1981;71(2):127–31.
3. Kerr EA, Heisler M, Krein SL, Kabeto M, Langa KM, Weir D, et al. Beyond comorbidity counts: how do comorbidity type and severity influence diabetes patients' treatment priorities and self-management? J Gen Intern Med. 2007;22(12):1635–40.
4. Laiteerapong N, Huang ES, Chin MH. Prioritization of care in adults with diabetes and comorbidity. Ann N Y Acad Sci. 2011;1243:69–87.
5. Zulman DM, Kerr EA, Hofer TP, Heisler M, Zikmund-Fisher BJ. Patient-provider concordance in the prioritization of health conditions among hypertensive diabetes patients. J Gen Intern Med. 2010;25(5):408–14.
6. Stewart MA, McWhinney IR, Buck CW. The doctor/patient relationship and its effect upon outcome. J R Coll Gen Pract. 1979;29(199):77–81.
7. Neuner-Jehle S, Zechmann S, Grundmann Maissen D, Rosemann T, Senn O. Patient-provider concordance in the perception of illness and disease: a cross-sectional study among multimorbid patients and their general practitioners in Switzerland. Patient Prefer Adherence. 2017;11:1451–8.
8. Voigt I, Wrede J, Diederichs-Egidi H, Dierks ML, Junius-Walker U. Priority setting in general practice: health priorities of older patients differ from treatment priorities of their physicians. Croat Med J. 2010;51(6):483–92.
9. Junius-Walker U, Stolberg D, Steinke P, Theile G, Hummers-Pradier E, Health DML. Treatment priorities of older patients and their general practitioners: a cross-sectional study. Qual Prim Care. 2011;19(2):67–76.
10. Fredericksen RJ, Edwards TC, Merlin JS, Gibbons LE, Rao D, Batey DS, et al. Patient and provider priorities for self-reported domains of HIV clinical care. AIDS Care. 2015;27(10):1255–64.
11. Deruaz-Luyet A, N'Goran AA, Tandjung R, Frey P, Zeller A, Haller DM, et al. Multimorbidity in primary care: protocol of a national cross-sectional study in Switzerland. BMJ Open. 2015;5(10):e009165.
12. Deruaz-Luyet A, N'Goran AA, Senn N, Bodenmann P, Pasquier J, Widmer D, et al. Multimorbidity and patterns of chronic conditions in a primary care population in Switzerland: a cross-sectional study. BMJ Open. 2017; 7(6):e013664.
13. N'Goran AA, Blaser J, Deruaz-Luyet A, Senn N, Frey P, Haller DM, et al. From chronic conditions to relevance in multimorbidity: a four-step study in family medicine. Family Practice. 2016:cmw030.
14. Hofmans-Okkes IM, Lamberts H. The international classification of primary care (ICPC): new applications in research and computer-based patient records in family practice. Fam Pract. 1996;13(3):294–302.
15. van den Bussche H, Koller D, Kolonko T, Hansen H, Wegscheider K, Glaeske G, et al. Which chronic diseases and disease combinations are specific to multimorbidity in the elderly? Results of a claims data based cross-sectional study in Germany. BMC Public Health. 2011;11:101.
16. Bentsen BG. International classification of primary care. Scand J Prim Health Care. 1986;4(1):43–50.
17. Kadam UT, Croft PR, North Staffordshire GPCG. Clinical multimorbidity and physical function in older adults: a record and health status linkage study in general practice. Fam Pract. 2007;24(5):412–9
18. Anden A, Andre M, Rudebeck CE. What happened? GPs' perceptions of consultation outcomes and a comparison with the experiences of their patients. Eur J Gen Pract. 2010;16(2):80–4.
19. Kroenke K, Wyrwich KW, Tierney WM, Babu AN, Wolinsky FD. Physician-estimated disease severity in patients with chronic heart or lung disease: a cross-sectional analysis. Health Qual Life Outcomes. 2006;4:60.
20. Lesho E, Foster L, Wang Z, Sarmiento D, Dennison S, Valley MT, et al. The accuracy of physicians' perceptions of patients' suffering: findings from two teaching hospitals. Acad Med. 2009;84(5):636–42.
21. Fried LP, Bandeen-Roche K, Kasper JD, Guralnik JM. Association of comorbidity with disability in older women: the Women's health and aging study. J Clin Epidemiol. 1999;52(1):27–37.
22. Fultz NH, Ofstedal MB, Herzog AR, Wallace RB. Additive and interactive effects of comorbid physical and mental conditions on functional health. J Aging Health. 2003;15(3):465–81.
23. Cheraghi-Sohi S, Bower P, Kennedy A, Morden A, Rogers A, Richardson J, et al. Patient priorities in osteoarthritis and comorbid conditions: a secondary analysis of qualitative data. Arthritis Care Res (Hoboken). 2013; 65(6):920–7.
24. Morris RL, Sanders C, Kennedy AP, Rogers A. Shifting priorities in multimorbidity: a longitudinal qualitative study of patient's prioritization of multiple conditions. Chronic Illn. 2011;7(2):147–61.
25. Fried TR, Tinetti ME, Iannone L, O'Leary JR, Towle V, Van Ness PH. Health outcome prioritization as a tool for decision making among older persons with multiple chronic conditions. Arch Intern Med. 2011;171(20):1854–6.

19

General practitioners' perceptions of population based bowel screening and their influence on practice

Greer Dawson[1,2*], Melanie Crane[3], Claudine Lyons[4], Anna Burnham[5], Tara Bowman[5], Donna Perez[5] and Joanne Travaglia[6]

Abstract

Background: Although largely preventable, Australia has one of the highest rates of bowel cancer in the world. General Practitioners (GPs) have an important role to play in prevention and early detection of bowel cancer, however in Australia this is yet to be optimised and participation remains low. This study sought to understand how GPs' perceptions of bowel screening influence their attitudes to, and promotion of the faecal occult blood test (FOBT), to identify opportunities to enhance their role.

Methods: Interviews were conducted with 31 GPs from metropolitan and regional New South Wales (NSW), Australia. Discussions canvassed GPs' perceptions of their role in bowel screening and the national screening program; perceptions of screening tests; practices regarding discussing screening with patients; and views on opportunities to enhance their role. Transcripts were coded using Nvivo and thematically analysed.

Results: The study revealed GPs' perceptions of screening did not always align with broader public health definitions of 'population screening'. While many GPs reportedly understood the purpose of population screening, notions of the role of asymptomatic screening for bowel cancer prevention were more limited. Descriptions of screening centred on two major uses: the use of a screening 'process' to identify individual patients at higher risk; and the use of screening 'tools', including the FOBT, to aid diagnosis. While the FOBT was perceived as useful for identifying patients requiring follow up, GPs expressed concerns about its reliability. Colonoscopy by comparison, was considered by many as the gold standard for both screening and diagnosis. This perception reflects a conceptualisation of the screening process and associated tools as an individualised method for risk assessment and diagnosis, rather than a public health strategy for prevention of bowel cancer.

Conclusion: The results show that GPs' perceptions of screening do not always align with broader public health definitions of 'population screening'. Furthermore, the way GPs understood screening was shown to impact their clinical practice, influencing their preferences for, and use of 'screening' tools such as FOBT. The findings suggest emphasising the preventative opportunity of FOBT screening would be beneficial, as would formally engaging GPs in the promotion of bowel screening.

Keywords: Bowel cancer, Bowel screening, FOBT, General practitioners, Qualitative, Cancer prevention, Early detection

* Correspondence: greer.dawson@saxinstitute.org.au
[1]Sax Institute, Level 13, Building 10, 235 Jones Street, Ultimo, NSW, Australia 2007
[2]School of Public Health and Community Medicine, Samuels Building, University of New South Wales, Sydney, NSW, Australia 2052
Full list of author information is available at the end of the article

Background

Although largely preventable, Australia has one of the highest rates of bowel cancer in the world [1]. Early diagnosis increases the likelihood of successful treatment, however fewer than 40% of bowel cancers are detected early [2]. A Faecal Occult Blood Test (FOBT) increases early detection of bowel cancer [3–6], while detection and removal of pre-cancerous lesions reduces overall incidence [7]. In Australia, *The Clinical Practice Guidelines for the Prevention, Early Detection and Management of Colorectal Cancer* (2005) recommend biennial FOBT screening in the average-risk population [8]. Population screening aims to reduce the burden of disease in the general population by increasing the likelihood of identifying individuals with the disease before symptoms develop [9]. It differs significantly from detecting symptomatic cases or 'individual case finding' in asymptomatic patients with certain risk factors [10].

The National Bowel Cancer Screening Program (NBCSP) commenced in Australia in 2006. The program uses an immunochemical FOBT and operates by mailing invitations and FOBT kits directly to eligible individuals' home addresses based on Medicare data [11]. Currently, FOBT screening is offered on a 5-yearly basis commencing from age 50, with progression to biennial screening by 2020 underway [11]. This differs from the bowel screening program in the United Kingdom, which offers biennial FOBT screening from age 60 [12], or Japan which offers annual screening from age 40 . The United States has no organised program, however screening with FOBT, sigmoidoscopy or colonoscopy (depending on individual risk factors) is promoted through guideline dissemination and media campaigns.

The success of population screening programs depends on high participation, yet suboptimal participation in bowel screening is common around the world [13]. In Australia, participation in the NBCSP is around 30% [11], although it should be noted that some individuals report screening outside of the NBCSP [14] and are therefore not captured in this figure. Poor participation may be attributable to a range of factors including poor knowledge and awareness [15–17], confusion regarding recommendations and eligible ages which have changed over time [15], and lack of General Practitioner (GP) endorsement [17]. There is however, potential to reduce bowel cancer incidence through a concerted approach to screening.

In Australia, GPs are the first point of contact that individuals have with the health system. On average, Australians visit their GP around five times per year [18]. At present, GPs have no formal role in recruiting individuals into the NBCSP however have considerable potential to encourage participation. GPs play a significant role in promoting breast and cervical screening in line with current recommendations and acknowledge this as part of their approach to preventative health [19]. In relation to bowel screening, research suggests GP endorsement substantially increases compliance [20–24], however in Australia there has not yet been a coordinated effort to optimise the role of GPs in promoting bowel-screening participation.

The importance of screening is gaining attention in primary care, with national calls for health promotion, prevention and screening to be recognised as core roles in general practice [25]. GPs also report feeling positive towards undertaking prevention and health promotion activities, however increasing expectations of GPs to undertake a range of preventative activities in addition to diagnosing and treating patients should be acknowledged. Discussions about screening can be inhibited by factors such as time, distractions during consultations, multiple health concerns, and uncertainty about particular screening recommendations [26]. Time pressures and high workload are cited as frequent barriers [19, 27–29]. GPs' attitudes and level of confidence to initiate health promotion interventions also influence the inclusion of such activities in their routine practice [27, 30].

Existing research suggests the success of population-based screening will largely be determined by GP attitudes and support of the FOBT [31, 32]. It has also been shown that some GPs have concerns about the efficacy of the FOBT [33], however it remains unclear as to how this fits with their understanding of population based screening and prevention, and to what extent this shapes their clinical practice. To date we have been unable to locate any studies that examine specifically how GPs' perceive population based bowel screening in relation to cancer prevention, and how this affects their use of the FOBT. To address this gap, we sought to understand how GPs' perceptions of bowel screening influence their attitudes to, and promotion of the FOBT.

Methods

This study was conducted in 2014, eight years after the commencement of the NBCSP. A qualitative approach was selected to enable a nuanced understanding of GPs perceptions and attitudes. Semi-structured interviews were conducted with 31 GPs from around NSW who were recruited through research panels. Research panels are groups of pre-screened respondents who have expressed a willingness to participate in research. Purposive sampling was used to ensure representation of GPs from a variety of metropolitan (*n* = 16) and regional (*n* = 15) locations in NSW. Proportions of males and females were approximately equal. The sample was structured to include GPs with a higher proportion of patients of eligible screening age (50 years and over). This was done via a screening question asked in the recruitment phase that excluded GPs who indicated they had a relatively low proportion of patients aged over 50.

Interviews were conducted once, either over the phone or in-person after hours in the clinic, and were approximately 30 min in duration. Two experienced independent interviewers from a specialised qualitative research firm were engaged to conduct the interviews. All members of the research team, including the external interviewers, were independent of the primary care sector and no prior relationship existed between the participants and the researchers/interviewers. Participants were not informed of the research topic in advance and were reimbursed for their time. The interviews followed a discussion guide developed by the authors (Table 1) and pilot tested by the interviewers. No new themes emerged following the last few interviews indicating thematic saturation was reached.

Interviews were transcribed verbatim and coded using NVivo by the first author, GD. A thematic analysis was developed around the research objectives and emergent trends in the data using the approach developed by Braun and Clarke (2006) [34]. Rigour was addressed through an iterative process of constant comparison and the analysis process was documented to ensure process auditability [35]. A second investigator (JT) reviewed a random sample of transcripts and analysis to check the interpretation then the final analysis was developed via a consultative process involving all authors. Reflexivity was facilitated through an iterative process of analysis, with assumptions underpinning interpretations exposed through comparisons between authors' interpretations and with existing evidence. Differences were resolved through discussion [36]. Participants were not recontacted or provided with copies of the transcripts for verification, however the authors crosschecked the final thematic analysis with the interviewers who had conducted a separate independent analysis.

Ethics approval was granted by the University of New South Wales Human Research Ethics Advisory Panel.

Table 1 Discussion guide

1. What do you see as your role as a GP in cancer screening (general)?
2. What do you see as your role as a GP in *bowel* screening?
3. What factors influence whether or not you discuss bowel screening with patients? (*Prompt for barriers and enablers*)
4. What advice do you give patients regarding bowel screening, and does this differ depending on the patient? Can you please elaborate?
5. What is your view of different bowel cancer screening tests (FOBT, colonoscopy, flexible sigmoidoscopy)?
6. From your perspective, how willing are patients to undertake bowel screening? What factors do you think affect this (patient willingness)?
7. What sources of information about bowel cancer / bowel cancer screening do you use?
8. What bowel cancer screening guidelines do you know about? What is available? How useful?
9. What do you know about the NBCSP?
10. What is your opinion of the NBCSP / Understanding of screening eligibility / The role of GPs in the program?
11. What is your experience of the NBCSP in your practice?
12. When you feel that a patient should have an FOBT, what do you do?
13. What do you do with patients not eligible for the NBCSP?
14. What could help enhance the role of primary care in bowel screening to improve screening and early detection?

Results

The results are presented in two sections. The first examines GPs' perceptions of screening, while the second section explores their preference for and use of different screening tools. The range of perspectives and opinions are illustrated in each section. Overall, GPs acknowledged they had a potentially important role to play in bowel screening, and support for the NBCSP was widespread despite confusion about its delivery. GPs articulated a range of interpretations of what their role might entail, including providing education, encouraging compliance, detecting patients who had been missed by the NBCSP, and facilitating alternative screening pathways. A few GPs observed that the existence of the NBCSP meant their role was limited. Although GPs saw their role in screening to be important, there was variation in how this translated in their everyday practice, with perceptions of screening observed to exert an important influence on both attitudes and practice.

Perceptions of 'screening'

GPs' perceptions of bowel screening were varied. A few GPs had a detailed understanding of the meaning of population screening and the importance of targeting the asymptomatic population to enable prevention and early detection of bowel cancer. The majority, however, referred to screening in terms of identifying risk factors and facilitating screening for those assessed to be at higher risk. GPs also referred to screening as part of the diagnostic process.

The screening 'process'

Most GPs discussed screening in terms of a diagnostic or risk assessment 'process'. GPs spoke about their role in identifying patients who *should* be screened due to pre-existing risk factors. Assessing whether an individual required screening was seen as the first step in the 'screening' process.

In accordance with the National Guidelines [8], age was a key factor in determining whether screening was a priority. Other risk factors GPs considered included, whether patients had a first-degree family history of bowel cancer, and the presence or history of gastrointestinal symptoms.

> *'My role is basically to find the right kind of patient to screen, so either age related or [if] they have a strong family history...'*
>
> Male, regional

Screening was also referred to as something that should be done to address symptoms. This GP was asked if she had a system for raising screening with patients. She responded:

> *'You ask them if they have any gastrointestinal symptoms and sure, if there was some suspicion, then I'd probably put an occult blood on the form'*
>
> Female, regional

Some GPs talked about bowel screening specifically in terms of aiding diagnosis. In these cases 'screening' was used to exclude certain conditions, including cancer, and hence formed part of the process of diagnosing rather than screening per se.

> *'There are acute triggers, like patients who present with painful motions, an unexplained change in bowel habits or new cases of anaemia, that lead me to recommend FOBT, not so much because I suspect cancer but more because I want to rule it out as a possible cause of the patient's symptoms.'*
>
> Male, regional

Screening for early detection and prevention

While the majority of GPs described screening in terms of an assessment and diagnosis process, a few spoke of its role in early detection and prevention.

> *'I think the studies so far have shown that if we do screen the population at certain ages, that it does seem to pick up some of the bowel cancers earlier and therefore it's a good thing to do.'*
>
> Male, metropolitan

> *'Look, we talk about prevention really. It's good to practice preventative medicine. So pap smears, mammograms, for cervical cancer and breast cancer ... and faecal occult blood for bowel cancer.'*
>
> Female, metropolitan

The role of population screening and the importance of targeting the asymptomatic population was also raised by some GPs.

> *'What I see is to pick up cancer in the asymptomatic population, and the higher the pick-up rate, the better the outcome because it's fixable in the early stages, it's treatable. So my role is to pick up [cancer] early, as soon as possible.'*
>
> Female, metropolitan

Use of screening tools

GPs perceptions of three types of bowel screening tools were explored, the colonoscopy, the FOBT and the flexible sigmoidoscopy, although the latter was reported as being used infrequently. GPs' attitudes and stated preferences tended to reflect their conceptualisation of screening and the perceived utility of specific methods as diagnostic tools.

For GPs who conceptualised screening in terms of identifying and assessing patients at higher risk (patients with a family history or symptoms), then, in accordance with the National Guidelines [8], colonoscopy was overwhelmingly the preferred methodology.

> *'We have to encourage a vigilant approach, especially in those with a change in bowel habits or close family history of bowel cancer, or for patients who have had polyps removed in the past ... These people need colonoscopy and I refer them to a gastroenterologist to check for bowel cancer.'*
>
> Male, regional

GPs who viewed screening in terms of its diagnostic end point (detection of cancer) also tended to perceive colonoscopy was the gold standard 'screening' tool as it enabled a definitive diagnosis to be made.

> *'Well, I think at the moment, that [colonscopy's] the best way or the gold standard to check for any bowel disease – bowel polyps and bowel cancer'*
>
> Male, metropolitan

> *'I mean, a screening test – it has to be valuable and diagnostic at the same time.'*
>
> Female, metropolitan

By the same token, owing to its limitations as a diagnostic test, the FOBT was perceived by some to be inferior.

'A faecal occult blood test is a very basic screening tool which does not necessarily pick up bowel cancer. ... I would only recommend it for the person who is not agreeable to go for a colonoscopy.'

Female, metropolitan

Several GPs questioned the accuracy of the FOBT, expressing concerns about the number of false positives.

'You only need a small amount of blood ... and it will come up positive in your stool, so I usually send them directly for a colonoscopy.'

Female, regional

Despite both its limitations as a diagnostic tool, and concerns regarding accuracy, many GPs still saw the FOBT as a useful tool that could indicate where further investigation was warranted.

'It's a good rough tool. Of course there's a significant rate of false positives, and no doubt a rate of false negatives as well, but it's not an unreasonable rough tool'

Male, regional

GPs tended to have more positive perceptions of the FOBT where their concept of screening was population based. For these GPs, FOBT was recognised as an economical, non-invasive tool for identifying individuals requiring further clinical investigation.

'It seems that there's really only one screening test: faecal occult blood testing, FOBT ... FOBT is the best population-screening tool just because it is cheap and zero-risk to the patient. Of course, it is not a perfect diagnostic test but it does help identify people for further investigation ...'

Female, metropolitan

Discussion

Increasing FOBT screening as a population measure is important given its potential to facilitate prevention and early detection of bowel cancer and reduce overall disease incidence. GPs have a key role to play in encouraging screening participation [20–23], therefore strategies to formally engage them in the promotion of routine asymptomatic screening to patients should be considered [37]. The present study provides important insight into how GPs both conceptualise screening and promote use of the FOBT in their clinical practice, pointing to both opportunities and strategies to enhance their role.

This study builds on previous research that has identified the importance of GPs' knowledge and attitudes in shaping their clinical practice in relation to bowel screening [38, 39] by exploring *how* these factors impact on their practice. A novel finding derived from this research shows that GPs' concepts of screening did not always align with broader public health definitions of 'population screening' [9]. In particular, many GPs did not appear to have a well-formed understanding of the role of asymptomatic bowel screening in detecting precancerous lesions and thus the role of screening in bowel cancer prevention. GPs frequently construed screening as either part of a diagnostic process, or reserved for patients with individualised risk factors or symptoms. These findings suggest GPs interpret 'screening' within their localised clinical context, rather than within the broader perspective of population level prevention. Conceptualising screening as either assessing risk or aiding diagnosis signifies that screening was often understood as opportunistic detection or individual case finding. Given clinicians generally operate within the patient-centric Hippocratic tradition, where how an intervention helps an individual patient is the most important determinant, it makes sense that they are less likely to think in terms of 'population' benefits [40]. The diagnostic emphasis of the medical model amalgamated with the pressures of time and workload further compound this [29, 38].

Moreover, we found that GPs' perceptions of screening influenced both their preferences for, and use of different screening tools, with the FOBT often mistakenly evaluated in terms of its diagnostic capabilities. For GPs who viewed screening as part of a diagnostic process, it seems logical that they might prefer a test such as colonoscopy, which can more effectively aid diagnosis. Similarly, for GPs who did not make a clear conceptual distinction between screening and diagnosis, the FOBT was often mistakenly evaluated in terms of its capabilities as a diagnostic test. As the FOBT is non-specific and thus limited in its diagnostic capabilities it follows that colonoscopy would be preferred. Concerns about false positives (where a cancer diagnosis does not follow), suggests that the FOBT seemed to be widely misunderstood as to its purpose. Such concerns amongst GPs have been reported previously by studies undertaken in the United States [41] and Australia [33]. FOBT is not a diagnostic test for bowel cancer; rather it is a test for blood in the stool for which it is very sensitive. Perceived in those terms, concerns about false positives should not be widespread. GPs tended to have a more positive view of the FOBT when it was perceived as a population-based screening tool to indicate where further investigation was required. Having a poor understanding of the role of screening in the prevention of disease is a barrier to the integration of routine asymptomatic bowel screening activities in general practice.

The findings from this study support existing research that has found the perceived efficacy of screening to be a determinant of clinical practice [32, 38]. To address these issues, we need strategies to engage and encourage GPs to adopt more preventive approaches within their current models of care. GPs need adequate information focused around the effectiveness of routine screening programs, including the proportion of false negatives and false positives, in order to effectively promote screening [42]. Targeted information around the natural history of bowel cancer including pre-cancerous lesions and the role of asymptomatic screening in prevention would also provide a useful framework from which to enhance GPs' understandings of population screening [37]. Formally engaging GPs in the promotion of bowel screening would likely raise the profile of the disease and reinforce the importance of prevention and early detection. In France, GPs are directly involved in administering the FOBT screening program, which has been shown to have implications for increased participation, particularly when the GP delivers the test [38]. The involvement of both GPs and patients in a shared care approach also provides an opportunity to facilitate awareness and promote the value of screening [38].

Practice-based strategies that prompt GPs to discuss screening with eligible patients should also be implemented [43, 44]. This could include establishing systems that enable GPs to identify patients who are eligible for screening and trigger a reminder at the time of consultation. Other strategies such as organising special clinics that focus on preventative activities or involving practice nurses in screening activities may assist in addressing some of the practical barriers faced by GPs in promoting screening to patients [45]. Engaging patients while they are waiting for a GP visit by asking them to complete a bowel screening self-assessment, may be another useful way to initiate discussions about screening and has the added advantage of fostering a shared decision-making approach.

Limitations

Although we sought diversity in our sample, it is possible that this may have been constrained by the recruitment of participants from research panels, which may limit the applicability of our findings to the broader population of GPs in NSW. Furthermore, self-report measures may not always reflect actual practice. Despite these limitations, the findings highlight important issues, which if adequately addressed may contribute to increasing bowel screening participation in NSW.

Conclusion

The results of this study show that GPs' interpretations of screening do not necessarily align with defined notions of population screening and the importance of FOBT screening may therefore be under realised. The findings illustrate how perceptions of screening influence attitudes and practice, and suggest a greater emphasis on the preventative opportunity of FOBT screening would be beneficial, as would formally engaging GPs in the promotion of bowel screening. This may assist in re-shaping how some GPs view the FOBT and utilise it in their clinical practice.

Abbreviations

FOBT: Faecal occult blood test; GP: General Practitioner; NBCSP: National Bowel Cancer Screening Program.

Acknowledgements

The authors wish to acknowledge Jennifer Crawford and John Sergeant from Curly Questions Pty Ltd who undertook the interviews and provided transcripts for analysis, and Professor Sanchia Aranda for reviewing and providing input into the manuscript.

Funding

This work was undertaken whilst Greer Dawson was employed as a trainee on the NSW Public Health Training Program funded by the NSW Ministry of Health. She completed this work whilst based at the Cancer Institute NSW. This study was funded internally by the Cancer Institute NSW.

Authors' contributions

GD, MC and DP designed the study with input from all the other authors. GD undertook the analysis of the interviews, which was crosschecked by JT and developed in consultation with MC, CL, AB and TB. The first draft of the manuscript was developed by GD and revised critically by MC, CL, AB, TB, JT and DP. All authors have read and approved the final version of this manuscript.

Competing interests

The authors declare that they have no competing interests.

Consent for publication

Not applicable.

Author details

[1]Sax Institute, Level 13, Building 10, 235 Jones Street, Ultimo, NSW, Australia 2007. [2]School of Public Health and Community Medicine, Samuels Building, University of New South Wales, Sydney, NSW, Australia 2052. [3]Prevention Research Collaboration, The Charles Perkins Centre, Level 6, The Hub, School of Public Health, University of Sydney, Sydney, NSW, Australia 2006. [4]NSW Department of Premier and Cabinet, 52 Martin Place, Sydney, NSW, Australia 2000. [5]Cancer Institute NSW, Australian Technology Park, Level 9, 8 Central Avenue, Sydney, NSW, Australia 2015. [6]Faculty of Health, University of Technology Sydney, Level 7, 235 Jones Street, Sydney, NSW, Australia 2007.

References

1. GLOBOCAN 2012 Estimated Cancer Incidence, Mortality and Prevalence Worldwide [http://globocan.iarc.fr/Pages/fact_sheets_cancer.aspx]
2. About bowel screening [http://www.cancerscreening.gov.au/internet/screening/publishing.nsf/Content/about-bowel-screening]
3. Heresbach D, Manfredi S, D'Halluin PN, Bretagne JF, Branger B. Review in depth and meta-analysis of controlled trials on colorectal cancer screening by faecal occult blood test. Eur J Gastroenterol Hepatol. 2006;18(4):427–33.
4. Hewitson P, Glasziou PP, Irwig L, Towler B, Watson E. Screening for colorectal cancer using the faecal occult blood test, Hemoccult. Cochrane Database Syst Rev. 2007;1:CD001216. doi:10.1002/14651858.CD001216.pub2.
5. Mandel JS, Bond JH, Church TR, Snover DC, Bradley GM, Schuman LM, Ederer F. Reducing mortality from colorectal cancer by screening for fecal occult blood. Minnesota Colon Cancer Control Study. N Engl J Med. 1993; 328(19):1365–71.
6. Hardcastle JD, Thomas WM, Chamberlain J, Pye G, Sheffield J, James PD, Balfour TW, Amar SS, Armitage NC, Moss SM. Randomised, controlled trial of faecal occult blood screening for colorectal cancer. Results for first 107,349 subjects. Lancet. 1989;1(8648):1160–4.
7. Leggett BA, Hewett DG. Colorectal cancer screening. Intern Med J. 2015; 45(1):6–15.
8. Australian Cancer Network Colorectal Cancer Guidelines Revision Committee. Guidelines for the Prevention, Early Detection and Management of Colorectal Cancer. Sydney: The Cancer Council Australia and Australian Cancer Network; 2005.
9. Population Based Screening Framework [http://www.cancerscreening.gov.au/internet/screening/publishing.nsf/Content/population-based-screening-framework]
10. Young GP. Population-based screening for colorectal cancer: Australian research and implementation. J Gastroenterol Hepatol. 2009;24 Suppl 3:S33–42.
11. Australian Institute of Health and Welfare: National Bowel Cancer Screening Program monitoring report: 2012–13. Cancer series No. 84 Cat. no. CAN 81. In. Edited by AIHW, Cat. no. CAN 81. edn. Canberra: AIHW; 2014.
12. NHS bowel cancer screening program [https://http://www.gov.uk/guidance/bowel-cancer-screening-programme-overview]
13. Bulliard JL, Garcia M, Blom J, Senore C, Mai V, Klabunde C. Sorting out measures and definitions of screening participation to improve comparability: the example of colorectal cancer. Eur J Cancer. 2014;50(2): 434–46.
14. Zajac IT, Flight I, Turnbull D, Young G, Cole S, Wilson C. Self-reported bowel screening rates in older Australians and the implications for public health screening programs. Australas Med J. 2013;6(8):411–7.
15. Dawson G, Crane M, Lyons C, Burnham A, Bowman T, Travaglia J. A qualitative investigation of factors influencing participation in bowel screening in New South Wales. Health Promot J Austr. 2016;27(1):48–53.
16. Keighley MR, O'Morain C, Giacosa A, Ashorn M, Burroughs A, Crespi M, Delvaux M, Faivre J, Hagenmuller F, Lamy V, et al. Public awareness of risk factors and screening for colorectal cancer in Europe. Eur J Cancer Prev. 2004;13(4):257–62.
17. Javanparast S, Ward PR, Carter SM, Wilson CJ. Barriers to and facilitators of colorectal cancer screening in different population subgroups in Adelaide, South Australia. Med J Aust. 2012;196(8):521–3.
18. Britt H, Miller G, Henderson J, Bayram C, Valenti L, Harrison C, Charles J, Pan Y, Zhang C, Pollack A, et al. General practice activity in Australia 2012–13. In: General practice series no33. Sydney: Sydney University Press; 2013.
19. McIlfatrick S, Keeney S, McKenna H, McCarley N, McElwee G. Investigating the role of the general practitioner in cancer prevention: a mixed methods study. BMC Fam Pract. 2013;14:58.
20. Myers RE, Sifri R, Hyslop T, Rosenthal M, Vernon SW, Cocroft J, Wolf T, Andrel J, Wender R. A randomized controlled trial of the impact of targeted and tailored interventions on colorectal cancer screening. Cancer. 2007; 110(9):2083–91.
21. Ferrante JM, McCarthy EP, Gonzalez EC, Lee JH, Chen R, Love-Jackson K, Roetzheim RG, Ferrante JM, McCarthy EP, Gonzalez EC, et al. Primary Care Utilization and Colorectal Cancer Outcomes Among Medicare Beneficiaries. Arch Intern Med. 2011;171(19):1747–57.
22. Ferreira MR, Dolan NC, Fitzgibbon ML, Davis TC, Gorby N, Ladewski L, Liu D, Rademaker AW, Medio F, Schmitt BP, et al. Health care provider-directed intervention to increase colorectal cancer screening among veterans: results of a randomized controlled trial. J Clin Oncol. 2005;23(7):1548–54.
23. Federici A, Giorgi Rossi P, Bartolozzi F, Farchi S, Borgia P, Guastcchi G. The role of GPs in increasing compliance to colorectal cancer screening: a randomised controlled trial (Italy). Cancer Causes Control. 2006;17(1):45–52.
24. Zajac IT, Whibley AH, Cole SR, Byrne D, Guy J, Morcom J, Young GP. Endorsement by the primary care practitioner consistently improves participation in screening for colorectal cancer: a longitudinal analysis. J Med Screen. 2010;17(1):19–24.
25. National Primary Health Care Strategic Framework [http://www.health.gov.au/internet/main/publishing.nsf/Content/6084A04118674329CA257BF0001A349E/$File/NPHCframe.pdf]
26. Miser WF. Cancer screening in the primary care setting: the role of the primary care physician in screening for breast, cervical, colorectal, lung, ovarian, and prostate cancers. Prim Care. 2007;34(1):137–67.
27. Brotons C, Bjorkelund C, Bulc M, Ciurana R, Godycki-Cwirko M, Jurgova E, Kloppe P, Lionis C, Mierzecki A, Pineiro R, et al. Prevention and health promotion in clinical practice: the views of general practitioners in Europe. Prev Med. 2005;40(5):595–601.
28. Yarnall KSH, Pollak KI, Ostbye T, Krause KM, Michener JL. Primary care: Is there enough time for prevention? Am J Public Health. 2003;93(4):635–41.
29. Rubio-Valera M, Pons-Vigués M, Martínez-Andrés M, Moreno-Peral P, Berenguera A, Fernández A. Barriers and Facilitators for the Implementation of Primary Prevention and Health Promotion Activities in Primary Care: A Synthesis through Meta-Ethnography. PLoS One. 2014;9(2):e89554.
30. McKinlay E, Plumridge L, McBain L, McLeod D, Pullon S, Brown S. "What sort of health promotion are you talking about?": a discourse analysis of the talk of general practitioners. Soc Sci Med. 2005;60(5):1099–106.
31. Turner GB, Chin MW, Foster NM, Emery J, Forbes GM. Attitudes of Western Australian general practitioners to colorectal cancer screening. Med J Aust. 2006;185(4):237.
32. Damery S, Clifford S, Wilson S. Colorectal cancer screening using the faecal occult blood test (FOBt): a survey of GP attitudes and practices in the UK. BMC Fam Pract. 2010;11:20–20.
33. Clavarino AM, Janda M, Hughes KL, Del Mar C, Tong S, Stanton WR, Aitken JF, Leggett BA, Newman B. The view from two sides: a qualitative study of community and medical perspectives on screening for colorectal cancer using FOBT. Prev Med. 2004;39(3):482–90.
34. Braun V, Clarke V. Using thematic analysis in psychology. Qual Res Psychol. 2006;3(2):77–101.
35. Miles MB, Huberman AM. Qualitative data analysis: An expanded sourcebook. Beverly Hills: Sage Publications; 1994.
36. Getrich CM, Bennett AM, Sussman AL, Solares A, Helitzer DL. Viewing Focus Groups Through a Critical Incident Lens. Qual Health Res. 2016;26(6):750–62.
37. Lionis C, Petelos E. Early detection of colorectal cancer: barriers to screening in the primary care setting. Fam Pract. 2011;28(6):589–91.
38. Aubin-Auger I, Mercier A, Lebeau JP, Baumann L, Peremans L, Van Royen P. Obstacles to colorectal screening in general practice: a qualitative study of GPs and patients. Fam Pract. 2011;28(6):670–6.
39. Thanapirom K, Treeprasertsuk S, Rerknimitr R. Awareness of colorectal cancer screening in primary care physicians. J Med Assoc Thai. 2012;95(7):859–65.
40. Lawrence DM. Priorities among recommended clinical preventive services. Am J Prev Med. 2001;21(1):66–7.
41. Dulai GS, Farmer MM, Ganz PA, Bernaards CA, Qi K, Dietrich AJ, Bastani R, Belman MJ, Kahn KL. Primary care provider perceptions of barriers to and facilitators of colorectal cancer screening in a managed care setting. Cancer. 2004;100(9):1843–52.
42. Woodrow C, Rozmovits L, Hewitson P, Rose P, Austoker J, Watson E. Bowel cancer screening in England: a qualitative study of GPs' attitudes and information needs. BMC Fam Pract. 2006;7(1):53.
43. Klabunde CN, Vernon SW, Nadel MR, Breen N, Seeff LC, Brown ML. Barriers to colorectal cancer screening: a comparison of reports from primary care physicians and average-risk adults. Med Care. 2005;43(9):939–44.
44. Guerra CE, Schwartz JS, Armstrong K, Brown JS, Halbert CH, Shea JA. Barriers of and Facilitators to Physician Recommendation of Colorectal Cancer Screening. J Gen Intern Med. 2007;22(12):1681–8.
45. Arroyave AM, Penaranda EK, Lewis CL. Organizational Change: A Way to Increase Colon, Breast and Cervical Cancer Screening in Primary Care Practices. J Community Health. 2011;36(2):281–8.

20

Procedures performed by general practitioners and general internal medicine physicians - a comparison based on routine data from Northern Germany

C. Strumann[1*], K. Flägel[1], T. Emcke[2] and J. Steinhäuser[1]

Abstract

Background: In response to a rising shortage of general practitioners (GPs), physicians in general internal medicine (GIM) have become part of the German primary care physician workforce. Previous studies have shown substantial differences in practice patterns between both specialties. The aim of this study was to analyse and compare the application of procedures by German GPs and GIM physicians based on routine data.

Methods: The Association of Statutory Health Insurance Physicians in the federal state Schleswig-Holstein (Northern Germany) provided invoicing data of the first quarters of 2013 and 2015. Differences between GPs and GIM physicians in the implementation rate of 46 selected primary care procedures were examined by means of the Pearson χ^2-test. The selection of procedures was based on international and own preliminary studies on primary care procedures.

Results: In the first quarter of 2013/2015 respectively, 1228/1227 GPs and 447/484 GIM physicians provided services in Schleswig-Holstein. Significant differences were found for 20 of the 46 procedures. GPs had higher application rates of procedures concerning health screening (e.g. adolescent health examination, well-child visits) and minor surgery. GIM physicians more often applied technology-oriented procedures, such as ultrasound scans, electrocardiograms (ECG), and 24-h ambulatory blood pressure measurements. The treatment patterns of both specialities did not vary much during the study period. Cardiac stress testing was the only significantly increased GP procedure in that time.

Conclusions: Our results suggest substantial differences in the application of procedures between GPs and GIM physicians with potential consequences for the overall primary healthcare provision. The findings could foster a discussion about training needs for procedures in primary care to ensure its comprehensiveness. The results reflect scope for changes in vocational training in the future for an effective and efficient re-allocation of primary healthcare.

Keywords: Procedural skills, Primary care, General internal medicine, General practitioner

Background

In most industrialised countries, the demand for healthcare is increasing due to an ageing population coinciding with a declining number of primary care physicians [1–3]. Primary care physicians are general practitioners (GPs), physicians in general internal medicine (GIM) or paediatricians who provide "care for the undifferentiated patient at the point of first contact" [4]. The range of services that primary care patients require is extensive [5]. However, according to previous studies, procedures differ considerably between GPs and GIM physicians, e.g. regarding the use of diagnostics [6], medical charges [7], prescribing [8], communication [9], provision of care for patients with common conditions [10], range of specific health needs covered [11] and patient outcomes [12].

In Germany, most primary care physicians are traditionally self-employed. However, they need an accreditation for service provision for patients within the statutory health insurance scheme that covers about 90% of the population. In 2016, around 79% of the German

* Correspondence: c.strumann@uni-luebeck.de
[1]Institute of Family Medicine, University Hospital Schleswig-Holstein, Campus Luebeck, Ratzeburger Allee 160, 23538 Luebeck, Germany

population visited a primary care physician at least once [13]. The distribution of physicians is regulated and allocated by the Association of Statutory Health Insurance Physicians (ASHIP), which is responsible for the accreditation process to maintain a sufficient and high-quality supply of physicians [14].

Whereas the international definition of primary care physicians includes paediatricians, the definition by the German ASHIP does not, so that the primary care physician workforce in Germany only consists of GPs and GIM physicians. By law, GPs are preferred in the accreditation process [15]. However, the declining number of GPs in the last decade has resulted in local shortages, especially in rural areas [16, 17]. In response to the rising shortage of GPs, a rise in the quota of GIM physicians providing primary care can be observed [18].

A previous study using self-assessment of GPs and GIM physicians [19] showed differences in the application of medical procedures and suggested implications for the quality and safety of primary care provision in Germany. In general, the use of survey data based on self-assessment can be problematic because of selection or response biases [20]. Influences on self-assessment such as gender, age, emotional status and recall bias have been described [21–24]. Moreover, studies based on survey data are prone to selection bias [25]. In contrast, routine data present a reliable source of information that avoid selection or recall bias [26, 27]. Findings of studies based on survey data can be crosschecked by analysing routine data.

The aim of this study was to analyse and compare, based on routine data, the application of procedures by German GPs and GIM physicians. The results may subsequently allow to deduce measures to promote an effective and efficient re-allocation of primary healthcare resources.

Methods

This study is based on the analysis of routine data from the ASHIP of the federal state Schleswig-Holstein located in Northern Germany. The concentration on a specific federal state of Germany allows to reduce practice variations based on regional differences and state-specific regulations [28].

Data selection

Based on a previously consented questionnaire comprising relevant procedures in German primary care [19, 25] the research team checked the doctor's fee scale 2015 [29] for codes addressing procedures or at least comprising procedures of the questionnaire. Both the routine data provided by the ASHIP and the data collected by the questionnaire refer to the first three months of the years 2013 and 2015 respectively. Data included the number of all billed codes of the doctor's fee scale by all GPs and GIM physicians in the federal state of Schleswig-Holstein. The analysis concentrated on codes reflecting services with high relevance in primary care [30–33]. Procedures were defined as discrete, diagnostic or therapeutic activities requiring knowledge and manual skills, performed on patients following the definition of Sylvester et al. [31]. Out of 90 possible physicians' procedures listed in the initial questionnaire [19, 25], 46 were identified that could be employed by both GPs and GIM physicians. Table 1 shows the codes for services and whether the respective procedure is part of the training curriculum of the respective specialty.

Statistical analysis

Differences in the application of a specific procedure by GPs and GIM physicians as well as differences between the two study periods were analysed by means of the Pearson χ^2-test. All tests of significance were two-tailed and were corrected using the Bonferroni method to counteract the problem of multiple comparisons [34]. A p-value < 0.05 was considered as statistically significant. Statistical analyses were performed with MATLAB software, version 9.4 (R2018a) (The MathWorks, Natick, MA, USA).

Results

In the first quarter of 2013, 1228 GPs and 447 GIM physicians provided services in Schleswig-Holstein. In 2015, the number of GPs remained unchanged (1227), while the number of GIM physicians had increased to 484. There are no substantial differences between the number of distinct fee scale codes submitted by GPs and GIM physicians. For both specialities the overall number of services invoiced and the physicians' average of services invoiced have increased over the time frame by 37.7% and 27.2%, respectively. The percentages of the total number of codes reflecting the selected procedures are relatively small and have declined slightly over the study period (2015: 2% (GP) and 2.7% (GIM)). Table 2 shows the number of physicians, the number of distinct service codes, the total number of codes invoiced and other statistics for both years and specialties.

There are several significant differences between GIM physicians and GPs with regard to the application of specific procedures. Of note are the higher GP figures for health screening services, especially adolescent health examination and well-child visits. The number of minor surgery procedures performed by GPs is also significantly higher. These include primary and secondary wound healing, excisions, treatment of ingrown toenails and phlebotomy. Procedures performed to a higher extent by GMI physicians are in general based on more technical approaches, i.e. services using ultrasound diagnostics

Table 1 Assignment of the procedures to the bill codes

Code	Bill code description [29]	Procedure [25]	Part of training [45]	
			GP	GIM
Well child visit				
01712	Well-child visit of the new-born during the 3rd to 10th day of life	Well-child visit	yes	no
01713	Well-child visit during the 4th and 5th week of life "(U3)"			
01714	Well-child visit during the 3rd and 4th month of life "(U4)"			
01715	Well-child visit during the 6th and 8th month of life "(U5)"			
01716	Well-child visit during the 10th and 12th month of life "(U6)"			
01717	Well-child visit during the 21st to 24th month of life "(U7)"			
01718	Well-child visit during the 46th to 48th month of life "(U8)"			
01719	Well-child visit during the 60th to 64th month of life "(U9)"			
01723	Well-child visit during the 36th to 43rd month of life "(U7a)"			
01720	Adolescent health examination "(J1)"	Adolescent health examination	yes	no
Minor surgery				
02301	Minor surgery II: primary wound closure with sutures	Surgical suture	yes	no
		Drainage of acute paronychia	yes	no
		Electrocautery of skin lesion	yes	no
		I&D of an abscess	yes	no
		I&D of a perianal abscess	yes	no
		Glueing of a wound	yes	no
02302	Minor surgery III: excisions, treatment of ingrown toenails, phlebotomy	Removal of foreign object	yes	no
		Excision of lipoma	yes	no
		Partial removal of toenail	yes	no
02310	Secondary healing wound care and/or decubital ulcer care	Wound debridement	yes	no
02311	Diabetic foot care			
02312	Treatment of single or multiple chronic venous ulcers			
02313	Compression therapy for chronic venous insufficiency, post-thrombotic syndrome, superficial and deep vein thrombosis and/or lymphoedema	Compression therapy	no	no
Injection and infusion				
02101	Infusion	Infusion	yes	yes
02321	Suprapubic catheter insertion	Suprapubic catheter insertion	yes	yes
02323	Transurethral catheter insertion	Transurethral catheter insertion	yes	yes
Paracentesis and insertion				
02340	Paracentesis	Ascites paracentesis	yes	yes
		Trepination of subungual haematoma	yes	no
		Paracentesis of knee joint	yes	yes
		Paracentesis of scapula joint	yes	yes
02343	Trephination of pleural cavity and non-surgical pleural drainage	Thoracentesis	yes	yes
		Trepination of tension pneumothorax	yes	yes
		Chest tube insertion	yes	yes
Treatment of musculoskeletal disorders				
02360	Treatment under local anaesthesia	Neural therapy	yes	no
31,910	Reduction of carpal or tarsal dislocation (distal)	Reduction of dislocated finger	no[a]	no
31,912	Reduction of dislocated cubital or knee joint (distal)	Reduction of displaced fracture of the radial head	no[a]	no
31,914	Reduction of dislocated cubital or knee joint (proximal)	Reduction of dislocated shoulder joint	no[a]	no

Table 1 Assignment of the procedures to the bill codes *(Continued)*

Code	Bill code description [29]	Procedure [25]	Part of training [45]	
			GP	GIM
Instrument-based procedures				
02500	Single inhalation therapy	Preparing a nebulizer for antiobstructive therapy	no	no
03321	Cardiac stress test	Cardiac stress test	yes	yes
03324	24-h ambulatory blood pressure monitoring	24-h ambulatory blood pressure monitoring	yes	yes
03330	Spirometry	Spirometry	yes	yes
03331	Proctoscopy	Proctoscopy	yes	yes
03335	Exploratory audiometry after previously documented, hearing test anomalies	Diagnostic audiometer test	no	no
33012	Thyroid sonography B-scan	Thyroid sonography thyroid	yes	yes
33042	Abdominal sonography B-scan	Abdominal sonography	yes	yes
33060	Sonographic examination of extracranial cerebral vessels, the periorbital arteries, subclavian arteries and vertebral arteries by CW-Doppler	Doppler ultrasound of brain-supplying vessels	yes	yes
33061	CW Doppler sonography of limb blood vessels, at least 3 transducer locations per limb	Compression sonography of lower extremities	yes	yes
33076	Limb vein B-scan sonography at least 8 transducer locations			
Laboratory diagnostic procedures				
32031	Microscopic urinalysis for morphological components	Microscopic urinalysis	yes	yes
32040	Faecal occult blood test in 3 samples	Faecal occult blood test	yes	yes
01734	Examination for faecal occult blood according to stage D.-III of the early detection of cancer-guideline, including costs			
32045	microscopic examination of bodily material	Examine a native sample for funghi	yes	yes
Emergency medicine				
01220	Resuscitation	Mask ventilation	yes	yes
01221	Supplement to Resuscitation (Coniotomy and / or Endotracheal Intubation)	Endotracheal intubation	yes	yes
01222	Supplement to Resuscitation (defibrillation)	Defibrillation	yes	yes
Gynaecology				
01830	Insertion of intrauterine device	insertion of intrauterine device	no	no
01730	Cancer screening for women	Gynaecological examination	no	no
01825	Cervical smear test	Cervical smear test	no	no

[a]These procedures are part of the mandatory 6-month surgical training during GP vocational training

Table 2 Descriptive Statistics

year	2013		2015		change (in %)	
specialty	GP	GIM	GP	GIM	GP	GIM
physicians	1228	447	1227	484	−0.1	8.3
number of fee scale codes invoiced	697	613	683	675	−2.0	10.1
total number of codes invoiced by all physicians	6,752,667	2,499,625	8,856,848	3,442,080	31.2	37.7
total number of codes invoiced per physician	5498.9	5592.0	7218.3	7111.7	31.3	27.2
total number of codes invoiced by all physicians reflecting selected procedures	179,095	85,413	180,779	93,286	0.9	9.2
percentage of the total number of codes reflecting selected procedures (in %)	2.7	3.4	2.0	2.7	−23.0	−20.7

or an electrocardiogram (ECG). Another service that is significantly more frequently performed by GIM physicians than GPs is the long-term blood pressure measurement. In general, the treatment patterns of both specialties did not vary much over the time frame. Cardiac stress testing was the only procedure by GPs that saw an increase in the study period. The proportions of GPs and GIM physicians performing a specific procedure in the study periods of 2013 and 2015 are shown in Tables 3 and 4 with the respective p-values for group differences. For ease of illustration, procedures which were applied by less than 1% of physicians are not shown.

Discussion

The comprehensiveness of general practice in the provision of primary healthcare [35] and its coordinating role in referring patients across the individual healthcare sectors [36, 37] determine the strength of primary care, since both factors have positive effects on health outcomes, equality and overall efficiency in healthcare systems [38–43]. Therefore, GPs traditionally received training focusing on treating the whole person through all stages of life [44]. The curriculum of GPs in Schleswig-Holstein includes working in primary care, i.e. private practices for at least 24 months. In contrast, the training of internal medicine physicians happens entirely in the hospital setting [45].

Table 3 Application rates of general practitioners (GPs) and general internal medicine (GIM) physicians for procedures performed to a greater extent by GPs (in %)

Code	Description	2013			2015		
		GP (n = 1228)	GIM (n = 447)	p-value*	GP (n = 1227)	GIM (n = 484)	p-value*
02310	Secondary healing wound care and/or decubital ulcer care	60.4	43.6	< 0.001	64.6	44.0	< 0.001
02301	Minor surgery II: primary wound closure with sutures	39.0	13.4	< 0.001	37.8	16.7	< 0.001
01734	Examination for faecal occult blood according to stage D.-III of the early detection of cancer-guideline, including costs	27.2	22.1	n.s.	27.9	24.8	n.s.
01720	Adolescent health examination "(J1)"	27.1	13.9	< 0.001	25.5	9.5	< 0.001
02312	Treatment of single or multiple chronic venous ulcers	23.2	17.4	n.s.	23.5	17.8	n.s.
01718	Well-child visit during the 46th to 48th month of life "(U8)"	13.8	2.5	< 0.001	12.2	1.2	< 0.001
01719	Well-child visit during the 60th to 64th month of life "(U9)"	13.6	2.0	< 0.001	13.9	1.4	< 0.001
02302	Minor surgery III: excisions, treatment of ingrown toenails, phlebotomy	13.0	2.0	< 0.001	12.1	2.1	< 0.001
01723	Well-child visit during the 43rd to 36th month of life "(U7a)"	10.9	1.6	< 0.001	11.8	1.7	< 0.001
01717	Well-child visit during the 21st to 24th month of life "(U7)"	10.6	0.9	< 0.001	10.2	1.0	< 0.001
01716	Well-child visit during the 10th and 12th month of life "(U6)"	10.3	1.8	< 0.001	8.6	1.2	< 0.001
01715	Well-child visit during the 6th and 8th month of life "(U5)"	8.3	1.3	< 0.001	8.2	1.2	< 0.001
01714	Well-child visit during the 3rd and 4th month of life "(U4)"	8.1	1.1	< 0.001	7.1	1.2	< 0.001
01713	Well-child visit during the 4th and 5th week of life "(U3)"	6.4	0.9	< 0.001	6.4	0.6	< 0.001
02500	Single inhalation therapy	5.3	2.5	n.s.	4.9	2.3	n.s.
03335	Exploratory audiometry after previously documented, hearing test anomalies	3.7	1.6	n.s.	3.1	0.8	n.s.
01730	Cancer screening for women	3.2	0.0	0.010	1.8	0.0	n.s.
01712	Well-child visit of the new-born during the 3rd to 10th day of life	2.5	0.0	n.s.	2.4	0.2	n.s.

*Bonferroni correction
only procedures with percentages larger than 1.0% for at least one specialty are shown
bold percentages indicate a significant difference between 2013 and 2015 (at the 5% level)
n.s. not significant (at the 5% level)

Table 4 Application rates of general practitioners (GPs) and general internal medicine (GIM) physicians for procedures performed to a greater extent by GIM physicians (in %)

Code	Description	2013			2015		
		GP ($n = 1228$)	GIM ($n = 447$)	p-value*	GP ($n = 1227$)	GIM ($n = 484$)	p-value*
03330	Spirometry	80.5	82.3	n.s.	80.1	83.7	n.s.
03324	24-h ambulatory blood pressure monitoring	72.2	82.8	< 0.001	74.2	82.9	0.011
32040	Faecal occult blood test in 3 samples	68.5	70.0	n.s.	66.0	66.9	n.s.
33042	Abdominal sonography B-scan	52.9	91.1	< 0.001	51.6	89.3	< 0.001
03321	Cardiac stress test	**45.5**	79.6	< 0.001	**52.6**	82.4	< 0.001
32031	Microscopic urinalysis for morphological components	37.8	41.6	n.s.	34.5	34.9	n.s.
33012	Thyroid sonography B-scan	21.4	73.6	< 0.001	21.5	75.4	< 0.001
02313	Compression therapy for chronic venous insufficiency, post-thrombotic syndrome, superficial and deep vein thrombosis and/or lymphoedema	15.8	16.1	n.s.	20.7	19.8	n.s.
03331	Proctoscopy	6.4	7.4	n.s.	5.2	7.2	n.s.
02311	Diabetic foot care	6.2	10.1	n.s.	5.5	9.9	n.s.
33061	CW Doppler sonography of limb blood vessels, at least 3 transducer locations per limb	1.6	8.5	< 0.001	1.5	7.2	< 0.001
33060	Sonographic examination of extracranial cerebral vessels, the periorbital arteries, subclavian arteries and vertebral arteries by CW-Doppler	1.1	3.6	0.036	1.1	3.3	n.s.
01220	Resuscitation	0.7	1.1	n.s.	1.1	0.0	n.s.
33076	Limb vein B-scan sonography at least 8 transducer locations	0.3	8.7	< 0.001	0.6	9.3	< 0.001

*Bonferroni correction
only procedures with percentages larger than 1.0% for at least one specialty are shown
bold percentages indicate a significant difference between 2013 and 2015 (at the 5% level)
n.s. not significant (at the 5% level)

We analysed differences in patterns of procedures performed by German GPs and GMI physicians based on routine data collected by ASHIP for the federal state of Schleswig-Holstein over two distinct time periods in 2013 and 2015. In total, 1227 GPs and 484 GIM physicians were looked at in 2015. This cohort represented about 3.5% of all GPs and GIM physicians practising in Germany in 2015 [18]. The ratio of codes billed per specialty (GPs: 72% (73%) and GIM physicians: 28% (27%) in 2015 (2013)) are nearly identical for both specialties and years to the respective nation-wide proportions of cases treated and codes billed in primary care [46, 47]. Furthermore, the differences over the time frame underline the rising significance of GIM physicians in the provision of primary care in Germany.

The results show substantial differences between GPs and GIM physicians in the application rates of most of the identified procedures. In general, procedures with higher application rates by GPs tend to be more advisory and concern the prevention of health problems. In contrast, procedures with higher application rates by GMI physicians are to a greater extent technically orientated. These results are consistent with findings of previous studies [7, 12, 19].

In 2015, for example, more than 25% of GPs performed health visits for adolescents. In contrast, less than 10% of GIM physicians performed this procedure. Well-child visits show similar differences. These figures reflect a wider range in the age of patients treated by GPs compared to GIM physicians. Health services for children are also provided by paediatricians [48]. In German rural areas, however, a shortage of paediatricians leads to children's healthcare services being delivered by GPs or GIM physicians [49]. Moreover, rural areas are particularly affected by the declining number of GPs. Therefore, GIM physicians stand a higher chance of accreditation in rural areas to counteract the shortage of GPs. Our results suggest that GMI physicians practising in rural areas need to get involved in children's and adolescents' healthcare services in order to safeguard a high quality of service provision.

Some of the procedures dealing with health screening of adults have also significantly higher application shares for GPs. This is in line with findings of previous studies, that GPs place more emphasis on preventive services [7, 12]. Recent studies highlight the positive effects of preventive care on the reduction of hospital admissions and emergency department visits [50–52]. In Germany, the increasing number of non-urgent emergency department visits has resulted in overstretched emergency facilities with negative effects on quality and effectiveness of the emergency care provision [53–55]. Especially in rural areas with relatively high proportions of elderly people [56] and limited public transport to gain access to primary healthcare provision [57] emergency departments tend to compensate for the lack of primary care physicians [58, 59]. This study found that a significantly smaller percentage of GIM physicians provided preventive services. Therefore, an increase in the overall number of GIM physicians is likely to result in a decrease in the provision of preventive services. This points to a need for the inclusion of preventive medicine in the curriculum for the future training of GIM physicians and postgraduate training for GIM physicians, especially for those practising in rural areas.

Most of the procedures involving minor surgery show significantly higher application rates for GPs. Minor surgery is largely part of the vocational training scheme of GPs as opposed to the training of GIM physicians [45]. Advantages of providing minor surgery in a primary care setting include improved access to surgical care for patients, reduced waiting times and improved patient satisfaction [60]. Although evidence about the quality and cost effectiveness is mixed [61], there are international studies that suggest lower referral rates to secondary care if minor surgery procedures had been performed by GPs [62]. Furthermore, only small differences have been observed between the quality of minor surgery procedures carried out in primary and secondary care setting. In any case, patient satisfaction for minor surgery procedures performed in primary care has been higher [63]. The data show a slightly but insignificant increase over time of GIM physicians offering minor surgery procedures, resulting in a narrowing of the gap between both specialties. However, in order to boost this development, a reassessment of GIM physicians' vocational training programmes should focus on minor surgical procedures.

Similar to previous findings [7, 12, 64] a more technical orientation of GIM physicians was observed in this study. Moreover, GIM physicians had significantly higher shares for procedures that, in Germany, are close to the specialty of internal medicine, e.g. ultrasound diagnostics, cardiac stress testing and 24-h blood pressure monitoring. This is not surprising due to the exclusive emphasis on internal medicine in the GIM physicians' training. A previous study showed that German GPs practising in rural areas perform a larger number of distinct procedures compared with GPs in urban areas [25], indicating that they may offset a lack of specialists. This is in line with the findings of Starfield et al. [11] that patients in the US who have a GP as their primary care physician see fewer specialists. The ability to perform a wider range of specialist procedures should be trained for both GPs and GIM physicians, especially for those who practise in rural areas.

In summary, our results suggest substantial differences in the application of procedures between GPs and GIM physicians with potential consequences for primary healthcare provision in general. Most of the differences correlate with differences in the training programmes. As only about 30% of the consultations in primary care practice relate to internal medicine [65], the findings could foster a discussion about training needs for procedures in primary care to ensure its comprehensiveness. The results reflect scope for changes in vocational training in the future. On the other hand, GIM physicians have the opportunity to train their procedural skills, e.g. by attending the educational seminars accompanying the post-graduate training for GPs. These seminars have been defined by the German College of General Practice and Family Physicians (DEGAM) as a core element to improve trainees' specific knowledge and competencies [66]. From the beginning, the trainees attend training courses preparing for the specific requirements of independent medical work, especially in rural regions.

Beyond training, economic incentives may also reduce the differences in the application of procedures between GPs and GIM physicians. In general, the use of financial incentives is considered to control the physician's behaviour [67, 68]. Improving the billing options and financial rewards for specific procedures (e.g. preventive care or minor surgeries) might encourage primary care physicians to perform these procedures more often. The explicit effect of changes in the reimbursement on the application of procedures is an interesting issue for future research.

Strengths and limitations

The study highlights the difference in services provided by GPs and GIM physicians and provides suggestions about emphases for residency trainings and future efforts for an effective and efficient re-allocation of primary healthcare.

The study has strengths as well as limitations. A strength of this study is that it relies on routine data collected for all GPs and GIM physicians in a specific region of Germany. There are no issues related to any selection or response bias, as might be the case when survey data are used [20]. Social desirability bias might play a particular role when surveying physicians about their services. On the one hand, focusing on the federal state of Schleswig-Holstein constrains the representativeness of the findings, on the other hand, this reduces practice variations based on regional differences and state-specific regulations [28]. Furthermore, this study shows only unconditional differences between both specialties. The age, gender, experience and regional characteristics of the physician may also determine the probability of specific services being provided [25]. Moreover, we cannot control for the patient mix. Unfortunately, for Germany there is no evidence available about the differences in the patient mix between GPs and GIM physicians. In Germany, patients can freely choose their doctor. Although an increasing use of physician-rating websites can be observed [69, 70] most patients consult the nearest primary care physician [66]. For example, in the US, only half of the primary care patients know whether their doctor has been trained as a GP or GIM physician [67]. Therefore, we conclude that the specialty of the primary care physician does not have a strong effect on the patient's physician choice in Germany either. Moreover, the study considered differences between the percentages of physicians performing a specific procedure even when only performed once. This measure will be relatively robust against moderate differences in the patient mix. However, future studies analysing practice style patterns of GIM physicians and GPs should be based on a country-wide dataset and take into account regional and personal characteristics, as well as patient mix information.

Another limitation is that most of the procedures applied by GIM physicians and GPs are not directly represented by the schedule of service codes. This has resulted in a limited number of procedures that were analysed. Moreover, opportunistic practices to increase the reimbursement might lead to billing of services that are not actually performed. Another limitation is given by potential differences between GPs and GIM physicians in their knowledge about how to bill specific procedures. Since GIM physicians do not necessarily need to pass through training in private practices, they may have different awareness or prioritisation in regard to billing. However, in comparison with the use of survey data about procedures applied and the related problems mentioned above, these issues may be negligible.

A further limitation is that the ASHIP is in charge only for the reimbursement of services that are provided to patients within the statutory health insurance system. Services provided to privately insured patients are not covered by the underlying dataset. There are large differences between the service provision for privately and statutorily insured patients [71]. Since the dataset covers 85% of the population of Schleswig-Holstein [72], this is regarded as a minor limitation. However, the effect of the health insurance status on service provision may represent an interesting topic for future research.

Conclusion

This study shows substantial differences in the application of procedures between GPs and GIM physicians with potential consequences for the overall primary healthcare provision. Most of the differences are explainable with differences in the training programmes between both specialties. These findings could foster a discussion that primary care physicians should uniformly master relevant procedures in primary care and reflect scope for changes in vocational training in the future.

Abbreviations

ASHIP: Association of Statutory Health Insurance Physicians; DEGAM: German College of General Practice and Family Physicians; ECG: Electrocardiograms; GIM: Physicians in general internal medicine; GP: General practitioner

Acknowledgements

We would like to thank Uwe Köppen and Andrea Strathausen for proofreading the manuscript.

Funding

No external funding was used for this study.

Authors' contributions

CS, KF and JS were involved in the conception and design of the study. KF assigned the procedures to the bill codes. TE extracted and cleaned the data. CS and KF carried out the statistical analysis. CS, KF and JS interpreted the data. CS produced the first draft of the manuscript. All authors contributed to and approved the final manuscript.

Consent for publication

Not applicable

Competing interests

JS is general practitioner; the other authors declare that they have no competing interests.

Author details

[1]Institute of Family Medicine, University Hospital Schleswig-Holstein, Campus Luebeck, Ratzeburger Allee 160, 23538 Luebeck, Germany. [2]Association of Statutory Health Insurance Physicians of the Federal State of Schleswig-Holstein, Bismarckallee 1-6, 23795 Bad Segeberg, Germany.

References

1. Dall T, West T, Chakrabarti R, Iacobucci W. The complexities of physician supply and demand: projections from 2013 to 2025. Washington: Association of American Medical Colleges; 2015.
2. Kaduszkiewicz H, Teichert U. Shortage of physicians in rural areas and in the public health service: a critical analysis of the evidence on the role of medical education and training. Bundesgesundheitsblatt, Gesundheitsforschung, Gesundheitsschutz 2017.
3. Petterson SM, Liaw WR, Tran C, Bazemore AW. Estimating the residency expansion required to avoid projected primary care physician shortages by 2035. Ann Fam Med. 2015;13(2):107–14.
4. American Academy of Family Physicians. Definition #3 - Primary Care Physician. https://www.aafp.org/about/policies/all/primary-care.html#3. (Accessed 19 Nov 2018).
5. Chan BT. The declining comprehensiveness of primary care. Can Med Assoc J. 2002;166(4):429–34.

6. Shackelton-Piccolo R, McKinlay JB, Marceau LD, Goroll AH, Link CL. Differences between internists and family practitioners in the diagnosis and management of the same patient with coronary heart disease. Med Care Res Rev. 2011;68(6):650–66.
7. Bertakis KD, Helms LJ, Azari R, Callahan EJ, Robbins JA, Miller J. Differences between family physicians' and general internists' medical charges. Med Care. 1999;37(1):78–82.
8. Brieler JA, Scherrer JF, Salas J. Differences in prescribing patterns for anxiety and depression between general internal medicine and family medicine. J Affect Disord. 2015;172:153–8.
9. Paasche-Orlow M, Roter D. The communication patterns of internal medicine and family practice physicians. J Am Board Fam Pract. 2003;16(6): 485–93.
10. Wiest FC, Ferris TG, Gokhale M, Campbell EG, Weissman JS, Blumenthal D. Preparedness of internal medicine and family practice residents for treating common conditions. JAMA. 2002;288(20):2609–14.
11. Starfield B, Chang H-Y, Lemke KW, Weiner JP. Ambulatory specialist use by nonhospitalized patients in US health plans: correlates and consequences. J Ambul Care Manage. 2009;32(3):216–25.
12. Bertakis KD, Callahan EJ, Helms LJ, Azari R, Robbins JA, Miller J. Physician practice styles and patient outcomes: differences between family practice and general internal medicine. Med Care. 1998;36(6):879–91.
13. Grobe TG, Steinmann S, Szecsenyi J. Arztreport 2018 - Schriftenreihe zur Gesundheitsanalyse Bd 7: Barmer GEK, Berlin; 2018.
14. Busse R, Blümel M, Knieps F, Bärnighausen T. Statutory health insurance in Germany: a health system shaped by 135 years of solidarity, self-governance, and competition. Lancet. 2017;390(10097):882–97.
15. Sozialgesetzbuch (SGB V), Fünftes Buch. Gesetzliche Krankenversicherung. https://www.sozialgesetzbuch-sgb.de/sgbv/73.html (Accessed 19 Nov 2018).
16. Steinhäuser J, Scheidt L, Szecsenyi J, Götz K, Joos S. Perceptions of the local government about the primary care physicians shortage-a survey among mayors in the Federal State of Baden-Wuerttemberg. Gesundheitswesen. 2012;74(10):612–7.
17. Kopetsch T. The German healthcare system is running out of physicians! A study on age structure and development of the number of physicians. Berlin: Bundesärztekammer und Kassenärztliche Bundesvereinigung; 2010.
18. Association of Statutory Health Insurance Physicians. Statistical information from the federal physician registry. Berlin: KBV; 2017.
19. Jaekel K, Brand B, Goetz K, Steinhaeuser J: Which procedures are performed by primary care physicians? - a comparison of specialists in family medicine and general internal medicine. In: WONCA Europe Conference 2016. Copenhagen, Denmark; 2016 (Conference Talk).
20. Davino C, Fabbris L: Survey data collection and integration: Springer; 2013.
21. Abadel FT, Hattab AS. How does the medical graduates' self-assessment of their clinical competency differ from experts' assessment? BMC Med Educ. 2013;13(1):24.
22. Colbert-Getz JM, Fleishman C, Jung J, Shilkofski N. How do gender and anxiety affect students' self-assessment and actual performance on a high-stakes clinical skills examination? Acad Med. 2013;88(1):44–8.
23. Minter RM, Gruppen LD, Napolitano KS, Gauger PG. Gender differences in the self-assessment of surgical residents. Am J Surg. 2005;189(6):647–50.
24. Coughlin SS. Recall bias in epidemiologic studies. J Clin Epidemiol. 1990; 43(1):87–91.
25. Steinhäuser J, Jäkel K, Szecsenyi J, Goetz K, Ledig T, Joos S. Procedures performed in general practice-a cross-sectional study. Gesundheitswesen. 2016.
26. Ohlmeier C, Frick J, Prütz F, Lampert T, Ziese T, Mikolajczyk R, Garbe E. Use of routine data from statutory health insurances for federal health monitoring purposes. Bundesgesundheitsblatt, Gesundheitsforschung, Gesundheitsschutz. 2014;57(4):464–72.
27. Powell AE, Davies HTO, Thomson RG. Using routine comparative data to assess the quality of health care: understanding and avoiding common pitfalls. BMJ Qual Saf. 2003;12(2):122–8.
28. Corallo AN, Croxford R, Goodman DC, Bryan EL, Srivastava D, Stukel TA. A systematic review of medical practice variation in OECD countries. Health Policy. 2014;114(1):5–14.
29. Kassenärztliche Bundesvereinigung: Einheitlicher Bewertungsmaßstab (EBM). http://www.kbv.de/html/online-ebm.php (Accessed 19 Nov 2018).
30. Kelly BF, Sicilia JM, Forman S, Ellert W, Nothnagle M. Advanced procedural training in family medicine: a group consensus statement. Fam Med. 2009; 41(6):398–404.
31. Sylvester S, Magin P, Sweeney K, Morgan S, Henderson K. Procedural skills in general practice vocational training: what should be taught? Aust Fam Physician. 2011;40(1/2):50.
32. Steinhaeuser J, Chenot J-F, Roos M, Ledig T, Joos S. Competence-based curriculum development for general practice in Germany: a stepwise peer-based approach instead of reinventing the wheel. BMC Res Notes. 2013;6(1): 314.
33. Wickstrom GC, Kelley DK, Keyserling TC, Kolar MM, Dixon JG, Xie SX, Lewis CL, Bognar BA, DuPre CT, Coxe DR, et al. Confidence of academic general internists and family physicians to teach ambulatory procedures. J Gen Intern Med. 2000;15(6):353–60.
34. Goeman JJ, Solari A. Multiple hypothesis testing in genomics. Stat Med. 2014;33(11):1946–78.
35. Van Lerberghe W. The world health report 2008: primary health care now more than ever. Geneva: World Health Organization; 2008.
36. Gottschalk A, Flocke SA. Time spent in face-to-face patient care and work outside the examination room. Ann Fam Med. 2005;3(6):488–93.
37. Bodenheimer T. Coordinating care—a perilous journey through the health care system. N Engl J Med. 2009;358(10):1064–71.
38. Starfield B, Shi L, Macinko J. Contribution of primary care to health systems and health. Milbank Q. 2005;83(3):457–502.
39. Shi L, Starfield B, Politzer R, Regan J. Primary care, self-rated health, and reductions in social disparities in health. Health Serv Res. 2002;37(3):529–50.
40. Lee A, Kiyu A, Milman HM, Jimenez J. Improving health and building human capital through an effective primary care system. J Urban Health. 2007;84(1):75–85.
41. Kringos DS, Boerma WG, Hutchinson A, van der Zee J, Groenewegen PP. The breadth of primary care: a systematic literature review of its core dimensions. BMC Health Serv Res. 2010;10(1):65.
42. Bazemore A, Petterson S, Peterson LE, Phillips RL. More comprehensive care among family physicians is associated with lower costs and fewer hospitalizations. Ann Fam Med. 2015;13(3):206–13.
43. Pavlič DR, Sever M, Klemenc-Ketiš Z, Švab I, Vainieri M, Seghieri C, Maksuti A. Strength of primary care service delivery: a comparative study of European countries, Australia, New Zealand, and Canada. Prim Health Care Res Dev. 2018;19(3):277–87.
44. Martin JCAR, Bowman MA, Bucholtz JR, Dickinson JR, Evans KL, Green LA, Henley DE, Jones WA, Matheny SC, Nevin JE, Panther SL, Puffer JC, Roberts RG, Rodgers DV, Sherwood RA, Stange KC, Weber CW. Future of family medicine project leadership committee: the future of family medicine: a collaborative project of the family medicine community. Ann Fam Med. 2004;2(suppl 1):S3–S32.
45. Ärztekammer Schleswig-Holstein: Weiterbildungsordnung. https://www.aeksh.de/system/files/documents/wbo_2011-05-25_idf_2017-04-19.pdf (Accessed 19 Nov 2018).
46. Grobe TG, Steinmann S, Szecsenyi J. Arztreport 2017 - Schriftenreihe zur Gesundheitsanalyse, Bd 1. Berlin: Barmer GEK; 2017.
47. Grobe TG, Klingenberg A, Steinmann S, Szecsenyi J. Arztreport 2015 - Schriftenreihe zur Gesundheitsanalyse, Bd. 30. Berlin: Barmer GEK; 2015.
48. Straßburg H-M: Herkömmliche und neue U-Untersuchungen beim Kleinkind. In: Kindergesundheit stärken: Vorschläge zur Optimierung von Prävention und Versorgung. edn. Bitzer EM, Walter U, Lingner H, Schwartz F-W. Berlin, Heidelberg: Springer Berlin Heidelberg; 2009: 91–99.
49. van den Berg N, Seidlitz G, Meinke-Franze C, Pieper C, Lode H, Hoffmann W: Auswirkungen des demografischen Wandels auf die kinder-und jugendmedizinische Versorgung in der Region Ostvorpommern. In: Think Rural! , Edn. Edited by Dünkel F, Herbst M, Schlegel T. Germany: Springer; 2014. 65–72.
50. Emery JCH, Zheng X. Would better access to preventive care reduce use of acute care? Evidence from a large-scale not-for-profit intervention in Alberta. Can Public Policy. 2018;44(1):13–24.
51. Heiwartz H, Klein N, Strumann C. Modelling hospital admission and length of stay by means of generalised count data models. J Appl Econ. 2016;31(6): 1159–82.
52. Büyükdurmus T, Kopetsch T, Schmitz H, Tauchmann H. On the interdependence of ambulatory and hospital care in the German health system. Health Econ Rev. 2017;7(1):2.
53. Carter EJ, Pouch SM, Larson EL. The relationship between emergency department crowding and patient outcomes: a systematic review. J Nurs Scholarsh. 2014;46(2):106–15.
54. Bernstein SL, Aronsky D, Duseja R, Epstein S, Handel D, Hwang U, McCarthy M, John McConnell K, Pines JM, Rathlev N, et al. The effect of emergency

department crowding on clinically oriented outcomes. Acad Emerg Med. 2009;16(1):1–10.
55. Johnson KD, Winkelman C. The effect of emergency department crowding on patient outcomes: a literature review. Adv Emerg Nurs J. 2011;33(1):39–54.
56. Haustein T, Mischke J, Schönfeeld F, Willand I. Ältere Menschen in Deutschland und der EU: Statistisches Bundesamt; 2016.
57. Stentzel U, Piegsa J, Fredrich D, Hoffmann W, Berg N. Accessibility of general practitioners and selected specialist physicians by car and by public transport in a rural region of Germany. BMC Health Serv Res. 2016;16(1):587.
58. Mathison DJ, Chamberlain JM, Cowan NM, Engstrom RN, Fu LY, Shoo A, Teach SJ. Primary care spatial density and nonurgent emergency department utilization: a new methodology for evaluating access to care. Acad Pediatr. 2013;13(3):278–85.
59. Fishman J, McLafferty S, Galanter W. Does spatial access to primary care affect emergency department utilization for nonemergent conditions? Health Serv Res. 2018;53(1):489–508.
60. Collins AM, Ridgway PF, Hassan MS, Chou CW, Hill AD, Kneafsey B. Surgical instruction for general practitioners: how, who and how often? J Plast Reconstr Aesthet Surg. 2010;63(7):1156–62.
61. Taneja A, Singh PP, Tan JP, Hill DG, Connolly AB, Hill AG. Efficacy of general practitioners with specialty interests for surgical procedures. ANZ J Surg. 2015;85(5):344–8.
62. van Dijk CE, Verheij RA, Spreeuwenberg P, Groenewegen PP, de Bakker DH. Minor surgery in general practice and effects on referrals to hospital care: observational study. BMC Health Serv Res. 2011;11(1):2.
63. George S, Pockney P, Primrose J, Smith H, Little P, Kinley H, Kneebone R, Lowy A, Leppard B, Jayatilleke N: A prospective randomised comparison of minor surgery in primary and secondary care. The MiSTIC trial. Technical Report Tunbridge Wells, Kent: Gray Publishing; 2008.
64. Bertakis KD, Robbins JA, Callahan EJ, Helms LJ, Azari R. Physician practice style patterns with established patients: determinants and differences between family practice and general internal medicine residents. Fam Med. 1999;31:187–94.
65. Steinhäuser J. Inhaltliche Verbesserung weiterbildungsbegleitender Lerngruppen durch Daten des CONTENT-Projekts. In: Laux G, Kühlein T, Gutscher A, Szecsenyi J, editors. Versorgungsforschung in der Hausarztpraxis. edn. München: Urban und Vogel; 2010. p. 76–9.
66. Flum E, Magez J, Aluttis F, Hoffmann M, Joos S, Ledig T, Oeljeklaus L, Simon M, Szecsenyi J, Steinhäuser J. Das Schulungsprogramm der Verbundweiterbildungplus Baden-Württemberg: Entwicklung und Implikationen für die Implementierung von Verbundweiterbildungsprogrammen in Deutschland. Zeitschrift für Evidenz, Fortbildung und Qualität im Gesundheitswesen. 2016;112:54–60.
67. Town R, Kane R, Johnson P, Butler M. Economic incentives and physicians' delivery of preventive care: a systematic review. Am J Prev Med. 2005;28(2): 234–40.
68. Armour BS, Pitts M, Maclean R, et al. The effect of explicit financial incentives on physician behavior. Arch Intern Med. 2001;161(10):1261–6.
69. Rothenfluh F, Schulz PJ. Content, quality, and assessment tools of physician-rating websites in 12 countries: quantitative analysis. J Med Internet Res. 2018;20(6):e212.
70. Emmert M, Hessemer S, Meszmer N, Sander U. Do German hospital report cards have the potential to improve the quality of care? Health Policy. 2014; 118(3):386–95.
71. Lüngen M, Gerber A, Stollenwerk B, Lauterbach KW. Ungleichheit der medizinischen Versorgung in Deutschland. Eine empirische Untersuchung in Hochschulambulanzen *Z Sozialreform.* 2005, 51(3):298–314.
72. Zentralinstitut für die kassenärztliche Versorgung in Deutschland (ZI): Zahl der Versicherten in der GKV gemäß KM6 - Statistiken des Bundesministeriums für Gesundheit (BMG). https://www.versorgungsatlas.de/fileadmin/pdf/Zi-IF_Publ-D%C3%84_vTabelle1_V5_20160609.pdf (Accessed 19 Nov 2018).
73. Ärztekammer Schleswig-Holstein: Berufsordnung. https://www.aeksh.de/system/files/documents/berufsordnung_final_3.pdf (Accessed 19 Nov 2018).

21

Who needs collaborative care treatment? A qualitative study exploring attitudes towards and experiences with mental healthcare among general practitioners and care managers

Marlene Christina Rosengaard Møller*, Anna Mygind and Flemming Bro

Abstract

Background: Collaborative care treatment is widely recognized as an effective approach to improve the quality of mental healthcare through enhanced and structured collaboration between general practice and specialized psychiatry. However, studies indicate that the complexity of collaborative care treatment interventions challenge the implementation in real-life general practice settings. Four Danish Collaborative Care Models were launched in 2014 for patients with mild/moderate anxiety and depression. These involved collaboration between general practitioners, care managers and consultant psychiatrists.

Taking a multi-practice bottom-up approach, this paper aims to explore the perceived barriers and enablers related to collaborative care for patients with mental health problems and to investigate the actual experiences with a Danish collaborative care model in a single-case study in order to identify enablers and barriers for successful implementation.

Methods: Combining interviews and observations of usual treatment practices, we conducted a multi-practice study among general practitioners who were not involved in the Danish collaborative care models to explore their perspectives on existing mental health treatment and to investigate (from a bottom-up approach) their perceptions of and need for collaborative care in mental health treatment. Additionally, by combining observations and qualitative interviews, we followed the implementation of a Danish collaborative care model in a single-case study to convey identified barriers and enablers of the collaborative care model.

Results: Experienced and perceived enablers of the Danish collaborative care model mainly consisted of a need for new treatment options to deal with mild/moderate anxiety and depression. The model was considered to meet the need for a free fast track to high-quality treatment. Experienced barriers included: poor adaptation of the model to the working conditions and needs in daily general practice, time consumption, unsustainable logistical set-up and unclear care manager role. General practitioners in the multi-practice study considered access to treatment and not collaboration with specialised psychiatry to be essential for this group of patients.

Conclusions: The study calls for increased attention to implementation processes and better adaptation of collaborative care models to the clinical reality of general practice. Future interventions should address the treatment needs of specific patient populations and should involve relevant stakeholders in the design and implementation processes.

* Correspondence: mcr.moller@ph.au.dk
Research Unit for General Practice & Section for General Medical Practice, Department of Public Health, Aarhus University, Bartholins Allé 2, 8000 Aarhus C, Denmark

Background

Collaborative care is a widely recognized approach to improve mental healthcare through enhanced and systematic collaboration between general practice and specialized psychiatry. Trials have shown better outcomes with collaborative care for patients with mental health problems when compared to usual care [1–10]. However, trial evidence seems difficult to translate into real-life care delivery [8, 11–17]. Danish Collaborative Care Models (DCCMs) for patients with mild/moderate depression and anxiety were launched in four (of five) Danish regions in 2014. The intervention designs of these DCCMs were in line with the recommendations in existing literature on collaborative care [18–21]. Gask et al. [22] defines CC treatment by four key components: (1) a multi-professional approach to patient care, (2) a structured management plan in the form of guidelines or protocols for interventions, e.g. antidepressant medication, patient screening, education, counselling, cognitive behavior therapy, (3) scheduled patient follow-up, and (4) enhanced inter-professional communication, e.g. team meetings, case conferences, individual consultation/supervision, shared medical records, patient-specific written or verbal feedback between caregivers.

The model explored in this study involved collaboration between general practitioner (GP) and care managers (often psychiatrically trained nurses) from specialized psychiatric units in the Central Denmark Region. Care managers offered a 12-week treatment course to patients in general practice. The course consisted of 5–6 individual Cognitive Behavioural Therapy-based sessions; first and last sessions were shared with the patient's GP. Other components were questionnaires for diagnosing and monitoring, group-based psycho-education, supervision and training of GPs, and weekly supervision of care managers by a psychiatrist. Each care manager collaborated with up to ten GPs.

The GPs were responsible for identifying eligible patients, arranging appointments with the care manager and the patient for a shared consultation and subsequently referring patients electronically through existing psychiatric visitation procedures by adding a reference to the specific care manager assigned the GP. Moreover, GPs held the treatment responsibility throughout the course of collaborative care treatment and provided a treatment room for the care manager. GPs were remunerated for the time spent on clinical conferences with the care managers.

The DCCM was designed by specialised psychiatry to engage GPs in a collaboration aiming to improve both the treatment of patients and the GPs' skills in psychiatric treatment through intensified cooperation across scientific disciplines and sector boundaries [23].

Aim

This paper aims to explore the experiences with current treatment practices among GPs, clinic staff and care managers and to examine their views on and perceptions of future collaborative care. The paper also aims to identify enablers and barriers for successful implementation of a specific DCCM. The study provides new knowledge on a sparsely researched topic by taking a qualitative approach to exploring experiences with and perceptions of collaborative care in a general practice setting.

Methods

Design and setting

We employed a qualitative approach and used a combined research design to conduct a multi-practice study among GPs together with a single-case study of the DCCM.

General practice clinics in Denmark are privately owned by GPs and organised in small units, either as single-handed practices (1 GP) or group practices (2–10 GPs) [24]. Most single-handed practices also have a medical receptionist and/or a nurse, whereas group practices usually have both types of clinic staff. More than 95% of the Danish population is listed with a specific GP (approximately 1600 patients per GP), and all inhabitants must obtain a referral from their GP to get specialist treatment. Treatment is tax-funded, and health services are divided into primary care (including general practice) and secondary care (including hospitals and specialised psychiatry) with separate organisations and different financial structures. Psychologists generally operate on a private basis, but GP-referred patients are entitled to partial reimbursement. Danish GPs treat patients with various degrees of mental health problems. For the larger patient population with mild/moderate anxiety and depression, usual care often consists of a limited number of conversational therapy consultations with the GP and in some cases medical treatment. Only in severe cases of mental health problems, GPs may refer patients to treatment in specialised psychiatry.

Sampling and recruitment

We conducted a multi-practice study to explore the experiences of GPs and their staff with current mental health treatment and to examine their perceptions of and need for collaborative care. The practices were selected among general practices that did not take part in the DCCM. To ensure diversity of opinion and broad general practice representation, we applied a purposive sampling strategy employing three main parameters: urban/rural location, practice size and proximity to specialised psychiatry. We thus identified clinics from three different geographic areas of the Central Denmark Region. We included a group practice located in an urban area in close vicinity of specialised psychiatry, a single-handed practice located in a rural area in long distance from specialised psychiatry, and a large group practice located in another rural area a bit closer to specialised psychiatry. Some GPs were known for their involvement in quality development and continuing education, whereas others were not. We included 10 GPs in our observational studies. Nine GPs participated in semi-structured interviews (Table 1). None of the GPs were personally or professionally acquainted with the anthropologist performing observations and interviews.

For the single-case study, we recruited a GP among the 15–20 GPs attending the information meeting hosted by the DCCM project managers in one of the participating municipalities. The recruited GP runs a single-handed practice located in an urban area with the assistance of a receptionist and a medical intern.

The care manager affiliated with the GP in the single-case study also agreed to participate in the single-case study. The care manager also collaborated with other GPs participating in the DCCM. Her participation was cleared with the DCCM management. A second care manager was recruited at the DCCM information meeting in the other DCCM participating municipality. The experiences of the second care manager helped qualify the findings in the single-case study and provided valuable insights into the workings of the DCCM. Moreover, since care managers involved in the DCCM collaborated with several general practitioners, the care manager in the single-case study was able to relate the single-case study experiences with her experiences with the DCCM in general.

Data collection

Observational studies

To explore current clinical practices and establish an understanding of the context of mental health treatment, we observed a number of GP-patient consultations and practice nurse-patient consultations in the multi-practice study and in the single case study before the launch of the DCCM. The first author (MM) spent 2–6 days in each included clinic to explore how GPs treat patients with various degrees of mental health problems. In the multi-practice study, we conducted a total of approximately 80 h of observations; these were evenly distributed between the GPs. Consequently, more hours of observations were done in clinics with more GPs.

To get insight into various DCCM components and to deepen our understanding of both the context and specific barriers and enablers, we followed one patient in the single-case study throughout the entire collaborative care treatment period through multiple observations and interviews with both GP and care manager. We conducted participant observations of their collaborative work through each step of the intervention, including their initial preparation meeting, the first shared consultation, the individual sessions between patient and care manager, and the final shared consultation between patient, GP and care manager. After each consultation, the care manager and/or the GP were asked to comment on

Table 1 Study participants and their participation in research activities

Participants	Practice type	Semi-structured interview	Follow-up interview	Ethnographic conversation	Direct observation	Participation in DCCM
Single-case study						
GP 1, practice 1	Single-handed, urban	x	x	x	x	x
Care manager 1		x	x	x	x	x
Care manager 2		x		x		x
Multi-practice study						
GP 2, practice 2	Group, rural	x		x	x	
GP 3, practice 2	Group, rural	x		x	x	
GP 4, practice 2	Group, rural	x		x	x	
GP 5, practice 2	Group, rural	Cancelled		x	x	
GP 6, practice 2	Group, rural	Left job		x	x	
GP 7, practice 3	Solo, rural	x		x	x	
GP 8, practice 4	Group, urban	x		x	x	
GP 9, practice 4	Group, urban	x		x	x	
GP 10	Group, urban	x				
GP 11	Group, urban	x				
Total		9	2	11	10	3

Abbreviations: *GP* general practitioner, *DCCM* Danish Collaborative Care Model it. The patients also agreed to participate in observations and interviews. Findings related to the patient perspective will be published elsewhere.

In both studies, observations of treatment practices included face-to-face encounters and consultations by phone or email. Observations focused on interactions/relations, treatment options, cross-sectorial cooperation, treatment decisions and GP-patient negotiation thereof.

All observations were initially jotted down and later extended into written field notes [25, 26]. To eliminate potential misunderstandings, observations were followed up by short ethnographic conversations with the GP, care manager or patient, and sometimes with all of them in individual informal conversations.

Interviews

For the multi-practice study, we developed separate interview guides for GPs and clinic staff for the semi-structured interviews. Interviews focused on experiences with and perspectives on existing treatment possibilities and limitations both in general practice and in collaboration with specialised psychiatric care. In the single-case study, we performed two semi-structured interviews with the GP and the care manager: one before initiating the DDCM and one follow-up interview to provide in-depth insight into their views on enablers and barriers for the implementation and function of the intervention. Furthermore, all GPs across the two studies were asked which kind of support and treatment options were needed to improve the treatment of patients with mental health problems and the role of collaborative care in this.

Interviews were conducted in the clinics during lunch break or after work. One practice nurse and one receptionist from the rural single-handed practice participated in a group interview. Two practice nurses from the other two practices participated in ethnographic conversations. Additional data was gathered and observations qualified by the GPs and the clinic staff through informal ethnographic conversations during the first author's presence in the practices, usually between patient consultations and during lunch break [25]. Interviews were recorded and transcribed verbatim. Practice nurse and secretary perspectives are not addressed in this paper.

Interviews with care managers centred on their experiences with usual treatment and usual cooperation with general practice (not related to the DCCM), on their expectations to the DCCM and their actual experiences with the DCCM. Both care managers collaborated with several different DCCM-participating practices; this offered additional, although second-hand, data on GP attitudes towards the DCCM. The care managers also provided their views on DCCM organization and implementation in various GP settings. Thus, the perspectives of the care manager in the single-case study are not exclusively related to the single-case study. Letting the care manager draw on the experiences with the DCCM across various general practice settings helped broaden the insight into barriers and enablers related to the DCCM. The same broadening of insights was gained by including the perspectives of the second care manager. Interview guides for interviews with care managers and GPs are shown as Additional file 1.

Analytic procedures

The analysis was conducted in an iterative process to closely connect data collection and analysis [26, 27]. The thematic analysis began from the initial review of literature and the preparation of research questions, over data collection, followed by pattern identification, interpretation and the final writing of this paper. Each interview transcript was read and reread to perform an initial coding. Key phrases and themes were compared across transcripts. Field notes based on observations in clinical settings and at DCCM recruitment meetings were included to provide a contextual framework for understanding the barriers. This procedure identified emerging insights and dominating themes [27], which were discussed and condensed by the research team. Scope and design of data collection were discussed throughout the course of fieldwork by the first and last authors. The first author conducted the initial coding and identification of themes. Final identification of themes, analytical choices and the framing of the paper were discussed by the research team before the writing of the first draft and in several iterations hereafter. All authors have contributed substantially to the writing of the manuscript.

Ethical considerations

The study followed the Code of Ethics by the American Anthropological Association [28]. The study was approved by the Danish Data Protection Agency (file number: 2014–41-3207), and data collection and data handling were performed in accordance with their guidelines. According to Danish law, no ethical approval from the regional Committee on Health Research Ethics was not needed for this study as no biomedical intervention was performed.

In accordance with existing guidelines and research ethics, all GPs, staff, and care managers received written information about the study and gave verbal consent before initiation of the study. All participants were informed about the purpose of the study, anonymity, that participation was voluntary, and that participants could withdraw from the study at any time. In addition, informal meetings before initiation of study activities were held with the participating general practices to inform

GPs and staff about the study and its implications. Written information about the study was posted in the waiting areas of the general practices.

The data material produced and analyzed as part of the study is not publicly available due to ethical considerations. We constantly strive to ensure the full anonymity of participants, and we respect the verbal agreements made with the participants. As they were not asked for permission to make entire raw data material publically available, we find it ethically inappropriate to make interview transcripts and observational study notes publicly available. Data material is available from the corresponding author on reasonable request.

Results

Three main sub-themes emerged from the analysis across the single-case study and the multi-practice study: 1) DCCM enablers, 2) DCCM barriers and 3) Who needs collaborative care? The relevance of target groups.

DCCM enablers

Access to "free" treatment and workload reduction

GPs in both studies were positive towards a new treatment model addressing the growing number of patients with mild/moderate depression and anxiety, as these patients are time-consuming:

> "*It would in fact be a relief to many general practices, no doubt about it, if you could* [refer patients]" (GP, multi-practice study).

> "*I could easily give up those conversations* [conversational therapy]*...because we are under quite a pressure staff-wise, so it* [treatment by a care manager] *would be a really nice relief. If I had lots of time I might not give it* [conversational therapy] *up*" (GP, multi-practice study).

Most GPs expressed frustration about limited referral options for these patients and long waiting lists for treatment by private practising psychologists. The care managers added that the DCCM meets a need in general practice for patients who are not sick enough for treatment in specialized psychiatric ambulatories. A care manager explained:

> "*There are certainly not any patients* [included in the DCCM] *with severe depression, and then they have no chance of being offered treatment in a psychiatric ambulatory. Alternatively, the GP should treat...and to my knowledge most GPs have done... these patients with conversational therapy, and now they have handed them over to the project* [the DCCM] *for a while*" (care manager).

Improved access to treatment and "free" treatment were important enablers among GPs and a reason for the single-case GP to join the DCCM:

> "*I joined the project to have an offer to patients who cannot afford a private psychologist and who are not sick enough for treatment at the psychiatric hospital ambulatories*" (GP, single-case study).

The DCCM also targeted another GP concern; the existing reimbursement structures for provision of conversational therapy to patients with mild/moderate anxiety and depression. Danish GPs receive reimbursement for conversational therapy only if the patient receives at least two consultations. If a patient does not return for a second conversational therapy consultation, the GP is not entitled to reimbursement for the time spent on the first consultation; this can have a negative impact on the motivation of some GPs:

> "*I allocate extra time and then maybe the problem is solved or the patient doesn't show up* [for the next appointment], *so I don't get the reimbursement for the extra time spent...so I think rather despondently that I won't engage in that*" (GP, single-case study).

The DCCM does not only accommodate workload issues concerning the many patients with mild/moderate anxiety and depression; it also tends to encompass the frustrations related to reimbursement structures.

Quality of treatment

In addition to workload issues, some GPs expected the CC treatment to improve the quality of care because the DCCM allowed more time for systematic cognitive conversational therapy. In the single-case study, the GP reported the impression that the care manager in fact improved the quality of care:

> "*Well, she* [care manager] *has more time, and I think she works more thoroughly than I do. I don't do it as thoroughly*" (GP, single-case study).

In line with this, a GP in the multi-practice study reflected on the advantages of collaborative care:

> "*It would be really nice to feel that they* [care managers] *are competent and hired directly to deal with this and to have allocated time slots, where this person* [care manager] *could offer half an hour... And this person* [care manager] *could reach some level of*

overview of our patients, and get some kind of knowledge about these patients and have a continuous relation to them...that would be fantastic, and it would take off some of the pressure" (GP, multi-practice study).

Most GPs across our studies agreed that the interest and expertise in mental health treatment vary immensely among GPs and that improved referral options would benefit both the GPs and their patients:

"When you open a referral option, most GPs who do not find it interesting to work with mental health treatment will hurry to refer [their patients]. *That is great, because everybody would be happy... And not everyone* [every GP] *has the competencies required in this field, or an interest..."* (GP, multi-practice study).

The lack of interest among some GPs combined with the need for improved quality in this field and the experience/knowhow of care managers could thus be another enabling factor for collaborative care.

Training and supervision by psychiatrist

GPs at the DCCM information meetings showed interest in the possibility for supervision and/or training by specialized psychiatrists. They especially requested brush-up courses on psychoactive drugs and regular supervision in peer groups lead by a psychiatrist. In the multi-practice study, GPs also stressed the importance of collaborating with a psychiatrist for specialised advice on patients who do not respond to the usual treatment in general practice. The same was expressed by the GP in the single-case study, but eight months after the DCCM launch she had not yet been introduced to brush-up courses or supervision by a psychiatrist.

The GPs' need for upgrading their psychiatric competencies might be an enabling factor of the DCCM if a psychiatrist facilitates training and supervision.

Care managers as implementers

The care managers proved to be translators of the overall idea of the DCCM. This task was not a described standardized element of the DCCM, which left the care managers to pragmatic maneuvering. Observations of GP-care manager interactions and interviews with the two care managers indicated that the care managers aimed to facilitate a smooth implementation of collaborative care, but they also acknowledged the challenge of entering general practice as outsiders:

"...it is about how you enter general practice, you enter their territory, and you come as a guest. So you have to tread cautiously ..." (care manager).

Approaching general practice in pragmatic ways and fitting the DCCM to the individual GP's preferences supported the implementation of the DCCM. The care managers had to adapt to different appointment systems, lack of office space, different therapeutic approaches and varying levels of engagement because they worked in many different clinics. The care managers also adjusted to the priorities of the GPs. For example, the GPs were to complete standard questionnaires with the patients, but the care managers took on this task when this did not happen although it deviated from DCCM "protocol" to get things done and avoid conflict:

"We [the care managers] *do take it* [the workload of GPs] *into consideration. Maybe it is overstated... I have defended this* [doing the GP's task] *to myself by thinking that it is extremely important that we get started well and that we get to know each other, and that I don't appear too rigid and too insisting"* (care manager).

The flexible and pragmatic approach taken by the care managers enabled implementation of the DCCM. The ability to juggle GP needs and adapt DCCM elements to different organisations made the care manager an asset in collaborative care.

DCCM barriers

Organizational and practical barriers

The DCCM caused several logistic and organizational problems that (although simple) caused trouble in the implementation. First, the referral procedures were inadequately described:

"It caused me trouble. The first few times I just referred [the patient] *to the psychiatric hospital with a note saying that this person wanted to participate in collaborative care, and then they declined because referral requires a scheduled time for consultation with the care manager...and I don't think I have been properly informed about that"* (GP, single-case study).

Second, there was lack of information about the practical procedures on how to obtain remuneration:

"We have these reimbursement options which I have tried to apply, and then they are rejected, apparently because I am not registered in the care manager project. Well. Who do I register with? So I just had to contact them again and claim to be registered in the project and then they accepted...I have contacted the project manager twice about this, and he hasn't replied...we need some follow-up on the information meeting" (Single-case GP).

Third, the DCCM increased the GP workload as it required shared consultations with the care manager, coordination and booking of consultations, and setting up appointments for patients. It also proved difficult to organise a consultation room for the care manager:

> "*Well, there is all the hassle; everything I have attended...information meetings, meetings* [with the care manager] *here and...yes, making sure the consultation room is ready. There is a lot I have to do extra...*" (GP, single-case study).

In line with this, a care manager stated:"*They don't have a spare room, so there is a lot of logistics and planning in it for us as care managers. My calendar, the patient's calendar and then the consultation room, the* [psycho-education] *classes, conferences. It is a huge logistic work. And some patients go to school and some go to work, which you must also show consideration for*" (care manager).

In the follow-up interview, the GP in the single-case study concluded that she might not want to volunteer and invest the extra resources in a similar future collaborative care model.

The findings indicate that the DCCM was inadequately prepared; the project did not get off to a smooth start, and this challenged successful implementation and continuation of the intervention.

Cross-sectorial collaboration

An important aim of the DCCM was to improve the cooperation and communication between primary and secondary care through facilitation by care managers. Although most GPs in both studies embraced the idea of collaboration with specialised psychiatry, several GPs at the recruitment meeting expressed a priori scepticism towards handing over their patients to care managers. Furthermore, some were reluctant to attend training courses facilitated by care managers. This a priori scepticism towards the role of care managers in cross-sectorial collaborative care can be interpreted as a mental barrier to the DCCM and as a sign of a lack of interprofessional respect. In line with this, a GP in the multi-practice study expressed a general frustration towards existing visitation procedures where psychiatric nurses assess whether a patient referred by a GP is eligible for specialized psychiatric care:

> "*It can be frustrating when you refer a patient who doesn't respond to the treatment, and then it is a nurse who assesses the patient and rejects the patient without having a psychiatrist involved*" (GP, multi-practice study).

The quote could be read as lack of confidence in the expertise of psychiatric nurses, but it also expresses a frustration in the GP towards what seems to be gatekeeping by psychiatric nurses when the GP needs assistance by a psychiatrist. This frustration was shared by most GPs in both the single-case study and the multi-practice study. Despite an a priori scepticism in some GPs, the GP in the single-case study expressed that her clinical cooperation with the care manager in the DCCM ran smoothly and that the care manager seemed to be competent. The care manager herself experienced a positive attitude towards her in most of the DCCM practices she collaborated with, and she found that the GPs actually welcomed interdisciplinary exchange:

> "*What I hear, at least from three of the GPs that I talked to, is simply a need for a professional back-and-forth; the dialogue, 'I see the case* [the patient] *like this and this: How do you see it?*" (care manager).

Despite the willingness in the GP to provide a professional back-and-forth, the DCCM set-up did not facilitate a closer cooperation according to the findings in the single-case study. Except for brief ad hoc exchanges of treatment plans and coordination of shared consultations, both the GP and the care manager considered it more as a *transfer* of the patient. In that sense, as also reported by the single-case GP, the collaborative care project facilitated only a shallow relationship across sectors and disciplines.

The GP stated:

> "*I don't cooperate a lot with the care manager in the sense that we exchange experiences and stuff ... I get to know the care manager a bit through the initial and last consultations. But proper exchange of knowledge and experience on how to handle these patients or sharing her tricks with me...that doesn't really happen*" (GP, single-case study).

Both care managers agreed. One care manager concluded:

> "*The way that our shared consultations worked meant that they actually had the characteristics of a transfer* [of the patient] *with the GP telling the patient, in my presence, that 'I have told this and this* [to the care manager] *about your situation'*" (care manager).

The other care manager said:

> "*...and my conclusion right now is that it is hard for me to see, in relation to these patients, why I should claim a need for a shared consultation*" (care manager).

The care managers and the GP agreed that written communication would have been sufficient to exchange the necessary information and that treatment of patients by care managers could have been conducted in a psychiatric outpatient ambulatory, but the collaborative care part would then have vanished. One care manager explained:

> "*They* [the patients] *might as well get treatment in the ambulatory, but then there would be no collaboration with general practitioners*" (care manager).

The GP in the single-case study acknowledged that increased cooperation across sectors was time consuming, and she was unsure if she would be willing to invest more time in it.

In addition to organisational and logistical issues, several other important barriers to the DCCM were identified: the unclear character and purpose of the cross-disciplinary cooperation, a priori scepticism in many GPs towards care manager-facilitated training, and limited actual exchange of knowledge and experience.

Sustainability

The single-case study revealed a number of organisational, practical, logistic and resource-related barriers to the DCCM when meeting the realities in general practice. The care managers were intended to provide treatment of patients in up to 10 general practices [23]. This set-up challenged both coordination and logistics, and the care managers experienced a considerable waste of time when commuting between different general practices. Due to these barriers and the lack of capacity in specialized psychiatric care, the care managers doubted that the model would be sustainable beyond the project period:

> "*There wouldn't be enough qualified nurses if you deploy this model everywhere. So I can't imagine how this model should be implemented permanently in its current form. I really don't*" (care manager).

The GPs in the multi-practice study appreciated the potential of the DCCM to free time, but some also feared that it might "steal time" due to planning and coordination with the care manager. The care managers found it time-consuming to get the DCCM model started and running (also after the run-in period).

The logistical problems of finding a vacant consultation room for the care manager were also mentioned as a potential barrier to the sustainability of the proposed DCCM by GPs in the multi-practice study:

> "*It* [treatment by care manager] *should not be done here. Then they* [the care managers] *would have to be here all the time. Then they* [the care managers] *would need their own consultation room, or we should receive some kind of reimbursement, or we should rent out* [the consultation room], *and then we would have the trouble with administrating their booking of consultations and things like that. So... otherwise, I would be the one paying for the patients' free treatment, and then we wouldn't do it. It* [collaborative care] *has to be solved* [done] *somewhere else, I think...then it would be really great, but yes... they should create an ambulatory for it because it would be swarmed with patients*" (GP, multi-practice study).
> the multi-practice study

One important barrier thus seems to be that the DCCM involved extra (rather than reduced) workload in general practice without compensating the GPs for this additional work.

Several barriers to the DCCM were experienced by the single-case GP and perceived by the GPs in the multi-practice study. Although the care managers played a central role in the treatment and collaboration related to the DCCM, none of the GPs in the multi-practice study requested elaborated cooperation with a care manager from specialised psychiatry for patients with mild/moderate anxiety and depression. The GPs seemed to expect benefits from collaborative care in terms of improved access to high-quality treatment rather than increased collaboration with external partners, including a care manager situated in the clinic. Consequently, the support gained by the DDCM was not considered to sufficiently justify the time spent.

Who needs collaborative care? The relevance of target group

DCCM enablers and barriers were partly related to the way that the GPs perceived mental healthcare for different patient groups, and how the GPs tended to divide these into categories according to the severity of the patients' mental illness and their treatments needs.

When asked which of patients with mental health problems they found the most challenging to treat, the GPs (across both studies) referred to specific diagnoses, and they categorised the patients into two main groups based on the severity of conditions: 1) a large group of patients with mild/moderate mental health problems and 2) a small group of patients with severe mental health problems (e.g. severe depression, schizophrenia and other psychotic conditions) and higher risk of somatic comorbidity and complex health problems:

> "*There are not as many patients with schizophrenia as patients with anxiety and depression so it is a matter of prioritising resources. The schizophrenic patients are left more to themselves; they are a more vulnerable*

group who rarely consult their GP. Patients with anxiety and depression consult their GP regularly. And often they have relatives who support them, whereas the schizophrenic patients are more socially isolated" (GP, multi-practice study).

The GPs considered treatment of mild/moderate mental health conditions to be a central GP task, but the number of patients is increasing, and the GPs do not have the capacity to handle the volume of patients. The GPs emphasized that the complexity of the mental/somatic/social problems in patients with severe mental health conditions makes them an especially vulnerable group; they are the most challenging to care for in general practice and have the highest need for improved treatment.

"Where are the schizophrenic patients now? The number of hospital beds have been cut back, they are discharged, and they disappear into nothing, and we are not in control of them...it happens too often" (GP, multi-practice study).

When asked about the potential of a collaborative care model that integrates psychiatric and general practice treatment, the GPs agreed that the patients with severe mental health problems and somatic comorbidity have the highest need for cross-disciplinary and collaborative treatment. The complexity of health conditions in these patients calls for new ways to ensure integrated mental healthcare that meets their somatic, psychiatric and social needs, whereas the GPs did not see a need for enhanced collaboration with specialised psychiatry on patients with mild/moderate mental problems. For this patient group, they requested a fast track to high-quality treatment in cases when usual care fails. This discordance between the target group of the DCCM and the actual and perceived needs of collaborative care suggests a major motivational barrier for successful implementation of the DCCM.

Discussion

Main findings

We did a purposeful sampling for the multi-practice study in order to include potential variations in GP perceptions and their need for collaborative care. However, we found very limited variation. Therefore, the analysis centred on the thematic trends across the two studies. The introduction of the DCCM for mild/moderate anxiety and depression was promoted by a need in the GPs for better access to free high-quality treatment and pragmatic manoeuvrings by the care managers. Major barriers to the implementation of the DCCM, as experienced by the single-case GP and the care managers, were organisational deficiencies concerning patient registration and reimbursement procedures, limited genuine collaboration and knowledge sharing, much GP time spent on practical issues and little availability of consultation rooms. Another barrier perceived by the GPs in the multi-practice study and, to some extent, by the single-case GP was the lack of confidence among GPs in the importance of investing time and resources for enhanced cooperation across sectors and disciplines on this patient group; most participants questioned the sustainability of the DCCM.

As an overall framework for treatment of patients with mental health problems, the DCCM fits well with the dominant discourse in modern western healthcare policy, which focuses on coherent, cross-disciplinary and cross-sectorial healthcare set-ups. However, it has been argued elsewhere that the societal focus on cooperation across traditional sector boundaries cannot be expected to be mirrored in everyday life [29, 30]. This may explain why carefully developed collaborative care models may work under experimental conditions but not in real-life situations, as we also found in this study. Such models collide with daily life in general practice, where GPs must make meaningful choices with limited resources; all activities are subject to standardised fee-for-service agreements, and all choices are influenced by competing tasks, different patient needs and individual preferences among GPs and patients.

If the GPs consider improved referral options and not collaboration with a care manager to be the most important for this patient group, the DCCM should reflect this. The logistic and financial constraints also need to be addressed. The GPs were not per se against the concept of collaboration, but they wanted cooperation and communication to fit with their practice life, and they were concerned about potential side effects in terms of increased workload. In particular, the introduction of an external care manager in general practice revealed logistic, practical and financial barriers.

The practical daily life of general practice should be taken as a starting point when a revised DCCM is developed and implemented. Marshall states that "improvement initiatives are sometimes planned on the hard high ground, but they are put into effect in the swampy lowlands" [31]. Therefore, central stakeholders, such as GPs and patients, need to be deeply involved in the development of new collaborative models to ensure that they are designed to meet the existing organisational, cultural and structural realities [32]. Our findings also indicate the importance of developing a DCCM in a systematic way, including pilot testing as described by the Medical Research Council in the guidance on the development of complex interventions, in order to adjust new intervention prototypes to the clinical reality of general practice before presenting a new model [33, 34].

The two-armed research design that combines the DCCM single-case study with a multi-practice study allows the discrepancies between model and reality to emerge. We wanted to take a bottom-up approach to the need for collaborative care in contrast to the top-down developed DCCM in order to discuss and problematise the introduction of new models without involving all relevant stakeholders.

Comparison with other studies

Our findings are consistent with other studies on the implementation of collaborative care in both the UK, the US and the Netherlands, which show that it can be challenging to implement research-designed collaborative care in real-life general practice settings [9, 12, 13, 16, 35, 36]. Other studies have found that collaborative care can be implemented if financial barriers are reduced, effective training and facilitation are provided, a common mental health model is developed, and new care processes are introduced [7]. The most important factors found in other studies using the Normalisation Process Theory as the analytical frame were shared understanding of mental illness between GPs and care managers and agreement on the division of tasks [4, 12]. Our findings support the crucial role of developing a common understanding of mental health conditions and their treatment as well as targeting logistic and financial barriers [37]. Adding to this, our study provides insight into the GPs' distinction between mild/moderate and severe mental illness. Treatment of mild/moderate conditions can be optimised within general practice and through more referral options to psychological therapy, whereas collaborative care is perceived to be more suitable for severe cases.

Strengths and limitations

The present study has limitations with regard to generalisability. The general practices in the study may not cover all types of practices, and the included GPs were known to be among the most progressive and active compared to other general practice clinics. Therefore, we would expect them to have a more positive attitude to new models of care delivery, such as a DCCM. Consequently, our findings may report a more positive attitude to the DCCM than would have been found in the general population of GPs.

Financial constraints allowed us to include only one GP clinic participating in the DCCM. Thus, the findings reflect the experiences from only one collaborative care setting and may not be representative of collaborative care experiences in other general practices. However, a broader perspective on the function of the model was ensured through the inclusion of two care managers as both of these interacted with several GPs across different general practice settings and with numerous patients during the first six months of the intervention. Moreover, the model was observed throughout the entire process (including information meetings, initial meetings between care manager and GP and the entire course of treatment) and through a combination of before and after interviews. This thorough exploration added strengths and depth to the study by providing broad and multi-facetted perspectives on the functioning of the model. Furthermore, many of the experiences from the single-case study accorded with the findings from the multi-practice study.

Conclusion

The increasing number of patients with mild/moderate anxiety and depression in general practice supports the implementation of collaborative care in mental health treatment. Additionally, the workload-reducing potential of care manager-led treatment did in fact constitute an actual and perceived enabling factor of the DCCM. Nevertheless, there are a number of experienced and suggested barriers to the sustainability of the DCCM in its current shape. Firstly, the GPs in this study did not request increased cooperation with specialised psychiatric care (represented by care managers) for patients with less severe mental conditions although they see a growing need for improved referral options for this patient group. Secondly, our single-case study suggests a number of practical and logistic barriers to the DCCM. Thus, the prospected barriers and concerns of GPs in the multi-practice study who had not experienced the implementation of the DCCM supplement the findings from the single-case study.

GPs and patients should be key in the development of future collaborative care models. The pragmatic reality of general practice, cross-sectorial differences in the perceptions of target groups, (lack of) needs for more cooperation, time constraints and identification of practical and logistical barriers should be considered to ensure successful implementation for all involved parties. Therefore, we argue that there is a need to ask: Who needs collaborative care?

Abbreviations

DCCM: Danish collaborative care model; GP: General practitioner

Acknowledgements

The authors wish to thank all the GPs and care managers who generously shared their time and experience for this study. We also owe thanks to the patients and clinic staff who participated in the study although their contributions do not form part of this paper. Finally, we thank the Lundbeck Foundation for funding the study.

Funding
The study was supported by an unrestricted grant from the Lundbeck Foundation (grant number: R155–2012-11280) and conducted in collaboration with the MEPRICA research group at the Research Unit for General Practice and Section for General Medical Practice, Department of Public Health, Aarhus University, Denmark.

Authors' contributions
MCRM designed the study, collected the data, analysed and interpreted the data, and drafted the manuscript. FB supervised the study and participated in the design of the study, the analysis of data and the drafting of the manuscript. AM contributed to the analysis of data and drafting of the manuscript. All authors have read and approved the final manuscript.

Ethics approval and consent to participate
The study followed the Code of Ethics by the American Anthropological Association [37]. The study was approved by the Danish Data Protection Agency (file number: 2014–41-3207), and data collection and data handling were performed in accordance with their guidelines. According to Danish law, no ethical approval from the regional Committee on Health Research Ethics was not needed for this study as no biomedical intervention was performed.
In accordance with existing guidelines and research ethics, all GPs, staff, and care managers received written information about the study and gave verbal consent before initiation of the study. All participants were informed about the purpose of the study, anonymity, that participation was voluntary, and that participants could withdraw from the study at any time. In addition, informal meetings before initiation of study activities were held with the participating general practices to inform GPs and staff about the study and its implications. Written information about the study was posted in the waiting areas of the general practices.
The data material produced and analyzed as part of the study is not publicly available due to ethical considerations. We constantly strive to ensure the full anonymity of participants, and we respect the verbal agreements made with the participants. As they were not asked for permission to make entire raw data material publically available, we find it ethically inappropriate to make interview transcripts and observational study notes publicly available. Data material is available from the corresponding author on reasonable request.

Competing interests
The authors declare to have no competing interests.

References
1. van der Feltz-Cornelis CM. Ten years of integrated care for mental disorders in the Netherlands. Int J Integr Care 2011;11 Spec Ed:e015.
2. Huijbregts KM, de Jong FJ, van Marwijk HW, Beekman AT, Ader HJ, Hakkaart-van Roijen L, et al. A target-driven collaborative care model for major depressive disorder is effective in primary care in the Netherlands. A randomized clinical trial from the depression initiative. J Affect Disord 2013;146(3):328–37.
3. Muntingh A, van der Feltz-Cornelis C, van Marwijk H, Spinhoven P, Assendelft W, de Waal M, et al. effectiveness of collaborative stepped care for anxiety disorders in primary care: a pragmatic cluster randomised controlled trial. Psychother Psychosom 2014;83(1):37–44.
4. Coupe N, Anderson E, Gask L, Sykes P, Richards DA, Chew-Graham C. Facilitating professional liaison in collaborative care for depression in UK primary care; a qualitative study utilising normalisation process theory. BMC Fam Pract. 2014;15:78.
5. Barley EA, Haddad M, Simmonds R, Fortune Z, Walters P, Murray J, et al. The UPBEAT depression and coronary heart disease programme: using the UK Medical Research Council framework to design a nurse-led complex intervention for use in primary care. BMC Fam Pract. 2012;13:119.
6. Katon WJ, Lin EH, Von Korff M, Ciechanowski P, Ludman EJ, Young B, et al. Collaborative care for patients with depression and chronic illnesses. N Engl J Med. 2010;363(27):2611–20.
7. Solberg LI, Crain AL, Jaeckels N, Ohnsorg KA, Margolis KL, Beck A, et al. The DIAMOND initiative: implementing collaborative care for depression in 75 primary care clinics. Implement Sci. 2013;8:135.
8. Byng R, Norman I, Redfern S, Jones R. Exposing the key functions of a complex intervention for shared care in mental health: case study of a process evaluation. BMC Health Serv Res. 2008;8:274.
9. Chwastiak L, Vanderlip E, Katon W. Treating complexity: collaborative care for multiple chronic conditions. Int Rev Psychiatry. 2014;26(6):638–47.
10. Archer J, Bower P, Gilbody S, Lovell K, Richards D, Gask L, et al. Collaborative care for depression and anxiety problems (review). Cochrane Database Syst Rev. 2012;10:CD006525.
11. Whitebird RR, Margolis KL, Asche SE, Trangle MA, Wineman AP. Barriers to improving general practice of depression. Perspectives of medical group leaders. Qual Health Res. 2013;23(6):805.
12. Knowles SE, Chew-Graham C, Coupe N, Adeyemi I, Keyworth C, Thampy H, et al. Better together? A naturalistic qualitative study of inter-professional working in collaborative care for co-morbid depression and physical health problems. Implement Sci. 2013;8:110.
13. Knowles SE, Chew-Graham C, Adeyemi I, Coupe N, Coventry PA. Managing depression in people with multimorbidity: a qualitative evaluation of an integrated collaborative care model. BMC Fam Pract. 2015;16:32.
14. Hermens ML, Muntingh A, Franx G, van Splunteren PT, Nuyen J. Stepped care for depression is easy to recommend, but harder to implement: results of an explorative study within primary care in the Netherlands. BMC Fam Pract. 2014;15:5.
15. Hauge-Helgestad A, Johansen KS, Hansen J. Behandling af mennesker med angst og depression. Kortlægning af behandlingsfeltet og diskussion af perspektiverne ved indførelse af collaborative care [Treatment of patients with anxiety and depression. A mapping of the field of treatment and a discussion of perspectives on the implementation of collaborative care. In Danish.]. DSI. 2012. https://www.kora.dk/media/763524/behandling-af-mennesker-med-angst-og-depression.pdf. Accessed 14 Dec 2017.
16. Overbeck G, Davidsen AS, Kousgaard MB. Enablers and barriers to implementing collaborative care for anxiety and depression: a systematic qualitative review. Implement Sci. 2016;11(1):165.
17. Katon W, Unutzer J. Collaborative care models for depression: time to move from evidence to practice. Arch Intern Med. 2006;166(21):2304–6.
18. Eplov LF, Lundsteen M, Birket-Smith M. Shared care for ikke-psykotiske sygdomme. Anbefalinger på baggrund af en systematisk litteraturundersøgelse [Shared care for non-psychotic mental illness. Recommendations based on a systematic review. In Danish]. Danish regions. 2009.
19. Richards DA, Hill JJ, Gask L, Lovell K, Chew-Graham C, Bower P, et al. Clinical effectiveness of collaborative care for depression in UK primary care (CADET): cluster randomised controlled trial. BMJ. 2013;347:f4913.
20. Brinck-Claussen UO, Curth NK, Davidsen AS, Mikkelsen JH, Lau ME, Lundsteen M, et al. Collaborative care for depression in general practice: study protocol for a randomised controlled trial. Trials. 2017;18(1):344.
21. Curth NK, Brinck-Claussen UO, Davidsen AS, Lau ME, Lundsteen M, Mikkelsen JH, et al. Collaborative care for panic disorder, generalised anxiety disorder and social phobia in general practice: study protocol for three cluster-randomised, superiority trials. Trials. 2017;18(1):382.
22. Gask L, Bower P, Lovell K, Escott D, Archer J, Gilbody S, et al. What work has to be done to implement collaborative care for depression? Process evaluation of a trial utilizing the normalization process model. Implement Sci. 2010;5:15.
23. Central Denmark Region. Revideret ansøgning til SATS puljen til styrket samarbejde mellem behandlingspsykiatrien og almen praksis (shared care). Projekt "Afprøvning af collaborative care-modellen i region Midtjylland" [revised grant application regarding increased collaboration between psychiatry and general practice (shared care). Project: "Test of the collaborative care model in the Central Denmark region. In Danish]. Central Denmark region. 2012. https://www.rm.dk/api/NewESDHBlock/DownloadFile?agendaPath=%5C%5CRMAPPS0221.onerm.dk%5Ccms01-ext%5CESDH%20Data%5CRM_Internet%5CDagsordener%5CUdvalg_vedroerende_nae%202013%5C08-01-2013%5CAaben_dagsorden&appendixId=39306. Accessed 14 Dec 2017.

24. Pedersen KM, Andersen JS, Sondergaard J. General practice and primary health care in Denmark. J Am Board Fam Med. 2012;25(Suppl 1):S34–8.
25. Bernard HR. Research methods in anthropology. Qualitative and quantitative approaches. Thousand Oaks: Sage; 1994.
26. Hammersley M, Ethnography AP. Principles in practice. New York: Routledge; 1995.
27. Pope C, Ziebland S, Mays N. Qualitative research in health care. Analysing qualitative data. BMJ. 2000;320(7227):114–6.
28. American Anthropological Association: Statement on Ethics. Principles of Professional Responsibility. 2012.http://ethics.americananthro.org/category/statement/. Accessed 30 Oct 2017.
29. De Certeau M. The practice of everyday life. Berkeley: University of California Press; 1988.
30. Jöhncke S, Svendsen MN, Whyte SR. Sociale teknologier som antropologisk arbejdsfelt [Social technologies as field of interest in anthropology. In Danish]. In: Hastrup K, editor. Viden om verden. En grundbog i antropologisk analyse [Knowledge about the world. A guide to anthropological analysis. In Danish]. Copenhagen: Hans Reitzels Forlag; 2004. p. 385–408.
31. Marshall M, de Silva D, Cruickshank L, Shand J, Wei L, Anderson J. What we know about designing an effective improvement intervention (but too often fail to put into practice). BMJ Qual Saf. 2017;26(7):578–82.
32. May CR, Johnson M, Finch T. Implementation, context and complexity. Implement Sci. 2016;11(1):141.
33. Craig P, Dieppe P, Macintyre S, Michie S, Nazareth I, Petticrew M. Developing and evaluating complex interventions: the new Medical Research Council guidance. BMJ. 2008;337:a1655.
34. Moore GF, Audrey S, Barker M, Bond L, Bonell C, Hardeman W, et al. Process evaluation of complex interventions: Medical Research Council guidance. BMJ. 2015;350:h1258.
35. Eghaneyan BH, Sanchez K, Mitschke DB. Implementation of a collaborative care model for the treatment of depression and anxiety in a community health center: results from a qualitative case study. J Multidiscip Healthc. 2014;7:503–13.
36. Speyer H, Christian Brix Norgaard H, Birk M, Karlsen M, Storch Jakobsen A, Pedersen K, et al. The CHANGE trial: no superiority of lifestyle coaching plus care coordination plus treatment as usual compared to treatment as usual alone in reducing risk of cardiovascular disease in adults with schizophrenia spectrum disorders and abdominal obesity. World Psychiatry. 2016;15(2):155–65.
37. Katon W. Collaborative depression care models: from development to dissemination. Am J Prev Med. 2012;42(5):550–2.

The value of an embedded qualitative study in a trial of a second antidepressant for people who had not responded to one antidepressant: understanding the perspectives of patients and general practitioners

Carolyn A. Chew-Graham[1*], Thomas Shepherd[1], Heather Burroughs[1], Katie Dixon[1] and David Kessler[2]

Abstract

Background: Depression is the leading cause of disability worldwide, and is a major contributor to the overall global burden of disease. The number of prescriptions for antidepressants has risen dramatically in recent years yet up to 50% of patients who are treated for depression with antidepressants do not report feeling better as a result of treatment, and do not show the desired improvement on depression measures. We report a qualitative study embedded in a trial of second antidepressant for people who had not responded to one antidepressant, exploring the acceptability of a combination of antidepressants from the perspectives of both patients and practitioners, together with experiences of participating in a clinical trial.

Methods: A qualitative study embedded in a randomized controlled trial investigating the effectiveness and cost-effectiveness of combining mirtazapine with Serotonin-Noradrenaline Reuptake Inhibitor (SNRI) or Selective Serotonin Reuptake Inhibitor (SSRI) antidepressants versus SNRI or SSRI therapy alone (the MIR trial). 59 interviews were conducted with people who declined to participate in the trial, people who completed the study and people who withdrew from the intervention, and 16 general practitioners.

Results: Across the data-sets, four main themes were identified: the hard work of managing depression, uncertainties over the value of a second antidepressant, help-seeking at a point of crisis, and attainment and maintenance of a hard-won equilibrium.

Conclusions: Exploring reasons for declining to participate in a trial of a second antidepressant in people who had not responded to one antidepressant suggests that people who are already taking one antidepressant may be reluctant to take a second, being wary of possible side-effects, but also being unconvinced of the logic behind such a combination. In addition, people describe being in a state of equilibrium and reluctant to make a change, reflecting that this equilibrium is 'hard-won' and they are unwilling to risk disturbing this. This makes some people reluctant to enrol in a clinical trial. Understanding a patient's view on medication is important for GPs when discussing antidepressants.

Keywords: depression, Antidepressants, Primary care, Qualitative methods

* Correspondence: c.a.chew-graham@keele.ac.uk
[1]Research Institute, Primary Care and Health Sciences, Keele University, Newcastle, Staffs ST5 5BG, UK
Full list of author information is available at the end of the article

Background

Depression is the leading cause of disability worldwide, and is a major contributor to the overall global burden of disease [1]. Currently, depression is thought to affect approximately one in ten of the population [2] and the prevalence of depressive symptoms may increase with age [3]·· Depression is more common in those people with long-term physical conditions [4].

GPs have been found to be good at recognizing moderate to severe depression [5], but they may be more likely to do so when patients present with psychosocial as opposed to somatic symptoms [6, 7]. A large WHO naturalistic study in 15 cities around the world (and in 11 languages), found that patients whose depression went unrecognized had milder depression at baseline and were not found to be at a disadvantage in terms of outcome [8]. Nevertheless a significant minority of people who might benefit from treatment remains undetected [9, 10].

People with depression are typically managed in primary care, and in the United Kingdom, depressive symptoms are the third most common reason to consult a general practitioner (GP) [11]. The National Institute for Health and Care Excellence (NICE) guideline on the treatment of depression [12] provides evidence-based guidance to primary and secondary care practitioners, in England, on the treatment of depression and promotes a stepped care model of treatment, recommending the least intensive therapies as a first line intervention. This is often a 'talking treatment' or psychological therapy [13] but referral to psychological therapists can be problematic due to waiting times for, and lack of availability of, appropriate and acceptable services [14]. The guideline suggests that where patients have moderate to severe, recurrent or chronic sub-threshold depression, antidepressants are indicated.

The number of prescriptions for antidepressants has risen dramatically in recent years; increasing by 7.2% (3.8 million items) between 2013 and 2014, in the NHS [15]. Indeed, antidepressants have shown a greater increase in the volume of prescribing in 2014 than drugs for any other therapeutic area, with over 57 million prescriptions being issued in England in 2014, at a cost of £265 million.

However, many patients do not respond to antidepressants. The STAR*D study (Sequenced Treatment Alternatives to Relieve Depression) found that half of those treated did not experience at least a 50% reduction in depressive symptoms following 12–14 weeks of treatment with a single antidepressant [16]. A substantial proportion of those who take their antidepressants in an adequate dose and for an adequate period, do not experience a clinically meaningful improvement in their depressive symptoms. This can be termed treatment resistant depression (TRD).

For patients who are deemed to have not responded to one antidepressant, the NICE guideline [12] suggests that General Practitioners (GPs) should re-consider the treatment option if there has been no response after 4 to 6 weeks of antidepressant monotherapy. The guideline describes a number of pharmacological strategies to attempt after inadequate response to initial treatments including combining antidepressants.

The 'MIR' trial evaluated the addition of mirtazapine to a Serotonin-Noradrenaline Reuptake Inhibitor (SNRI) or Selective Serotonin Reuptake Inhibitor (SSRI) antidepressant over placebo in primary care patients with TRD [17]. The embedded qualitative study, embedded in the MIR trial, reported here aimed to explore patients' perspectives on being invited to participate in a trial [17] of a second antidepressant for TRD and the acceptability of combination drug treatments for depression to patients and GPs.

Patients' health beliefs are central to reaching agreement about treatment between patient and practitioner, requiring a discussion which is inclusive of and considers the views and beliefs of both parties [18]. Furthermore, Patient beliefs and attitudes also influence adherence to antidepressant medication [19, 20]. Previous literature reporting patients' views on the management of depression suggest that some patients prefer psychological treatments to medication, [21, 22] but these preferences vary depending on a number of factors including age, gender and their own understanding of depression [23, 24]. Negative views on antidepressants include concerns that they are addictive [25], and older people may be particularly reluctant to take antidepressants [26, 27].

It cannot be assumed that patients already on antidepressant medications will have either a positive attitude to, or a good understanding of, that treatment or will therefore be willing to take another antidepressant if their depressive symptoms remain. Evidence suggests that some patients using SSRI antidepressants would prefer to stop but are afraid to do so [20] and that when considering stopping the use of SSRIs, patients have a number of concerns about cessation which clinicians should attend to. [28, 29] In a meta-ethnographic synthesis of qualitative evidence it was found that patients were heavily engaged in negotiating a 'medication career' or 'moral career' [30] making choices about how to proceed with treatment and sense-making around their illness. This study also emphasizes the vital role that GPs play in facilitating patient decision-making, through discussion to aid understanding and meaning-making around depression and treatment experiences.

The views of patients who decline to take part in research can highlight salient attitudes about interventions. Barnes et al. [31] reported, in their qualitative study exploring views of people who had declined to participate in a trial of cognitive behavioural therapy (CBT) for Treatment Resistant Depression, that the acceptability of the trial intervention was an important factor in determining whether patients chose to participate in the trial.

O'Caithain, Thomas & Drabble et al. (2014) emphasises that the value of qualitative research to randomized controlled trials includes 'improving the external validity of trials and facilitating interpretation of trial findings' [32]. This paper reports a qualitative study embedded in the MIR trial, and aims to contribute to the understanding of TRD, as well as the acceptability of a combination of antidepressants from the perspectives of both patients and practitioners, with implications for how the intervention may be received more widely by patients and GPs in primary care.

Methods

Ethical approval was obtained from the South East Wales Research Ethics Committee (12/WA/0353).

We conducted semi-structured interviews with people who were invited to participate in the MIR trial [17], but declined, trial participants (those who completed the trial, and who withdrew) to generate in-depth data on perspectives of participating in the trial, reasons for completion or withdrawal. In addition, we interviewed GPs to explore their experiences of participating in the MIR trial, perspectives on managing people with depression, with a focus on perspectives of antidepressant prescribing.

Participants were recruited to the MIR trial [17] from 106 general practices in Bristol, North Staffordshire and Shropshire, Hull, York and Exeter. A screening questionnaire was posted to 2299 potential participants. Respondents who declined to participate could give a reason on a form which provided closed questions to indicate their reason(s) for declining. There was also a free text response box for respondents to give additional details about or alternative reasons for declining. Respondents were also given an option to indicate their willingness to be contacted to be interviewed about their reasons for declining. The questionnaire was brief, to maximise the likely response. These data were collected throughout the recruitment period.

Recruitment

If respondents indicated that they were willing to be contacted about their reasons for declining participation, this data was stored on a database, accessed by the trial team to invite a sample of willing respondents, categorized as 'decliners' to participate in a semi-structured interview. Sampling from within the 'decliner' population was purposive, on the basis of gender, age, geographic location and reasons for declining to participate, to gain maximum variation within the sample. Free text responses were also used to direct sampling when respondents had selected 'other' as a closed response and when details were given in the free text box which would indicate their suitability or unsuitability to be contacted about their reasons for declining. Once identified as suitable for contact, the research assistant (KD) made telephone contact with the respondent, gave details about the purpose of the call, the relationship of the qualitative study within the MIR trial and their rights as a potential participant of the study to confidentiality and to withdraw their consent at any time. They were then asked whether they had further questions and whether they would be willing to participate in a telephone interview. If verbal consent was given these interviews were usually conducted at the time of the initial phone call or arrangements were made to call the respondent at a more convenient time.

Sampling of trial participants was carried out at 12 weeks (once primary outcome measures assessed), taking gender, age and geographical location to gain maximum possible variation within the available sample. Participants were advised at the12 week assessment by the researcher that they may be contacted by study team to discuss their experiences of participation in the trial. The research assistant (KD) received regular reports from the trial teams on participants who had reached the primary outcome measure, and following review of the participant record, would attempt to contact participants, where the contact notes suggested it was appropriate to do so. Where there had been any serious or adverse events or where the participant had declined further contact after the primary outcome measure, these individuals were not invited to participate in the qualitative study. Participants were initially contacted by telephone and asked whether they would be willing to take part in an interview to discuss their experiences of being in the trial. If a trial participant agreed, an information sheet with further details of the study was sent to the participant and a provisional date for a face-to-face interview was made (usually 1–2 weeks after the date of the phone call to allow the information sheet time to arrive and the participant to consider the content).

When a participant withdrew from the trial, KD reviewed the participant record with the researcher or research nurse who had visited the participant, and contacted the 'withdrawer' to gain consent to an interview. If the person agreed, an information sheet was sent and a provisional date for a telephone interview was made. 'Withdrawers' were asked to send their consent forms back to the research team prior to the interview which was conducted by telephone.

GPs were recruited from the 106 practices participating with the MIR trial. Sampling of GP practices was purposive and selection based on the geographical location of the practice, gender and experience of the GP, to give maximum variation in the available population. Sampling was also contingent on whether the practice had patients who had been randomized to the MIR trial.

GPs and practice managers were initially contacted by email, with the information sheet as an attachment, inviting them to discuss their experiences of managing people with depression and views of using a combination of anti-depressants. If there was no response to the email, telephone calls were made to the practice. If a GP expressed interest in participating in an interview, the research assistant (KD) arranged a telephone interview at a time that was convenient to the GP.

Data generation

Informed consent to participate in the qualitative study was obtained from all participants in the study. People invited to take part in interviews about their reasons for declining to participate in the MIR trial, were provided with a short questionnaire during the trial recruitment phase on which to indicate consent to be contacted about their reasons for non-participation. When these patients were contacted by telephone, they were asked to confirm that they had consented to taking part in a telephone interview and for their verbal consent to record the telephone interview. Participants were reminded about their rights as a participant to confidentiality and to withdraw their consent at the beginning and the end of the conversation respectively. This procedure for gaining consent to conduct and record telephone interviews was also followed when contacting GPs for telephone interviews for the study. Interviews with GP participants and decliners were conducted via telephone.

Patients participating in the trial were sent an information sheet in the post after their 12 week outcome measure had been taken by the researcher or research nurse, outlining information about participation in the qualitative study. For those participants who agreed to an interview, each participant was asked to sign a written consent form to indicate their consent to participate, and the researcher confirmed this consent further verbally before commencing the interview. The majority of interviews with patient participants were held face to face with the participant, in their own homes.

Data were generated using semi-structured interviews with participants conducted either via the telephone (patients who declined participation in the trial and general practitioners) or during face to face interviews (patients who completed or withdrew from the trial).

Topic guides for each group of participants (decliners, patients and GPs) were produced prior to the commencement of the first interviews and were amended and adapted in response to initial analysis of interviews and after discussion within the research team. The process was iterative throughout the period of data generation to better explore the concepts and themes which emerged as being important to the interviewees and required more in depth examination during subsequent interviews.

Data generated from each of these data sets were collected during each interview by the qualitative research assistant, using a digital audio recorder. Audio files were transcribed verbatim by an authorized transcription company and transcripts were stored securely by the research assistant in accordance with standard operating procedures. Each interview was checked against the audio-recording, cleaned and anonymized prior to analysis.

Data generation was continued until data saturation within each data-set was considered, by the research team, to have been achieved.

Data analysis

Thematic analysis of the data [33] was conducted independently by authors CCG, HB and KD in the first instance. Subsequently the three members of the qualitative research team discussed their individual analysis and themes were agreed through discussion [33]. The three researchers were from different professional backgrounds (academic primary care, health services research and anthropology) which increases trustworthiness of analysis. [34]. Transcripts were read and re-read, themes arising during data generation and analysis within the team, and the topic guides modified iteratively as data collection and analysis progressed.

The qualitative research team met regularly to discuss and agree coding, revisiting the data from each dataset (and from analysis of other data-sets) in an iterative manner to verify coding and themes generated from these codes. This process was repeated until it was agreed that each individual data-set had reached saturation. Analysis was initially conducted within each data-set, then comparisons carried out across the datasets, in order to identify similarities and differences (disconfirmatory evidence). Discussion was continued until consensus was reached amongst the larger research team and PPIE group. NVIVO 10 [35] was used to store data and aid analysis.

The qualitative research team worked with a Patient and Public Involvement and Engagement (PPIE) group to discuss transcripts from the data-sets. The aim was to add value to the analysis with the lay partners adding value to the analysis by bringing their own perspectives and identifying further areas for the researcher to look for in the interviews [36]. Four meetings were held with the PPIE group over the course of data generation and analysis.

Members of the study PPIE group were recruited from members of the Keele Research User Group (RUG) which consists of over 100 members who contribute to all stages of development of studies. The study team invited people to participate in the study PPIE group if they had personal experience, or experience as a carer, of depression.

Two or three interview transcripts, or extracts of transcripts, were circulated prior to the PPIE meeting, and then the transcripts were discussed during the meeting, exploring what meaning the PPIE members gave to certain data extracts, and the research team offering their interpretations and checking this out with the PPIE group. The PPIE group members were supported by a RUG Advisor at each meeting.

Results

We will present reasons given by people invited but who declined to participate in the MIR trial.

We will then describe the participants in the qualitative study, followed by key themes across the data-sets.

Reasons given for declining to participate in the MIR trial:

The reasons that people gave for not wanting to participate in the MIR trial are listed in Table 1.

The commonest reason for declining was not wanting to take part in a trial (49%). 36% of people invited indicated that they did not want to take mirtazapine; it is not known if this was because of prior experience of being prescribed this anti-depressant. Not wanting to take more than one antidepressant was given by 20% people invited to participate in the MIR trial. Interestingly, 17% of people suggested that they were not taking an antidepressant – even though they were being prescribed and SSRI or SNRI according to their GP records; 39% people said they planned to stop taking the current antidepressant.

Table 1 Reasons for declining participation in the MIR trial

	Reason	N = 4702 (25%)[a]
a	I do not want to take part in a research study	2298 (49%)
b	I plan to stop taking my current antidepressant	1822 (39%)
c	I do not want to take mirtazapine	1692 (36%)
d	I do not want to take a placebo	1328 (28%)
e	I only want to take one antidepressant	936 (20%)
f	I'm not taking antidepressants	818 (17%)
g	I am too busy	463 (10%)
h	I am not depressed	323 (7%)
i	Other reason(s)	1321 (28%)

[a] Individuals were able to indicate more than one reason, thus percentages do not add up to 100%

Qualitative study participants

A total of 59 interviews were conducted; 23 with decliners (Mean duration = 11 min 27 s) (Table 2); 23 completers and withdrawers (Mean duration = 47 min 35 s) (Table 3), and 14 with General Practitioners (mean duration 19 min 31 s) (Table 4).

Key themes across the data-sets

Key themes presented in this manuscript include 'the hard work of managing depression', uncertainties over the value of a second antidepressant, help-seeking at a point of crisis, and attainment and maintenance of a hard-won equilibrium.

Illustrative data will be presented with the gender and age of the patient participant given as identifiers in the case of trial participants (completers and withdrawers) and those who declined to participate (decliners). Data from GP transcripts will be identified with numbers reflecting the chronological order in which the interviews were conducted.

The hard work of managing depression

Respondents reflected on the history of their depressive symptoms, and there were rich descriptions of endeavours to manage their mental-health, including a broad range of self-management strategies and help-seeking.

Many respondents described delays in recognizing the cause of their depression, outlining repeated investigation for physical problems until a diagnosis of depression was achieved by default:

> *"Erm, what it went back to was – I think it was postnatal depression, it started, and I didn't realise what it was. Erm, that was [...] so that was 20 years ago and I thought I'd got ME or, or MS or something, because I, I, physically, couldn't walk. I wasn't particularly unhappy, but I, I was physically fatigued really, really fatigued. And I struggled with that for years, going for tests, and one thing and another, and it never came to anything, because it was depression."*[Female, 55, decliner].

Once recognized as depression, respondents reported that they had tried numerous strategies and life-style

Table 2 Decliners

Site	Participant total	Gender Male	Gender Female	Age Range (years)
Bristol	7	1	6	27–66
Exeter	6	2	4	40–54
Keele	6	3	3	32–76
Hull/York	4	2	2	35–68
Totals	**23**	**8**	**15**	

Table 3 Completers and Withdrawers

Site	Participant total	Gender Male	Gender Female	Age range (years)
Bristol	11	5	6	32–63
Exeter	3	2	1	56–83
Keele	5	2	3	38–69
Hull/York	4	0	4	49–52
Total	**23**	**9**	**14**	

changes to manage their own symptoms, including exercise and diet, seeking support from family and friends, taking steps to ease the pressure on themselves, and pursuing psychological and alternative therapies:

> *"Well I'd been on websites to look at the condition….to look at what I could do, such as the omega-3, eating well, exercising, getting as much light as you can…all those sort of things."* [Male, 57, decliner].

Respondents described the effort involved in 'carrying on':

> *"you feel as if you don't have as much confidence and you don't feel erm what – erm like you don't want to participate in things that you did want to participate in and you're not really bothered about things. Obviously you are, but that's how it makes you feel, you know. And also, like you haven't got as much energy as you did have and you keep putting things off… 'Oh yeah, I'll do it tomorrow.' And yet, I mean, I'm a very busy person. I have a full-time job and I work at least 40 h a week, so I mean I do hide it well, it's on the inside I would say."* [Female 59, completer].

All respondents indicated the hard work involved in trying to manage their symptoms and endeavouring to find something that might help:

> *"…I've been doing a lot of meditation and, sort of, pursuing the mindfulness route […] I think to get out of depression, you have to probably put in a lot of different things in place to be able to tackle the things that have got you there, [okay] and exercise and eating well or trying to eat well even though I didn't have an appetite."* [Female, 37, decliner].

Table 4 General Practitioners

Site	Participant total	Gender Male	Gender Female
Bristol	5	4	1
Exeter	5	4	1
Keele/ N Staffs/Shropshire	2	2	0
Hull/York	2	1	1
Total	**14**	**11**	**3**

> *"there's a group called* (names third sector group*), to get in contact with them, and see what they would suggest, as well, and what they could do to help. And also, er, through work, I contacted, hmm, another similar group…and they directed me to, like, er, a series of one-to-ones or just, sort of, counselling, sort of soft counselling, or something [okay], just talking to somebody, talking therapy [uh-huh]. Er, a via* (a different third sector group*), I ended up doing a, erm, what was it called, which is more to do with, sort of, the food and overeating side of things, and I ended up having cognitive behavioural therapy with somebody, as well. Erm that was more along the line to control eating, which was, as opposed to dealing with depression in a particular way [okay]. But, yeah, I came away that day, from the doctor's, with antidepressants."* [Male, 55, completer].

Some respondents described an initial reluctance to take anti-depressants, but having got over this, suggested that they had come to terms with the need to use drugs to manage their mood. However, many respondents expressed concerns over the length of time that they would have to take their current antidepressant and were resistant taking a second antidepressant.

> *"I felt […] that I didn't wanna get involved in taking tablets for six, nine, 12 months. I'm already six months into taking them now [hmm], which is longer than I thought I would be…I thought, 'Oh, I'll get rid of it. I'll be okay. I'll have a few months or I'll have a couple of months off. I'll be back to my normal self,' but it hasn't worked like that..Erm, and whether another antidepressant would help I really don't know."* [Male, 55, decliner].

Such reluctance was sometimes due to a fear of (additional) side-effects:

> *"I didn't want to start with the side effects what I got from the first one [uh-huh]. I didn't want to start with new side effects and things."* [Female, 4, decliner].

Whilst GPs described managing people with depression as 'the bread and butter of general practice,' they reflected on the complexity of the work involved in the assessment of a patient:

> *"I mean all of it is history taking initially, finding out a little bit about the, the, the physical problems, social*

problems and obviously their mental health problems. There might be more significant social connotations. So they might have alcohol related problems or drug use problems and things like that so that can make things a bit more challenging" [GP04].

"you can't give a global answer to that actually because it's incredibly tailored individual ...to individual patient circumstances and patient beliefs [...] so I'm - you know, I just think it's - it's just very individual I think we all adopt different consultation styles for different patients, don't we?" [GP02].

This multifaceted and individual assessment of patients who presented with depressive symptoms or ongoing depression, described by some GPs as a large component of their workload, was also described as one that can feel like a 'battle' and at times overwhelming:

"Erm, so it's, it's inevitably a battle [yeah]. Well, not a battle, it's a challenge to, to relate to the patient in the way that they understand. That's what we do for a living, isn't it? [Hmm] I suppose." [GP12].

In addition, GPs described the complexity in negotiating management of depression with patients:

"erm I think it's - some of it's about previous response or lack of previous depression, really. [okay] Erm the, the - I think then that's looking at the broader context of what the patient's like, whether it's a personality disorder erm and whether it's err circumstantial, you know, whether it's - there's, there's - it - there's quite a few things that feed into that, really" [GP10].

Maintaining equilibrium

The invitation to participate in a trial was described as posing a challenge, as managing depression was already seen as a series of complex decisions, with continued reflection and self-monitoring required. Respondents indicated that they were declining to take part because they feared disturbing the sense of balance they had achieved with their current antidepressant medication. The potential work involved in participation was felt to be a challenge to current stability:

"Because you know when you suddenly drop and you don't know why? [Hmm] Erm, I've had a drop recently, so that, I don't know what that was, but I had a drop recently, and I had to, sort of, look again at what I was doing [yeah]. Erm, so, adding something, changing something, is a bit scary for me [uh-huh] because I was feeling good, and I like feeling okay." [Female, 53, decliner].

"but for me, taking something, erm, potentially taking something that could disrupt the way I am when I'm, you know, feel I'm on a steady level, I, I didn't really want to, to take that risk." [Female, 27, completer].

Other respondents, whilst recognizing that something else may be necessary to help them manage their symptoms, expressed a preference for talking treatments:

"....I'm on quite a low dose really, 20 milligrams of, erm, Citalopram, and I think it was doing the job it needed to do [...] to get me to point where I could look at some issues." [Female, 39, decliner].

A number of interview participants who had declined to consent to participate in the trial stated that, had they been offered combination treatment at a point of crisis, when they felt out of balance and unable to cope, they might have agreed to take part in the trial because of their desperation to overcome their depression. In the following extract, the decliner participant is responding to a question from the researcher about whether they would have considered taking two antidepressants if they hadn't felt better on one tablet. Their response suggests that if they had been 'at rock bottom' taking two tablets would not have been an issue if it offered the chance of getting better.

"...I needed to do whatever it took to, you know, get well again, quite simply. So I, I would do whatever it takes. When you - I think when you really hit rock bottom you are prepared to do whatever it takes and I have absolute faith in my doctor" [Female, 42, decliner].

One participant makes an extreme comparison, but makes the same point about being willing to accept whatever was necessary to escape being depressed.

"I think, I think if you'd caught me when I was depressed, I would have taken anything to be honest, I would have done anything to get out of it [...] in the first instance I struggled for a few weeks erm, thinking oh I can get out of this and it's alright, it's temporary and then it gets to a point where two, three weeks down the line, I just thought, I can't deal with this, I'm on a sinking ship, so I think if the study had been then, and someone had offered me, you know, I don't know, a shot of heroin a day to get out of it, I would have done it!" [Female, 38, completer].

Why would another tablet help?

Some respondents expressed scepticism about the 'chemical imbalance' story that they felt had been told to them, to explain why a tablet would help their mood. Why a second anti-depressant would help if the first had not was questioned:

> ***(I)***: *"...would you have had any concerns about taking two antidepressants?"*
>
> ***(P)***: *"Erm, no, I don't think so...but I should wonder why I suppose I hadn't had any, er, sort of beneficial reaction and maybe had to go to the doctors again and say it doesn't seem to be working terribly well, what else can we do"* [Male, 76, decliner].

Respondents described the protracted sequence of trying out other antidepressants, increases in the dosage of their medication which had been either been ineffective or had worked for a limited time, then seemed to stop working, and referrals to talking therapies. Hoping that this trial would be another option for them to regain a sense of wellbeing was prevalent in accounts of these participants' experiences:

> *"I felt that the antidepressants, I'd already been on, you know, I was given 20 milligrams, and then they were increased to 40 [uh-huh], and yet I still wasn't feeling, I wasn't really feeling, er, 100% [uh-huh]. So I just felt that that [taking part in the trial] could be a different way of trying to get things, trying to get me a bit more better, you know"* [Male, 54, completer].

Participants in the trial were keen to get back to a level of coping and wellbeing they had experienced previously. They described that they were no longer feeling a beneficial effect from their medication and in some cases had sought out another option from their GP. The participant in the following extract gives an account of approaching her GP asking for them to 'do something':

> *"I was taking sertraline erm probably from quite a while, really; about four months or so. And I felt they hadn't made enough difference. [okay] Erm so I went back to the doctor and I was really worried and I said, 'Look, I need some - either to up this medication or change it, do something"* [Female, 49, completer].

The opportunity to participate in the MIR trial came at a time when they were seeking an alternative option to help them manage their depression.

Patients who withdrew from the trial did so either because of side-effects of because they felt that they had regained their equilibrium:

> *"I think the medication that I was on, got me, you know, on an acceptable level, you know. I'm not as bad as I was [...] And then you get to a stage where yeah, things are acceptable. You just accept things and you just carry on"* [Female, 69, withdrawer].

> *"Had my weight gain not been so severe I would've gone on longer taking the drug – and I told her* (the researcher) *that. I said to her that I couldn't warrant having great thoughts and then dying of a cardiac arrest [laughs] because I'd put on so much weight. I have weight issues anyway, so it was just like the balance wasn't right for me by the end of it"* [Female, 36, completer - withdrew after un blinding].

Although some GPs described a level of confidence in prescribing two antidepressants, all expressed caution about how long such a combination should be continued. Some speculated on how they might try to reduce one anti-depressant in a combination, but none of the GPs interviewed reported experience of stopping one in the combination:

> *"I daresay we'd reduce one to zero, first of all, and see how it goes, and then reduce the other to zero [uh-huh]. I don't think I would stop them both at the same time [yeah]. I don't know [uh-huh], but I think I would, I'm sure I would do that, actually. I'd, I'd choose one and say, 'Well, how are you doing?' And, 'We're gonna have to start reducing these now [yeah], and I would suggest that,' er, 'we get you off one first of all, for a few weeks, and see how you feel, and then withdraw the other one slowly."*[GP 12].

All GPs expressed concern about patients remaining on two anti-depressants, suggesting that patients were commonly prescribed SSRIs without a plan to withdraw:

> *"it's all right initiating it, isn't it, and - but then I think then there becomes a bit more of a long-term issue about if you - how long do they stay on them both? [huh-huh] Do you - which one do you tail off first? [huh-huh] And erm you don't - you wouldn't necessary want people stuck on both antidepressants for time immemorial, which sometimes happens with SSRI, doesn't it?"* [GP102].

Thus, GPs described a future dilemma if antidepressants were combined.

Help-seeking at a point of crisis

Those people who felt they were approached to participate in the MIR trial when they were at a point of crisis, described seeing the trial as an opportunity to deal with that crisis. Thus, participants detailed the current impact of their depression on their ability to cope and to the point where they recognized they needed help:

"I had a lot of work stress going on as well [uh-huh], er, and it all got on top of me[...]. I was massively, er, overeating, erm, oversleeping, permanent low mood, just generally unwell [...] So, er, at, sort of, that point, I went to the doctor and said, 'Look, this is what's going on. I need some help with this.'"[Male, 52, completer].

Another patient reflects on how his feelings of desperation had led him to accepting referral into the trial by his GP, in the hope that it would offer alleviation of his current condition:

"Well I think I was desperate enough to take her advice that it was more likely to be helpful than anything, than a hindrance, it wasn't going to do any harm and it might do some good" [Male, 83, completer].

GPs' accounts reflected the perspectives of patients – that often help-seeking was at a point of crisis:

"And, and if somebody's depressed they really - if they're, you know, if they're at a watershed and they've actually come to the doctor's about it [...] because it's often a crisis really when they've - or it's been a huge step to actually come and do something about it." [GP102].

"but a lot of the time, when people come and see us, er, it's normally at the crisis point" [GP08],

"I think a lot of people by the time they've got to us they're probably quite sort of... you know, er, they're needing some help really." [GP03].

Such help-seeking at crisis point was not just described in new presentations, GPs described how patients with long-standing mood problems, would often re-present at a time of crisis:

"Erm, clearly there's a, quite an imperative to prescribe in some people, people who have been unwell for years. Some people want medication and don't have the time or the inclination, or the enthusiasm to go for counselling, for a long period of time, and wait. They just want something done now, please." [GP114].

Discussion

Summary of findings

This qualitative study, embedded within a trial of a combination of two anti-depressants for people with treatment-resistant depression illustrates patients and GPs descriptions of the hard work involved in managing depression; patients described the need to maintain themselves at an equilibrium, and the importance of a 'crisis point' in the precipitation of help-seeking. People who declined to participate in the MIR trial [17] described feeling that they were at an equilibrium, and feared that participating in the trial would disturb that hard-won equilibrium. Experiencing a crisis-point seemed to be a motivator to make a change in management, and the offer of trying a second antidepressant within a trial could act as that motivator to change. Some 'decliners' expressed uncertainties about the role of medication in the management of depression (even though they were already taking one antidepressant) and feared that a second tablet would not help, or could not see the logic of a second medication.

Those people who participated in the trial (whether they completed or withdrew) described the persistent hope that something would help their mood, and this was something that the participation in the trial offered. The narratives of GP respondents reflected the patient data – describing the 'hard work' needed to manage people with depression, how 'treatment resistance' was about more than a poor response to an antidepressant, but rather about a complex patient presenting the GP a challenge in management. GPs described how patients often present at a crisis-point and how the MIR trial offered an option for them to help manage such patients.

Comparison with previous literature

Qualitative research can address questions in trial recruitment that are not easily addressed by quantitative methods, by providing in-depth information on the experiences of participants and recruiters. [37] The commonest reason for people to decline to participate in the MIR trial [17] was not wanting to take part in a research study, as described in Barnes et al. qualitative study [31] nested in a trail of Cognitive Behavioural Therapy (CBT)for 'treatment-resistant depression'. But, in contrast to Barnes' qualitative study, where the 'decliners' expressed negative feelings about the treatment offered (CBT) in the trial, in our study 'decliners' who were interviewed, described how they were at an equilibrium which would be disturbed if they chose to participate in the trial, although a second antidepressant was not thought to be logical by a number of the 'decliners' interviewed. The patient may be perceived to be resistant to make a further change, having tried out various strategies and reached a position they were satisfied with, and feared losing. This illustrates the difficulty of the term 'treatment resistant depression' – the individual rather than the depression needs to be considered.

Hughes-Morley et al. [38] described how individuals declined to participate in a trial because they judged themselves ineligible or not in need of the trial therapy. Similarly, our analysis suggests that the 'decliners' we interviewed did not feel that they were in need of the trial intervention, a second antidepressant. MIR trial participants described experiencing a crisis as a motivator to participate in the trial, which resonates with Schofield et al. (2011) who reported that participants described their first course of antidepressants as typically occurring when they had 'hit rock bottom', having exhausted all other possibilities [39]. Schofield reported that participants described periods of experimentation where it was usual to stop and restart medication, often several times. Ultimately, these recurring cycles lead to participants becoming more expert about their condition and better able to make an informed decision about medication, yet still asking their GP for help. This description of patient expertise resonates with our analysis. Schofield also reported that for older people there was often an acceptance that their condition, and medication use, would be long term. [39] This acceptance might resonate with the concept of 'equilibrium' we describe in this study. In a meta-ethnography [30] Malpass and colleagues (2008) outline the role of the general practitioner in supporting decision-making about anti-depressant use, facilitating concordant relationships with patients regarding antidepressant use. Not having this discussion at entry into the trial may account for some people declining to participate. Malpass et al. [30] recommend that GPs are aware of the competing demands that patients experience at a decision-making juncture. We identified the importance of a 'crisis' in influencing a decision to try something new, or a sense of equilibrium in resisting change.

Strengths and limitations

Exploring the reasons for non-participation in trials is still unusual (and difficult), and this study describes how such interviews can be incorporated into a trial recruitment procedure. A limitation of the study is that people who responded to the decliner questionnaire, and invitation to participate in a telephone interview about their reasons for declining to participate in the MIR trial, were a self-selected group, which may limit the generalisability of the findings. Perhaps people with stronger opinions about the trial might be more likely to respond. In addition, the telephone interviews were relatively short (mean duration less than 12 min). A strength of this study was involvement of the PPIE group in the analysis [36], although some challenges arose, including difficulties in recruiting a diverse range of members of the public to participate in the PPIE group, and the research team sometimes experienced difficulties keeping the PPIE members on track within meetings.

Implications

Collecting information about those who decline to take part in research is a key way to learn about the acceptability of treatments being studied. In pilot studies for large-scale RCTs, gathering such information may be useful in refining recruitment estimates. Researchers recruiting to trials need to be sensitive to the patients' prior experience of the same (or a similar) intervention being studied, their feelings about the intervention, and their views on their potential eligibility.

Similarly, when recruitment takes place with a primary care consultation, GPs need to explore patients' reasons for declining to address any concerns or misconceptions about the research. This could increase recruitment to studies and thus ultimately contribute to increasing the evidence base.

Exploring reasons for declining to participate in a trial of a second antidepressant for depression suggests that people who are already taking one antidepressant may be reluctant to take a second, being wary of possible side-effects, but also being unconvinced of the logic behind such a combination. In addition, people describe being in a state of equilibrium and reluctant to make a change, reflecting that this equilibrium is 'hard-won' and they are unwilling to risk disturbing this.

The importance of achieving and maintaining an 'equilibrium' is a key finding of this qualitative study and should be incorporated into recruitment strategies in future trials of treatments for patients with depression not responding to an antidepressant, and for whom the addition of a second antidepressant, or switching an antidepressant, as suggested by the NICE guideline [12].

A crisis seemed to be the motivator for a patient with depression to try something new, including agreeing to take a combination of antidepressants, and this is the point at which people often consult their GP for help in routine practice. If a patient receives an invitation to participate in a trial when they are at such a point, they may be more willing to participate in the study. Whilst the MIR trial [17] evaluating the addition of mirtazapine to an SSRI, did not find convincing evidence of a clinically important benefit for mirtazapine in addition to an SSRI or SNRI antidepressant over placebo in primary care patients who were already on one antidepressant but remained depressed, it is likely that clinicians will continue to offer the addition of a second antidepressant, including mirtazapine, to patients with so called 'treatment-resistant depression'. It is vital that the GP explores with the patient their views on antidepressants, what other strategies they have tried to manage their symptoms, and whether the patient feels they are at a point of crisis or equilibrium. This has implications for the education and training of GPs about the management of depression in primary care, and the importance of regular review and monitoring for people with depression.

Conclusions

Understanding a patient's view on medication is important for GPs when discussing antidepressants in the routine primary care consultation when a diagnosis of depression has been made and agreed. Understanding patients' self-management strategies and what has precipitated their consultation is key to negotiating appropriate and acceptable management strategies.

Abbreviations

CBT: Cognitive Behavioural Therapy; GP : General Practitioner; MIR trial: Mirtazapine added to SSRIs or SNRIs for treatment resistant depression in primary care: phase III randomised controlled trial; UK: United Kingdom

Acknowledgements

The authors would like to thank the participants who took part in this study, for their time and valuable contributions. The authors would like to thank the rest of the MIR trial team, participating practice, and the PPIE group.

Funding

This study was funded by the National Institute for Health Research Health Technology Assessment programme (project number 11/129/76). The views and opinions expressed here are those of the authors and do not necessarily reflect those of the HTA programme, NIHR, NHS or the Department of Health.

Authors' contributions

KD conducted interviews with participants. KD, HB and CACG participated in data analysis.

CACG drafted the manuscript, and all authors contributed to draft versions of the manuscript, and approved the final version.

Consent for publication

Consent was received from all participants to publish the findings from this study. Consent was also received for the publication of pseudonymised direct quotes.

Competing interests

The authors declare that they have no competing interests.

Author details

[1]Research Institute, Primary Care and Health Sciences, Keele University, Newcastle, Staffs ST5 5BG, UK. [2]Centre for Academic Primary Care, Oakfield House, Oakfield Grove, Clifton, Bristol BS8 2BN, UK.

References

1. Global Burden of Disease Study 2015. Global Burden of Disease Study 2015 (GBD 2015) Reference Life Table. Seattle: United States: Institute for Health Metrics and Evaluation (IHME); 2016.
2. Evans DL, Charney DS, Lewis L, Golden RN, Gorman JM, Krishnan KRR, et al. Mood disorders in the medically ill: scientific review and recommendations. Biol Psychiatry [Internet]. Elsevier; 2005 Aug 1 [cited 2014 May 26];58(3):175–89. Available from: http://www.biologicalpsychiatryjournal.com/article/S0006322305005743/fulltext.
3. van't Veer-Tazelaar PJ, van Marwijk HWJ, Jansen APD, Rijmen F, Kostense PJ, van Oppen P, et al. Depression in old age (75+), the PIKO study. J Affect Disord [Internet]. 2008 Mar [cited 2014 May 27];106(3):295–9. Available from: http://www.sciencedirect.com/science/article/pii/S016503270700256X.
4. Katon W, Ciechanowski P. Impact of major depression on chronic medical illness. J Psychosom Res [Internet]. 2002 Oct [cited 2014 May 27];53(4):859–63. Available from: http://www.sciencedirect.com/science/article/pii/S0022399902003136.
5. Thompson C, Ostler K, Peveler RC, et al. Dimensional perspective on the recognition of depressive symptoms in primary care. Br J Psychiatry. 2001; 179:317–23.
6. Kirmayer LJ, Robbins JM, Dworkind M, et al. Somatization and the recognition of depression and anxiety in primary care. Am J Psychiatr. 1993; 150:734–41.
7. Tylee A, Freeling P, Kerry S, et al. How does the content of consultations affect the recognition by general practitioners of major depression in women? Br J Gen Pract. 1995;45:575–8.
8. Goldberg D, Privett M, Ustun B, et al. The effects of detection and treatment on the outcome of major depression in primary care: a naturalistic study in 15 cities. Br J Gen Pract. 1998;48:1840–4.
9. Kessler D, Bennewith O, Lewis G, et al. Detection of depression and anxiety in primary care: follow up study. BMJ. 2002;325:1016–7.
10. Lancet Global Mental Health Group. Scale up services for mental disorders: a call for action. Lancet. 2007;370:1241–52.
11. Mental Health Foundation. (2016). Fundamental facts about mental health 2016. Mental Health Foundation: London. https://www.mentalhealth.org.uk/publications/fundamental-facts-about-mental-health-2016. (accessed 06/11/2018).
12. National Institute for Health and Clinical Excellence, editor. THE NICE GUIDELINE ON THE TREATMENT AND DEPRESSION THE TREATMENT AND MANAGEMENT OF DEPRESSION IN ADULTS UPDATED EDITION. Updated Ed. London: The British Psychological Society and the Royal College of Psychiatrists; 2009.
13. Philp FMPWAR. Primary care-based guided self-help for depression provided by a nurse practitioner: a pilot evaluation. Prim Care Ment Heal Jul. 2006; 4(3):159.
14. Yohannes AM. General practitioners views and experiences in managing depression in patients with chronic obstructive pulmonary disease. Expert Rev Respir Med [Internet]. Informa HealthcareLondon; 2012 Dec 9 [cited 2014 May 27];6(6):589–95. Available from: http://informahealthcare.com/doi/abs/10.1586/ers.12.64.
15. Prescribing and Medicines Team. Health and Social Care Information Centre. Prescriptions dispensed in the Community: England; 2015. p. 2004–14.
16. Trivedi M, Rush A, Wisniewski S, Nierenberg A, Warden D, Ritz L, et al. Evaluation of outcomes with citalopram for depression using measurement-based care in STAR*D: implications for clinical practice. Am J Psychiatry. 2006;163:28–40.
17. Kessler D, Macneill Tallon D, Lewis G, Peters TJ, Hollingworth W, Round J, Burns A, Chew-Graham CA, Anderson IN, Shepherd T, Campbell J, Dickens CM, Carter M, Jenkinson C, Macleod U, Gibdson S, Wiles NJ. Mirtazapine added to SSRIs or SNRIs for treatment resistant depression in primary care: phase III randomised controlled trial (MIR). BMJ. 2018;363:k1218.
18. Snowden A, Marland G. No decision about me without me: concordance operationalised. J Clin Nurs [Internet]. 2013 May [cited 2013 Oct 21];22(9-10):1353–60. Available from: http://www.ncbi.nlm.nih.gov/pubmed/23121664.
19. Moradveisi L, Huibers M, Renner F, Arntz A. The influence of patients' preference/attitude towards psychotherapy and antidepressant medication on the treatment of major depressive disorder. J Behav Ther Exp Psychiatry [Internet]. 2014 Mar [cited 2014 Jan 28];45(1):170–7. Available from: http://www.sciencedirect.com/science/article/pii/S0005791613000773.
20. Brown C, Battista DR, Bruehlman R, Sereika SS, Thase ME, Dunbar-Jacob J. Beliefs about antidepressant medications in primary care patients: relationship to self-reported adherence. Med Care [Internet]. 2005 Dec [cited

2014 Dec 9];43(12):1203–7. Available from: http://www.ncbi.nlm.nih.gov/pubmed/16299431.
21. Lam RW. Patients' preferences and counselling for depression in primary care. Lancet [Internet]. 2001 24 [cited 2014 Dec 9];357(9256):575–6. Available from: http://www.sciencedirect.com/science/article/pii/S0140673600040769.
22. Van Schaik DJF, Klijn AFJ, van Hout HPJ, van Marwijk HWJ, Beekman ATF, de Haan M, et al. Patients' preferences in the treatment of depressive disorder in primary care. Gen Hosp Psychiatry [Internet]. [cited 2014 Nov 28];26 (3): 184–9. Available from: http://www.ncbi.nlm.nih.gov/pubmed/15121346.
23. Prins M A, Verhaak PFM, Bensing JM, van der Meer K. Health beliefs and perceived need for mental health care of anxiety and depression--the patients' perspective explored. Clin Psychol Rev [Internet]. 2008 Jul [cited 2013 Nov 20];28(6):1038–58. Available from: http://www.ncbi.nlm.nih.gov/pubmed/18420323.
24. Houle J, Villaggi B, Beaulieu M-D, Lespérance F, Rondeau G, Lambert J. Treatment preferences in patients with first episode depression. J Affect Disord [Internet]. 2013 May [cited 2013 Nov 20];147(1–3):94–100. Available from: http://www.ncbi.nlm.nih.gov/pubmed/23167975.
25. Gum AM, Arean PA, Hunkeler E, Tang L, Katon W, Hitchcock P, et al. Depression Treatment Preferences in Older Primary Care Patients. Gerontologist [Internet]. 2006 1 [cited 2014 May 28];46(1):14–22. Available from: http://gerontologist.oxfordjournals.org/content/46/1/14.full.
26. Givens JL, Datto CJ, Ruckdeschel K, Knott K, Zubritsky C, Oslin DW, et al. Older patients' aversion to antidepressants. A qualitative study. J Gen Intern Med [Internet]. 2006 Feb [cited 2013 Oct 24];21(2):146–51. Available from: http://www.pubmedcentral.nih.gov/articlerender.fcgi?artid=1484662&tool=pmcentrez&rendertype=abstract.
27. Verbeek-Heida PM, Mathot EF. Better safe than sorry — why patients prefer to stop using selective serotonin reuptake inhibitor (SSRI) antidepressants but are afraid to do so: results of a qualitative study. Chronic Illn [Internet]. 2006 1 [cited 2014 May 29];2(2):133–42. Available from: https://www.ncbi.nlm.nih.gov/pubmed/17175656.
28. Van Geffen ECG, Hermsen JHCMJHCM, Heerdink ER, Egberts ACG, Verbeek-Heida PM, Van Hulten R. The decision to continue or discontinue treatment: Experiences and beliefs of users of selective serotonin-reuptake inhibitors in the initial months-A qualitative study. Res Soc Adm Pharm [Internet]. Division of Pharmacoepidemiology and Pharmacotherapy, Faculty of Science, Utrecht Institute for Pharmaceutical Sciences (UIPS), Utrecht University, PO Box 80082, 3508 TB, Utrecht, Netherlands: Elsevier Inc; 2011 Jun [cited 2014 May 28];7(2):134–50. Available from: http://www.ncbi.nlm.nih.gov/pubmed/21272543.
29. Leydon GM, Rodgers L, Kendrick T. A qualitative study of patient views on discontinuing long-term selective serotonin reuptake inhibitors. Fam Pract [Internet]. 2007 [cited 2014 Dec 9];24(6):570–5. Available from: http://www.ncbi.nlm.nih.gov/pubmed/18032401.
30. Malpass A, Shaw A, Sharp D, Walter F, Feder G, Ridd M, et al. "Medication career" or "moral career"? The two sides of managing antidepressants: a meta-ethnography of patients' experience of antidepressants. Soc Sci Med [Internet]. 2009 [cited 2013 Oct 24];68(1):154–68. Available from: http://www.ncbi.nlm.nih.gov/pubmed/19013702.
31. Barnes M, Wiles N, Morrison J, Kessler D, Williams C, Kuyken W, et al. Exploring patients' reasons for declining contact in a cognitive behavioural therapy randomised controlled trial in primary care. Br J Gen Pract [Internet]. 2012 May [cited 2014 May 28];62(598):e371–7. Available from: http://www.pubmedcentral.nih.gov/articlerender.fcgi?artid=3338059&tool=pmcentrez&rendertype=abstract.
32. O'Cathain A, Thomas KJ, Drabble SJ, Rudolph A, Goode J, Hewison J. Maximising the value of combining qualitative research and randomised controlled trials in health research: the QUAlitative Research in Trials (QUART) study – a mixed methods study. Health Technol Assess. 18(38):1–197.
33. Braun V, Clarke V. Using thematic analysis in psychology. Qual Res Psychol. 2006;3(2):77–101.
34. Henwood KL, Pidgeon NF. Qualitative research and psychological theorizing. Br J Psychol. 1992;83:97–111.
35. NVivo. qualitative data analysis Software: QSR International Pty Ltd. Version 10; 2012. https://www.qsrinternational.com/nvivo/what-is-nvivo.
36. Garfield S, Jheeta S, Husson F, Jackline A, Bischler A, Norton C, Franklin BD. Lay involvement in the analysis of qualitative data in health services research: a descriptive study. Res Involv Engagem. 2016;2:29. https://doi.org/10.1186/s40900-016-0041-z.
37. Hennessy M, Hunter A, Healy P, Galvin S, Houghton C. Improving trial recruitment processes: how qualitative methodologies can be used to address the top 10 research priorities identifiedwithin the PRioRiTy study. Trials. 2018;19(584). https://doi.org/10.1186/s13063-018-2964-1.
38. Hughes-Morley A, Young B, Hempel RJ, Russell I, Waheed W, Bower P. What can we learn from trial decliners about improving recruitment? Qualitative study. BMC Trials. 2016;17:494 https://www.ncbi.nlm.nih.gov/pubmed/27733181.
39. Schofield P, Crosland A, Waheed W, Aseem S, Gask L, Wallace A, Dickens A, Tylee A. Patients' views of antidepressants: From first experiences to becoming expert. British Journal of General Practice. 2011;61(252–253). https://doi.org/10.3399/bjgp11X567045.

23

Understanding type 2 diabetes mellitus screening practices among primary care physicians: a qualitative chart-stimulated recall study

Dina Hafez[1,2,3,4*], Daniel B. Nelson[3], Evan G. Martin[3], Alicia J. Cohen[2,3,4], Rebecca Northway[3] and Jeffrey T. Kullgren[1,3,4]

Abstract

Background: Early diagnosis and treatment of prediabetes and type 2 diabetes mellitus (T2DM) can prevent future health problems, yet many individuals with these conditions are undiagnosed. This could be due, in part, to primary care physicians' (PCP) screening practices, about which little is known. The objectives of this study were to identify factors that influence PCPs' decisions to screen patients for T2DM and to characterize their interpretation and communication of screening test results to patients.

Methods: We conducted semi-structured chart-stimulated recall interviews with 20 University of Michigan Health System (UMHS) primary care physicians. PCPs were asked about their recent decisions to screen or not screen 134 purposively sampled non-diabetic patients who met American Diabetes Association criteria for screening for T2DM. Interviews were audio-recorded, transcribed, and analyzed using qualitative directed content analysis. Data on patient demographic characteristics and comorbidities were abstracted from the electronic health record.

Results: The most common reasons PCPs gave for not screening 63 patients for T2DM were knowledge of a previously normal screening test (49%) and a visit for reasons other than a health maintenance examination (48%). The most common reasons PCPs gave for screening 71 patients for T2DM were knowledge of a previously abnormal screening test (49%), and patients' weight (42%) and age (38%). PCPs correctly interpreted 89% of screening test results and communicated 95% of test results to patients. Among 24 patients found to have prediabetes, PCPs usually (58%) recommended weight loss and increased physical activity but never recommended participation in a Diabetes Prevention Program or use of metformin.

Conclusions: Previous screening test results, visit types, and patients' weight and age influenced PCPs' decisions to screen for T2DM. When patients were screened, test results were generally correctly interpreted and consistently communicated. Recommendations to patients with prediabetes could better reflect evidence-based strategies to prevent T2DM.

Keywords: Type 2 diabetes mellitus, Prediabetes, Diabetes prevention, Primary care, Preventive care, Communication, lifestyle counselling

* Correspondence: dhafez@med.umich.edu
[1]VA Ann Arbor Healthcare System, 2800 Plymouth Road, Building 14, Room G100-36, Ann Arbor, MI 48109-2800, USA
[2]Robert Wood Johnson Foundation Clinical Scholars Program, University of Michigan, Ann Arbor, MI, USA
Full list of author information is available at the end of the article

Background

Type 2 diabetes mellitus (T2DM) affects 25.1 million US adults and is a major cause of cardiovascular disease, kidney disease, blindness, and lower extremity amputation [1]. An additional 86 million individuals – one third of the US adult population – are estimated to have prediabetes [1], which if left untreated will result in 5–10% of these individuals progressing to T2DM each year [2].

Fortunately, T2DM and its complications can often be prevented through early detection and treatment of T2DM [3] and prediabetes [4, 5]. Several national initiatives are now aiming to identify more individuals with these conditions and connect them to evidence-based treatments. For example, in 2015 the US Centers for Disease Control and Prevention (CDC) and the American Medical Association (AMA) launched "Prevent Diabetes STAT: Screen/ Test / Act Today," a joint initiative that encourages diabetes prevention through screening for T2DM and referral to a Diabetes Prevention Program (DPP) [6]. Also in 2015, the United States Preventive Services Task Force (USPSTF) updated its recommendation for screening of adults for T2DM to include behavioral counseling interventions for those with abnormal results [7]. Most recently, the Centers for Medicare and Medicaid Services announced Medicare would cover the DPP for beneficiaries with prediabetes [8], joining the growing numbers of private insurers already doing so [9].

The promise of these national initiatives to improve population health hinges on the early identification and management of T2DM and prediabetes, which often begins in primary care practices through tests to screen for T2DM and communication of these test results to patients. Therefore, decisions primary care physicians make about whom to screen for T2DM, interpretation of screening test results, and communication of these results to patients can have important implications. For example, if clinicians do not accurately perceive risk factors for T2DM or if they incorrectly interpret screening test results, they may fail to identify at-risk patients. Further, clinicians may not communicate T2DM screening test results to patients or they may not provide evidence-based treatment recommendations, which can affect patients' perceptions of risk and their decisions about preventive behaviors [10]. If these deficiencies are widespread, they could help explain why more than 80 million individuals with T2DM and prediabetes are unaware they have these conditions [11].

Despite the population health implications of primary care physicians' T2DM screening practices, little is known about how primary care physicians decide which patients to screen for T2DM, what screening tests they choose, how they interpret screening test results, and what they communicate to patients about these results. The objective of our study was to identify factors that influence primary care physicians' decisions to screen patients for T2DM and to characterize primary care physicians' interpretation and communication of screening test results to patients.

Methods

Study design

Our team, which consisted of 3 primary care physician health services researchers, 1 fulltime primary care clinician, and 2 preclinical medical students, invited Internal Medicine physicians ($n = 50$), Family Medicine physicians ($n = 39$), nurse practitioners ($n = 2$), and physician assistants ($n = 5$) from 14 UMHS primary care practices to participate in a study about T2DM screening practices. We excluded trainees and clinicians with less than 0.5 full time equivalents devoted to outpatient clinical practice. Study invitation letters were sent by email, and informed providers that the primary aim of this study was to explore the factors that influence providers' decisions to screen for T2DM.

Among clinicians who consented to study participation we conducted chart-stimulated recall (CSR) interviews, a methodology used to assess clinical decision-making processes [12, 13]. During CSR interviews, a clinician uses his or her own documentation to answer questions and explain the rationale for specific clinical decisions. A significant strength of this approach – which has been used to examine physician decisions about screening for colorectal cancer [14] and screening for prostate cancer [15] – is that it examines a physician's own recent clinical decisions, which could provide more valid data on their clinical decision making than assessments of how they might respond to hypothetical clinical scenarios.

Sample

Twenty-five physicians responded to our recruitment e-mail and agreed to participate in our study. We planned to conduct a minimum of 20 interviews with additional interviews to be conducted only if data saturation was not achieved at this point. Prior to each CSR interview, one investigator (DH) reviewed in the electronic health record (EHR) each physician's clinical encounters from the previous 2 weeks to identify visits for non-diabetic patients 45 years of age and older who were candidates for screening for T2DM at their visit and thus eligible for inclusion in the CSR interviews. We focused on patients 45 years of age and older for 2 reasons. First, the American Diabetes Association (ADA) recommends screening all individuals over the age of 45 for T2DM regardless of other risk factors; therefore an age-based focus allowed us to easily identify patients for whom the ADA recommends periodic T2DM screening. Second, this age-based criterion was more feasible to implement in the context of the EHR than other more detailed criteria for which the ADA recommends screening for T2DM, such as being less than 45 years of age and overweight with at least one additional risk factor for T2DM [16].

While both the ADA and the USPSTF recommend routine screening for T2DM among at-risk individuals, we used the ADA's screening criteria because at the time of our interviews they were broader than the 2008 USPSTF criteria [17]. The USPSTF has since issued revised screening guidelines (disseminated in October 2015), but these were released after completion of all CSR interviews. We did not sample patients who had already been screened for T2DM within the previous year, as most non-diabetic patients do not need to be screened more than annually [16] and this study was not designed to explore reasons for over-screening.

To facilitate discussion of the range of factors that influence physicians' decisions to screen for T2DM, we selected in approximately equal numbers encounters in which patients appeared (using the available information in the EHR) to have been screened for T2DM or not screened for T2DM. We classified the following as screening tests for T2DM, based on the ADA guidelines: hemoglobin A1c (HbA1c) tests, oral glucose tolerance tests (OGTTs), and fasting blood glucose (FBG) tests [16]. Because blood glucose tests at our institution are not routinely labeled as "fasting," we classified blood glucose tests (drawn either in isolation or as part of a metabolic panel) as being fasting if they were obtained before 11 a.m. or drawn at the same time as a lipid panel that had been labeled in the EHR as fasting.

We also sampled in approximately equal numbers encounters in which patients were seen for either health maintenance examinations (HMEs) or return visits (RVs). We focused on both HMEs and RVs because there is debate about the utility of annual HMEs [18–20] and physicians have been encouraged to consider providing opportunistic preventive screenings at non-HME visits [21–23]. We excluded urgent care visits because in our institution these are typically focused, single-problem visits in which patients are commonly seen by clinicians other than their own primary care clinician.

Using this approach, for each clinician we aimed to select 12 encounters (i.e., roughly 3 each for HMEs with screening, HMEs without screening, RVs with screening, and RVs without screening) from the previous 2 weeks to potentially be discussed during the CSR interview. A goal of 12 encounters for each physician provided the opportunity to skip a particular encounter during the interview in the event that the clinician did not recall the encounter, while still permitting discussion of at least 6 separate patient encounters which has previously been shown sufficient to yield a valid and reliable assessment of practice patterns [24].

Interviews were conducted by trained preclinical medical students (DN, EM) and lasted approximately 30 min in duration. During the CSR interviews, physicians were first asked whether they screened each patient for T2DM and what factors influenced this decision. Our questions about reasons for the physician's decision were guided by whether the physician stated they had or had not screened the patient for T2DM, rather than how the patient had been classified in our purposive sampling. For example, if it appeared from the EHR that the physician had screened the patient for T2DM, but the physician stated that they had not screened the patient for T2DM, then the physician was asked why they had not screened the patient for T2DM. Conversely, if a patient had been sampled as having not been screened (e.g., because they had a random glucose), but the physician said they had screened the patient for T2DM, we asked the physician why they screened the patient (even though the test chosen was not an ADA-recommended test). This approach allowed us to focus on physicians' decision making processes irrespective of the outcome of that process.

When a screening test result was available for review (i.e., there was a lab result for a screening test that had been ordered at that visit), physicians were asked how they interpreted the result, whether and how they communicated the result to the patient, and what they communicated to the patient about the result. Following the CSR interview, physicians were also asked general questions regarding barriers to T2DM screening. Physicians had access to their EHR documentation during the interview. The interview guide was derived from previous CSR studies [14, 15] and is provided in the Additional file 1.

For each interview, physicians received a $50 gift card. The study was approved by the Institutional Review Board at the University of Michigan Medical School.

Analysis

All interviews were audio-recorded and transcribed verbatim. Three members of the research team (DH, DN, JK) independently reviewed a subset of transcripts. The transcripts were de-identified prior to data analysis to minimize the potential for biased interpretation of the data. Codes and definitions were generated during consensus conferences using directed content analysis [25]. Specifically, initial codes were created to reflect the main topics in the interview guide (e.g. decision to screen or not screen patients for T2DM), and additional codes were subsequently generated to reflect the patterns and themes that emerged from the data [26]. Once the coding scheme was established, two investigators (DH, DN) independently coded each transcript. These investigators then met to review their coding and resolve all differences. Few new themes emerged after coding 12 transcripts and no new themes emerged after coding 16 transcripts. Given that we reached data saturation [27, 28], we did not conduct additional interviews following the 20 interviews. All transcripts were coded in Dedoose, a software program for qualitative analysis.

The following data were abstracted from the EHR for each patient after the interviews were completed: age; sex; race; ethnicity; BMI; risk factors for T2DM documented in the patient's problem list such as hypertension, hyperlipidemia, cardiovascular disease, prediabetes, history of gestational diabetes or polycystic ovarian disease.

Results

Twenty primary care physicians (14 Internal Medicine and 6 Family Medicine) across 10 clinic sites participated in the study. There were no nurse practitioners or physician assistants who responded to our invitation.

These 20 physicians discussed a total of 156 patients who met our study inclusion criteria (mean 7.8 patients per physician) during the CSR interviews we conducted between January 2015 and July 2015. We then limited our analyses to the 63 patients who physicians stated they did not screen for T2DM and the 71 patients who physicians stated they screened for T2DM. We excluded 22 patients from our analyses because at the sampling stage they appeared to have been screened for T2DM with a blood glucose drawn prior to 11 a.m., but during the interview physicians indicated they did not screen the patient for T2DM and rather had ordered the blood glucose as part of an electrolyte panel to monitor kidney function.

A total of 134 patients were included in our analysis. In general, the patients who were screened for T2DM were had a higher BMI and a greater prevalence of prediabetes compared to patients who were not screened. Additionally, screening was more likely to occur during HMEs than RVs. Patient characteristics, stratified according to whether they had been screened for T2DM during the discussed encounter, are summarized in Table 1.

Table 1 Patient characteristics ($n = 134$)

Characteristics	Screened for T2DM ($n = 71$)	Not screened for T2DM ($n = 63$)	p-value[a]
	Mean (SD) or n (%)		
Age (years)	57.5 (9.6)	61.4 (12.2)	0.041
BMI (kg/m^2)	31.4 (6.6)	28.6 (5.7)	0.012
Female	34 (47.9)	39 (61.9)	0.10
Race[b]			
White	57 (80.3)	57 (90.5)	0.23
Black	7 (9.9)	2 (3.2)	
Asian	3 (4.2)	1 (1.6)	
Hispanic ethnicity[c]	3 (4.23)	1 (1.6)	0.37
Visit type[d]			
Health maintenance examination	48 (67.6)	19 (30.2)	<0.001
Return visit	23 (32.4)	44 (69.8)	
Comorbidities[e]			
Hyperlipidemia	38 (53.2)	25 (39.7)	0.11
Hypertension	28 (39.4)	21 (33.3)	0.46
Cardiovascular disease	3 (4.2)	3 (4.8)	0.88
Prediabetes[f]	15 (21.1)	2 (3.2)	0.002

[a] p-values were derived using logistic regression for continuous variables and Chi-squared test for categorical variables
[b] Race was listed in the EHR as "other" or "not reported" for 6 patients (4.5%)
[c] Ethnicity was listed in the EHR as "unknown" or "not reported" for 12 patients (9.0%)
[d] "Return visits" refer to problem-focused visits that range from 15 to 30 min in duration. "Health maintenance examinations" refer to prevention-focused visits that range from 40 to 45 min in duration
[e] The list of co-morbidities was selected based on the American Diabetes Association's criteria for screening for type 2 diabetes mellitus. There were no patients in our sample who had a documented history of 2 other ADA criteria for screening: polycystic ovarian syndrome and gestational diabetes mellitus
[f] Patients were classified as having prediabetes if they had one or more of the following diagnoses listed on their EHR problem list: prediabetes, impaired glucose tolerance, impaired fasting glucose, or borderline diabetes

Screening decisions

For the 63 patients who were not screened for T2DM, the most common reasons for not screening that physicians cited were knowledge of a previous normal screening test (49%) and the visit being for a reason other than a health maintenance examination (48%). Clinicians frequently cited more than one reason for not screening, and additional reasons are shown in Table 2.

For the 71 patients who were screened for T2DM, the most common reasons for screening that physicians cited were knowledge of a previously abnormal screening test for T2DM (49%), the patient being overweight or obese (42%), and patient age (38%). Two physicians specifically mentioned age ≥ 45 years as a screening criterion; others referenced the patient's actual age (e.g. "she is 60 years old") or noted that "the risk of diabetes goes up as we get older." Clinicians often cited multiple reasons for screening, and these additional reasons are shown in Table 3.

Among the 71 patients who were screened for T2DM, the most commonly ordered screening tests were a laboratory HbA1c ($n = 29$, 40.8%) and a fasting blood glucose ($n = 23$, 32.4%). Four patients (5%) were screened with a point-of-care HbA1c, and 8 patients were screened with a random blood glucose (i.e., a blood glucose drawn after 11 a.m.). Seven patients (9.9%) had more than one screening test ordered (i.e., both a fasting blood glucose and an HbA1c). No physician ordered an OGTT to screen for T2DM. Physicians reported ordering an HbA1c test for reasons such as: "it is more familiar and comfortable," "it is a little more reliable," "patients don't need to be fasting" and "it gives a better

Table 2 Physician-identified reasons for not screening for type 2 diabetes mellitus ($n = 63$)

Reasons	n (%)[a]
Previously normal T2DM screening test result(s)	31 (49.2)
Return visit	30 (47.6)
Normal weight	6 (9.5)
Future health maintenance examination	4 (6.4)
Normal blood pressure	2 (3.2)
Did not believe screening indicated based on guidelines	2 (3.2)
Younger age	2 (3.2)
Other[b]	12 (19.1)

[a]Number of times code occurred and frequency of occurrence among the 63 patients who were not screened. Codes were not mutually exclusive and therefore the percentages sum to more than 100
[b]Includes physician not being the patient's primary care physician; patient reported recent normal labs obtained elsewhere; patient preference to avoid a blood draw; patient enrolled in hospice

[overall] picture." Physicians ordered a fasting blood glucose – either in isolation or as part of a metabolic panel – if the patient had already been fasting for another test (e.g., a fasting lipid panel) or if the physician wanted to concurrently evaluate other components of the metabolic panel (e.g., electrolytes or renal function).

Interpretation of screening test results

Of the 71 patients for whom screening tests for T2DM were ordered, 50 had screening test results available in the EHR for review at the time of the interview. Based on the ADA guidelines,[29] 24 patients had screening test results that showed prediabetes, and 26 patients had screening test results that were normal. None of the sampled patients were found to have a new diagnosis of T2DM. Physicians discussed 47 of the 50 available test results, and of these correctly classified the majority (42, 89%) of the screening test results.

Table 3 Physician-identified reasons to screen for type 2 diabetes mellitus ($n = 71$)

Reasons	n (%)[a]
Previously abnormal screening test result(s)	35 (49.3)
Overweight or obesity	30 (42.3)
"Older age"	27 (38.0)
Hypertension	18 (25.4)
Hyperlipidemia	11 (15.5)
Health maintenance examination	8 (11.3)
Family history of T2DM	6 (8.5)
Sedentary lifestyle	4 (5.6)
History of cardiovascular disease	3 (4.2)
Race/ethnicity	3 (4.2)
Tobacco use	3 (4.2)

[a]Number of interviews in which the theme emerged and the frequency of occurrence using total number patients who physicians intended to screen (71) in the denominator

Communication of screening test results

Physicians communicated 95% of screening test results to patients. Most communications occurred by mailed letter or secure electronic messaging through the health system's patient portal (69%). Communication occurred by phone when either the screening test or another laboratory study was abnormal (16%); such telephone communications were always performed by a nurse. Communication occurred during an office visit only if the patient had laboratory tests performed prior to the encounter (15%).

Among patients found to have prediabetes, the content of communications focused mostly on diet and exercise, often with offers of referral to a nutritionist. For example, one physician stated, "I told her...diet and exercise would be the key. [We] can also offer referral to our nutritionist for pre-diabetes counseling, if she would like." In many cases, physicians' recommendations to patients were general and lacked specific goals or targets. An example of this was a physician who recommended, "just to continue with, what we call...lifestyle modifications. You know, a little bit of exercise, healthy diet, stuff like that." Some physicians minimized the significance of screening test results if they were at the lower end of the prediabetic range. For example, one physician said, "[The blood glucose] is slightly high at 101. What I told [him] is that he is just out normal range, but not in a concerning...urgent way, and that we'll talk about it in his next visit." Another said, "[The HbA1c] is stable from a year ago at 6.2%, which I feel is consistent with pre-diabetes and puts her at a high risk of developing diabetes...[I told her] that the lab looks stable...I kept it very short and sweet. I probably could have said something more about lifestyle."

Communications to patients with prediabetes never included specific, evidence-based treatment recommendations such as DPP participation or pharmacotherapy with metformin [30]. One physician said that "we talked about the diabetes prevention trial, and we set 150 min of exercise for her goal [per] week," but she did not specifically recommend or refer the patient to a DPP. None of the physicians started metformin for patients whose test results were in the prediabetic range, although one mentioned that a patient with prediabetes was already using metformin and a few acknowledged that metformin might be an option for such patients. One physician said, "I know there is some data talking about using metformin early on people like this. I don't like to add more medications than I have [to]. So I don't typically do that until the A1C starts to get up to closer to 6.5."

Discussion

Through CSR interviews among primary care physicians of a large academic medical center we found that screening for T2DM was appropriately targeted to patients with major risk factors for T2DM, including a history of prediabetes, older age, and being overweight or obese. The main reasons for not screening for T2DM included physicians' knowledge of previously normal results of a screening test for T2DM and clinical encounters for reasons other than an HME. While physicians usually interpreted screening results correctly and consistently communicated these results to patients, they never recommended evidence-based treatments to patients with prediabetes, such as Diabetes Prevention Program participation or use of metformin.

One contributor to high rates of undiagnosed prediabetes and T2DM may be screening among only patients with certain risk factors. Consistent with prior studies [31], physicians in our study targeted screening to individuals with certain major risk factors for T2DM such as obesity or a previously abnormal screening test result. However, our findings suggest that physicians may miss opportunities to screen older individuals who lack other risk factors for T2DM. Specifically, although "older age" was cited as reason for screening in over one-third of the discussed encounters, all of the patients discussed during the CSR interviews were old enough to meet ADA criteria for screening for T2DM. Further, in our sample the mean age was actually lower among patients who were screened for T2DM compared with patients who were not screened (58 years versus 61 years). One practical strategy to help clinicians consistently identify patients with major risk factors for T2DM would be to integrate age-based clinical reminders into the EHRs, an approach that has been shown to improve targeting of other types of clinical preventive services [32, 33].

A clinical encounter for a reason other than an HME was a common reason why physicians did not screen for T2DM, which suggests additional missed opportunities to screen at-risk patients for T2DM. While some physicians mentioned intentionally deferring screening to future HMEs, others felt they simply did not have the time to address preventive health issues in the context of problem-focused encounters. Primary care clinicians have been increasingly encouraged to perform opportunistic screenings during problem-focused and urgent care encounters [23, 28], and practice innovations could offer opportunities for other members of primary care teams to share responsibility for screening patients for T2DM when they seek primary care for a broader range of reasons [34].

While the primary care physicians we interviewed nearly always correctly interpreted results of screening tests for T2DM, their responses to these screening tests suggest many patients may not be receiving evidence-based preventive recommendations and treatments. Specifically, physicians never referred patients with prediabetes to a DPP or initiated treatment with metformin. This is consistent with prior studies, which show that physicians often fail to respond to abnormal screening test results [27, 35]. For example, one previous study found less than 1% of patients with prediabetes were prescribed metformin, and only 5% were referred to or attended health education, wellness, or lifestyle programs [35, 36]. Educational initiatives to increase physician awareness of the benefits of the DPP and metformin could be considered. However, because primary care physicians often report being overburdened with preventive health tasks [37] an alternative strategy might be to reflexively target patients with prediabetes for education about strategies to prevent T2DM.

Limitations

First, we conducted our study in a single academic center and our findings may not generalize to all clinical environments. Second, it is possible that physicians with a particular interest in screening for T2DM may have been more likely to participate in the study, and there were no nurse practitioners or physician assistants who chose to participate. Third, none of the patients discussed in the CSR interviews were found to have T2DM through screening, thus limiting our insight into how physicians interpret and respond to such results. Fourth, physicians' responses could have been influenced by recall or social desirability biases, though physician use of the EHR during interviews and our inquiries about recent visits by preclinical medical students aimed to mitigate the potential for such biases. Further, although physician access to the EHR at the time of the interview was intended to prompt recall of the encounter, it is possible that some physicians may have used EHR data to justify their decisions to screen or not screen a patient for T2DM. Finally, the USPSTF issued an updated recommendation for screening for T2DM following our study period, which could lead to changes in physician screening practices that we could not capture during this study.

Conclusions

Our study provides new insight into T2DM screening practices among primary care physicians. We identified factors that may contribute to high rates of undiagnosed T2DM and prediabetes and thus could limit the impact of recent national initiatives aimed at reducing the public health burden of T2DM and its complications. These factors could be addressed through systems-based strategies to increase the early identification and evidence-based treatment of patients with abnormal screening tests for T2DM. More research is needed to determine whether such strategies can increase the early identification of at-risk patients and better connect these patients with evidence-based treatments.

Abbreviations

ADA: American Diabetes Association; AMA: American Medical Association; CDC: Centers for Disease Control and Prevention; CSR: Chart-Stimulated Recall; EHR: Electronic Health Record; FBG: Fasting Blood Glucose; HbA1c: Hemoglobin A1c; HME: Health Maintenance Examination; OGTT: Oral Glucose Tolerance Test; PCP: Primary Care Provider; RV: Return Visit; T2DM: Type 2 Diabetes Mellitus; UMHS: University of Michigan Healthcare System; USPSTF: United States Preventive Services Task Force

Acknowledgements

The authors would like to thank all the primary care physicians who participated agreed to be interviewed for this study.

Funding

This research was supported by The National Med/Peds Residency Association. Support was also provided by the Department of Veterans Affairs, Veterans Health Administration, Health Services Research and Development Service. Dr. Kullgren is a VA HSR&D Career Development awardee at the Ann Arbor VA. The views expressed in this article are those of the authors and do not necessarily reflect the position or policy of the Department of Veterans Affairs or the United States government.

Authors' contributions

All authors (DH, DN, EM, AC, RN, JK) participated in the design of the study. EM and DN performed the interviews. JK, DH, and DN performed the data analysis. All authors read and approved the final manuscript.

Competing interests

Dr. Kullgren has received consulting fees from SeeChange Health and HealthMine. The other authors have no conflicts of interest to report.

Consent for publication

Not applicable.

Author details

[1]VA Ann Arbor Healthcare System, 2800 Plymouth Road, Building 14, Room G100-36, Ann Arbor, MI 48109-2800, USA. [2]Robert Wood Johnson Foundation Clinical Scholars Program, University of Michigan, Ann Arbor, MI, USA. [3]University of Michigan Medical School, Ann Arbor, MI, USA. [4]University of Michigan Institute for Healthcare Policy and Innovation, Ann Arbor, MI, USA.

References

1. 2014 Diabetes Report Card - diabetesreportcard2014.pdf [Internet]. [cited 2016 May 27]. Available from: http://www.cdc.gov/diabetes/pdfs/library/diabetesreportcard2014.pdf
2. Gerstein HC, Santaguida P, Raina P, Morrison KM, Balion C, Hunt D, et al. Annual incidence and relative risk of diabetes in people with various categories of dysglycemia: A systematic overview and meta-analysis of prospective studies. Diabetes Res Clin Pract. 2007;78:305–12.
3. Holman RR, Paul SK, Bethel MA, Matthews DR, Neil HAW. 10-year follow-up of intensive glucose control in type 2 diabetes. N Engl J Med. 2008;359:1577–89.
4. Group DPPR, et al. Reduction in the incidence of type 2 diabetes with lifestyle intervention or metformin. N Engl J Med. 2002;346:393.
5. Perreault L, Temprosa M, Mather KJ, Horton E, Kitabchi A, Larkin M, et al. Regression From Prediabetes to Normal Glucose Regulation Is Associated With Reduction in Cardiovascular Risk: Results From the Diabetes Prevention Program Outcomes Study. Diabetes Care [Internet]. 2014 [cited 2014 Jul 27]; Available from: http://care.diabetesjournals.org/cgi/doi/10.2337/dc14-0656
6. Prevent Diabetes STAT | General Public [Internet]. Prev. Diabetes STAT. [cited 2016 May 27]. Available from: http://www.preventdiabetesstat.org
7. Final Recommendation Statement: Abnormal Blood Glucose and Type 2 Diabetes Mellitus: Screening - US Preventive Services Task Force [Internet]. [cited 2016 May 27]. Available from: http://www.uspreventiveservicestaskforce.org/Page/Document/RecommendationStatementFinal/screening-for-abnormal-blood-glucose-and-type-2-diabetes
8. Alex ADA 1701 NBS, ria, 1-800-Diabetes V 22311. National Diabetes Prevention Program Named the First Preventive Health Initiative Eligible for Medicare Coverage via CMMI Expansion [Internet]. Am. Diabetes Assoc. [cited 2016 May 27]. Available from: http://www.diabetes.org/newsroom/press-releases/2016/national-dpp-named-first-preventive-health-initiative-eligible-for-medicare.html
9. Health Plans Preventing Diabetes and Improving Well-Being [Internet]. AHIP. 2016 [cited 2016 May 27]. Available from: https://www.ahip.org/diabetes/
10. Gopalan A, Lorincz IS, Wirtalla C, Marcus SC, Long JA. Awareness of Prediabetes and Engagement in Diabetes Risk–Reducing Behaviors. Am J Prev Med. 2015;49:512–9.
11. Centers for Disease Control and Prevention. National Diabetes Statistics Report: Estimates and Its Burden in the United States [Internet]. [cited 2016 May 27]. Available from: http://www.cdc.gov/diabetes/pubs/statsreport14/national-diabetes-report-web.pdf
12. Reddy ST, Endo J, Gupta S, Tekian A, Park YS. A Case for Caution: Chart-Stimulated Recall. J Grad Med Educ. 2015;7:531–5.
13. Goulet F, Jacques A, Gagnon R, Racette P, Sieber W. Assessment of Family Physicians' Performance Using Patient Charts: Interrater Reliability and Concordance With Chart-Stimulated Recall Interview. Eval Health Prof. 2007;30:376–92.
14. Guerra CE, Schwartz JS, Armstrong K, Brown JS, Halbert CH, Shea JA. Barriers of and Facilitators to Physician Recommendation of Colorectal Cancer Screening. J Gen Intern Med. 2007;22:1681–8.
15. Guerra CE, Jacobs SE, Holmes JH, Shea JA. Are Physicians Discussing Prostate Cancer Screening with Their Patients and Why or Why Not? A Pilot Study. J Gen Intern Med. 2007;22:901–7.
16. American Diabetes Association. Standards of Medical Care in Diabetes–2014. Diabetes Care. 2014;37:S14–80.
17. Dall TM, Narayan KM, Gillespie KB, Gallo PD, Blanchard TD, Solcan M, et al. Detecting type 2 diabetes and prediabetes among asymptomatic adults in the United States: modeling American Diabetes Association versus US Preventive Services Task Force diabetes screening guidelines. Popul Health Metr. 2014;12:12.
18. Laine C. The annual physical examination: needless ritual or necessary routine? Ann Intern Med. 2002;136:701–3.
19. Mitka M. Studies continue to show no benefit from annual physicals in healthy adults. JAMA. 2012;308:2321–2.
20. Flocke SA, Stange KC, Goodwin MA. Patient and visit characteristics associated with opportunistic preventive services delivery. J Fam Pract. 1998;47(3):202-08. PMID 9752372.
21. Stange KC, Flocke SA, Goodwin MA. Opportunistic preventive services delivery. Are time limitations and patient satisfaction barriers? J Fam Pract. 1998;46(5):419–24.
22. Kikano GE, Flocke SA, Gotler RS, Stange KC. Are you practicing 'opportunistic' prevention? Fam Pract Manag. 2000;7(3):56.
23. Klein Woolthuis EP, de Grauw WJC, van Gerwen WHEM, van den Hoogen HJM, van de Lisdonk EH, Metsemakers JFM, et al. Yield of Opportunistic Targeted Screening for Type 2 Diabetes in Primary Care: The Diabscreen Study. Ann Fam Med. 2009;7:422–30.
24. Jennett P, Affleck L. Chart audit and chart stimulated recall as methods of needs assessment in continuing professional health education. The Journal of Continuing Education in Health Professions. 1998;18:163–71.
25. Hsieh H F, Shannon SE. Three Approaches to Qualitative Content Analysis. Qual Health Res. 2005;15:1277–88.
26. Potter WJ, Levine-Donnerstein D. Rethinking validity and reliability in content analysis. J Appl Commun Res. 1999;27:258–84.
27. Thomas J, Harden A. Methods for thematic synthesis of qualitative research in systematic reviews. BMC Medical Research Methodology. 2008;8:45.
28. Francis JJ, Johnston M, Robertson C, Glidewell L, Entwistle V, Eccles MP, et al. What is an adequate sample size? Operationalising data saturation for theory-based interview studies. Psychol Health. 2010;25:1229–45.
29. Standards of Medical Care in Diabetes—2014 [Internet]. [cited 2014 Jul 28]. Available from: http://care.diabetesjournals.org/content/37/Supplement_1/S14.full.pdf+html

30. national-diabetes-report-web.pdf [Internet]. [cited 2016 Mar 31]. Available from: http://www.cdc.gov/diabetes/pubs/statsreport14/national-diabetes-report-web.pdf
31. Ealovega MW, Tabaei BP, Brandle M, Burke R, Herman WH. Opportunistic screening for diabetes in routine clinical practice. Diabetes Care. 2004;27:9–12.
32. Dexheimer JW, Talbot TR, Sanders DL, Rosenbloom ST, Aronsky D. Prompting Clinicians about Preventive Care Measures: A Systematic Review of Randomized Controlled Trials. J Am Med Inform Assoc. 2008;15:311–20.
33. Reminder Systems for Immunizations and Preventive Services [Internet]. [cited 2016 May 27]. Available from: http://www.ahrq.gov/cahps/quality-improvement/improvement-guide/6-strategies-for-improving/health-promotion-education/strategy6r-reminder-systems.html
34. Davis K, Schoenbaum SC, Audet A-M. A 2020 vision of patient-centered primary care. J Gen Intern Med. 2005;20:953–7.
35. Schmittdiel JA, Adams SR, Segal J, Griffin MR, Roumie CL, Ohnsorg K, et al. Novel Use and Utility of Integrated Electronic Health Records to Assess Rates of Prediabetes Recognition and Treatment: Brief Report From an Integrated Electronic Health Records Pilot Study. Diabetes Care. 2014;37:565–8.
36. Moin T, Li J, Duru OK, Ettner S, Turk N, Keckhafer A, et al. Metformin Prescription for Insured Adults With Prediabetes From 2010 to 2012: A Retrospective Cohort Study. Ann Intern Med. 2015;162:542.
37. Yarnall KS, Pollak KI, Østbye T, Krause KM, Michener JL. Primary care: is there enough time for prevention? Am J Public Health. 2003;93:635–41.

Permissions

All chapters in this book were first published in FP, by BioMed Central; hereby published with permission under the Creative Commons Attribution License or equivalent. Every chapter published in this book has been scrutinized by our experts. Their significance has been extensively debated. The topics covered herein carry significant findings which will fuel the growth of the discipline. They may even be implemented as practical applications or may be referred to as a beginning point for another development.

The contributors of this book come from diverse backgrounds, making this book a truly international effort. This book will bring forth new frontiers with its revolutionizing research information and detailed analysis of the nascent developments around the world.

We would like to thank all the contributing authors for lending their expertise to make the book truly unique. They have played a crucial role in the development of this book. Without their invaluable contributions this book wouldn't have been possible. They have made vital efforts to compile up to date information on the varied aspects of this subject to make this book a valuable addition to the collection of many professionals and students.

This book was conceptualized with the vision of imparting up-to-date information and advanced data in this field. To ensure the same, a matchless editorial board was set up. Every individual on the board went through rigorous rounds of assessment to prove their worth. After which they invested a large part of their time researching and compiling the most relevant data for our readers.

The editorial board has been involved in producing this book since its inception. They have spent rigorous hours researching and exploring the diverse topics which have resulted in the successful publishing of this book. They have passed on their knowledge of decades through this book. To expedite this challenging task, the publisher supported the team at every step. A small team of assistant editors was also appointed to further simplify the editing procedure and attain best results for the readers.

Apart from the editorial board, the designing team has also invested a significant amount of their time in understanding the subject and creating the most relevant covers. They scrutinized every image to scout for the most suitable representation of the subject and create an appropriate cover for the book.

The publishing team has been an ardent support to the editorial, designing and production team. Their endless efforts to recruit the best for this project, has resulted in the accomplishment of this book. They are a veteran in the field of academics and their pool of knowledge is as vast as their experience in printing. Their expertise and guidance has proved useful at every step. Their uncompromising quality standards have made this book an exceptional effort. Their encouragement from time to time has been an inspiration for everyone.

The publisher and the editorial board hope that this book will prove to be a valuable piece of knowledge for researchers, students, practitioners and scholars across the globe.

List of Contributors

Guri Aarseth and Bård Natvig
Department of General Practice, University of Oslo, Faculty of Medicine, Institute of Health and Society, Blindern 0318, OSLO, Norway

Eivind Engebretsen
Department of Health Science, University of Oslo, Faculty of Medicine, Institute of Health and Society, Blindern 0318, OSLO, Norway

Anne Kveim Lie
Departement of Community Medicine and Global Health, University of Oslo, Faculty of Medicine; Institute of Health and Society, Blindern 0318, OSLO, Norway

J. Westman
Division for Family Medicine, Department of Neurobiology, Care Sciences and Society, Karolinska Institutet, Stockholm, Sweden

M. E. H. Larsson
Region Västra Götaland, Närhälsan Research and Development Primary Health Care, Gothenburg, Sweden
Department of Health and Rehabilitation, Unit of Physiotherapy, Institute of Neuroscience and Physiology, University of Gothenburg, Gothenburg, Sweden

M. André
Department of Public Health and Caring Sciences - Family Medicine and Preventive Medicine, Uppsala University, Uppsala, Sweden

H. Ågren
Institute of Neuroscience and Physiology, University of Gothenburg, Gothenburg, Sweden

Chris F. Johnson
Pharmacy and Prescribing Support Unit, NHS Greater Glasgow and Clyde, 2nd Floor, Main Building, West Glasgow Ambulatory Care Hospital, Dalnair Street, Yorkhill, Glasgow G3 8SJ, UK

Brian Williams and Nadine J. Dougall
School of Health and Social Care, Edinburgh Napier University, Sighthill Court, Edinburgh EH11 4BN, UK

Stephen A. MacGillivray
School of Nursing and Health Sciences, University of Dundee, Airlie Place, Dundee DD1 4HN, UK

Margaret Maxwell
Nursing Midwifery and Allied Health Professionals Research Unit, University of Stirling, Unit 13 Scion House, Stirling University Innovation Park, Stirling FK9 4NF, UK

Sylvain Le Calvé
Unité de Soins de Longue Durée, Centre Hospitalier de Saint Malo, La Briantais, 78, boulevard du rosais, 35400 Saint-Malo, France

Dominique Somme
CHU de Rennes, Service de gériatrie, Rennes, France
Université Rennes 1, Faculté de Médecine, Rennes, France
Centre de recherche sur l'action politique en Europe, UMR 6051, Rennes, France

Joaquim Prud'homm and Aline Corvol
CHU de Rennes, Service de gériatrie, Rennes, France
Centre de recherche sur l'action politique en Europe, UMR 6051, Rennes, France

Marion Eisele, Sigrid Boczor, Anja Rakebrandt, Eva Blozik and Martin Scherer
Department of Primary Medical Care, Center for Psychosocial Medicine, University Medical Center Hamburg-Eppendorf, Martinistraße 52, 20246 Hamburg, Germany

Jens-Martin Träder
Department of Primary Medical Care, University of Luebeck, Ratzeburger Allee 160, 23538 Luebeck, Germany

Stefan Störk
Comprehensive Heart Failure Center Würzburg, University and University Hospital Würzburg, Straubmühlweg 2a, 97078 Würzburg, Germany

Christoph Herrmann-Lingen
University of Göttingen Medical Center, and German Center for Cardiovascular Research, partner site Göttingen, von-Siebold-Str. 5, D-37099 Göttingen, Germany

Ingrid V. F. van den Broek
Epidemiology and Surveillance Unit, Centre for Infectious Diseases Control, RIVM, Bilthoven, The Netherlands

Gé A. Donker
NIVEL Primary Care Database, Sentinel Practices, Utrecht, The Netherlands

Karin Hek
NIVEL Primary Care database, Utrecht, The Netherlands

Birgit H. B. van Benthem
Epidemiology and Surveillance Unit, Centre for Infectious Diseases Control, RIVM, Bilthoven, The Netherlands

Jan E. A. M. van Bergen
Epidemiology and Surveillance Unit, Centre for Infectious Diseases Control, RIVM, Bilthoven, The Netherlands
Department of General Practice, Academic Medical Center, Amsterdam; STI AIDS Netherlands, Amsterdam, The Netherlands

Hannelore M. Götz
Epidemiology and Surveillance Unit, Centre for Infectious Diseases Control, RIVM, Bilthoven, The Netherlands
Department of Infectious Disease Control, Municipal Public Health Service Rotterdam-Rijnmond, Rotterdam, The Netherlands

Klaus B. von Pressentin and Robert J. Mash
Division of Family Medicine and Primary Care, Faculty of Medicine and Health Sciences, Stellenbosch University, Cape Town 8000, South Africa

Laurel Baldwin-Ragaven
Department of Family Medicine, School of Clinical Medicine, University of the Witwatersrand, Johannesburg, South Africa

Roelf Petrus Gerhardus Botha
Department of Family Medicine, University of Pretoria, Pretoria, South Africa

Indiran Govender
Family Medicine, Sefako Makgatho Health Sciences University, Pretoria, South Africa

Wilhelm Johannes Steinberg
Family Medicine, University of the Free State, Bloemfontein, South Africa

Tonya M. Esterhuizen
Biostatistics Unit, Centre for Evidence-based Health Care, Department of Global Health, Stellenbosch University, Cape Town, South Africa

Khic-Houy Prang, Rachel Canaway, Marie Bismark, David Dunt and Margaret Kelaher
Centre for Health Policy, Melbourne School of Population and Global Health, The University of Melbourne, Level 4, 207 Bouverie Street, Carlton, VIC 3010, Australia

Esmée Botman, Johannes C. van der Wouden and Otto R. Maarsingh
Department of General Practice & Elderly Care Medicine and Amsterdam Public Health research institute, VU University Medical Center, Van der Boechorststraat 7, 1081, BT, Amsterdam, The Netherlands

C. Wim Ang
Department of Medical Microbiology & Infection Control, VU University Medical Center, Amsterdam, The Netherlands

Pauline Slottje
Department of General Practice & Elderly Care Medicine and Amsterdam Public Health research institute, VU University Medical Center, Van der Boechorststraat 7, 1081, BT, Amsterdam, The Netherlands
Academic Network of General Practice, Department of General Practice & Elderly Care Medicine, VU University Medical Center (ANH VUmc), Amsterdam, The Netherlands

Johanna H. K. Joosten
Academic Network of General Practice, Department of General Practice & Elderly Care Medicine, VU University Medical Center (ANH VUmc), Amsterdam, The Netherlands

W. A. de Graaf-Ruizendaal and L. van der Hoek
NIVEL: Netherlands Institute for Health Service Research, 3500, BN, Utrecht, The Netherlands

D. H. de Bakker
NIVEL: Netherlands Institute for Health Service Research, 3500, BN, Utrecht, The Netherlands
Scientific centre for care and welfare, Tranzo, Tilburg University, 5000, LE, Tilburg, The Netherlands

Jacques Cornuz
Department of Ambulatory Care and Community Medicine, Lausanne University, Rue du Bugnon 44, 1011 Lausanne, Switzerland

Christine Cohidon
Department of Ambulatory Care and Community Medicine, Lausanne University, Rue du Bugnon 44, 1011 Lausanne, Switzerland
Institute of Family Medicine, Department of ambulatory care and community medicine, University of Lausanne, Lausanne, Switzerland

Julian Jakob
Department of Ambulatory Care and Community Medicine, Lausanne University, Rue du Bugnon 44, 1011 Lausanne, Switzerland
Institute of Primary Health Care (BIHAM), University of Bern, Bern, Switzerland
Policlinique Médicale Universitaire, Rue du Bugnon 44, CH-1011 Lausanne, Switzerland

Kevin Selby
Department of Ambulatory Care and Community Medicine, Lausanne University, Rue du Bugnon 44, 1011 Lausanne, Switzerland
Kaiser Permanente Division of Research, 2000 Broadway, Oakland, USA

Clara Korenvain and Ida-Maisie Famiyeh
Women's College Hospital, 76 Grenville Street, Toronto, ON, Canada
Leslie Dan Faculty of Pharmacy, University of Toronto, 144 College Street, Toronto, ON, Canada

Lisa M. McCarthy
Women's College Hospital, 76 Grenville Street, Toronto, ON, Canada
Leslie Dan Faculty of Pharmacy, University of Toronto, 144 College Street, Toronto, ON, Canada
Faculty of Medicine, University of Toronto, 1 King's College Circle, Toronto, ON, Canada
The Wilson Centre, University Health Network, 200 Elizabeth Street, Toronto, ON, Canada

Sheila Dunn
Women's College Hospital, 76 Grenville Street, Toronto, ON, Canada
Faculty of Medicine, University of Toronto, 1 King's College Circle, Toronto, ON, Canada
The Wilson Centre, University Health Network, 200 Elizabeth Street, Toronto, ON, Canada

Cynthia R. Whitehead
Women's College Hospital, 76 Grenville Street, Toronto, ON, Canada
Faculty of Medicine, University of Toronto, 1 King's College Circle, Toronto, ON, Canada
Women's College Research Institute, 76 Grenville St, Toronto, ON M5S 1B2, Canada

Paula A. Rochon
Women's College Hospital, 76 Grenville Street, Toronto, ON, Canada
Faculty of Medicine, University of Toronto, 1 King's College Circle, Toronto, ON, Canada
The Wilson Centre, University Health Network, 200 Elizabeth Street, Toronto, ON, Canada

Erik Børve Rasmussen
Centre for the study of professions, OsloMet - Oslo Metropolitan University, St. Olavs plass, N-0130 Oslo, Norway

Karin Isaksson Rø
LEFO, Institute for studies of the medical profession, Oslo, Norway

Gloria Córdoba, Anne Holm, Lars Bjerrum, Volkert Siersma and Håkon Sandholdt
The Research Unit for General Practice and Section of General Practice, Department of Public Health, University of Copenhagen, Øster Farimagsgade 5, 1014 Copenhagen, Denmark

Tina Møller Sørensen
Department of Veterinary Clinical Sciences, University of Copenhagen, Copenhagen, Denmark

Marjukka Makela
Finnish Office for Health Technology Assessment (FINOHTA) - National Institute for Health and Welfare, Helsinki, Finland

Niels Frimodt-Møller
Department of Clinical Microbiology, Rigshospitalet, Copenhagen, Denmark

C. Wikberg and C. Björkelund
Department of Primary Health Care/Public Health and Community Medicine, Institute of Medicine, Sahlgrenska Academy, University of Gothenburg, Gothenburg, Sweden

Marlene Christina Rosengaard Møller, Anna Mygind and Flemming Bro
Research Unit for General Practice & Section for General Medical Practice, Department of Public Health, Aarhus University, Bartholins Allé 2, 8000 Aarhus C, Denmark

Anouk Déruaz-Luyet, Alexandra A. N'Goran, Nicolas Senn, Daniel Widmer and Lilli Herzig
Institute of Family Medicine, University of Lausanne, 44 rue du Bugnon, 1011 Lausanne, Switzerland

Jérôme Pasquier and Bernard Burnand
Institute of Social and Preventive Medicine, Lausanne University Hospital, Lausanne, Switzerland

Patrick Bodenmann
Department of Ambulatory Care and Community Medicine, Lausanne University Hospital, Lausanne, Switzerland

Stefan Zechmann and Stefan Neuner-Jehle
Institute of Primary Care, University of Zurich, Zurich, Switzerland

Sven Streit
Institute of Primary Health Care (BIHAM), University of Berne, Berne, Switzerland

Andreas Zeller
Centre for Primary Health Care, University of Basel, Basel, Switzerland

Dagmar M. Haller
Primary Care Unit, Faculty of Medicine, University of Geneva, Geneva, Switzerland

Angela Xiao Han
University of Alberta, 116 St & 85 Ave, Edmonton, AB T6G 2R3, Canada

Sandy Rosalie Whitehouse and Steve Tsai
University of British Columbia, 2329 West Mall, Vancouver, BC V6T 1Z4, Canada

Sandy Hwang
Child Family Research Institute, 950 W 28th Ave, Vancouver, BC V5Z 4H4, Canada

Sally Thorne
University of British Columbia School of Nursing, T201-2211 Wesbrook Mall, Vancouver, BC V6T 2B5, Canada

K. Flägel, C. Strumann and J. Steinhäuser
Institute of Family Medicine, University Hospital Schleswig-Holstein, Campus Luebeck, Ratzeburger Allee 160, 23538 Luebeck, Germany

T. Emcke
Association of Statutory Health Insurance Physicians of the Federal State of Schleswig-Holstein, Bismarckallee 1-6, 23795 Bad Segeberg, Germany

Maria Noonan
Department of Nursing and Midwifery, Faculty of Education & Health Sciences, Health Sciences Building, University of Limerick, Limerick, Ireland

Owen Doody
Department of Nursing and Midwifery, Faculty of Education & Health Sciences, Health Sciences Building, University of Limerick, Limerick, Ireland

Andrew O'Regan
Graduate Entry Medical School, Faculty of Education & Health Sciences, University of Limerick, Limerick, Ireland

Julie Jomeen
Faculty of Health and Social Care, University of Hull, Hull, UK

Rose Galvin
School of Allied Health, Faculty of Education & Health Sciences, Health Sciences Building, University of Limerick, Limerick, Ireland

Carolyn A. Chew-Graham, Thomas Shepherd, Heather Burroughs and Katie Dixon
Research Institute, Primary Care and Health Sciences, Keele University, Newcastle, Staffs ST5 5BG, UK

David Kessler
Centre for Academic Primary Care, Oakfield House, Oakfield Grove, Clifton, Bristol BS8 2BN, UK

E-L. Petersson, R. Eggertsen and J. Thorn
Department of Primary Health Care/Public Health and Community Medicine, Institute of Medicine, Sahlgrenska Academy, University of Gothenburg, Gothenburg, Sweden
Region Västra Götaland, Närhälsan Research and Development Primary Health Care, Gothenburg, Sweden

Section for General Medical Practice, Department of Public Health, Aarhus University, Bartholins Allé 2, Aarhus DK-8000, Denmark

Peter Vedsted
Research Unit for General Practice, Department of Public Health, Aarhus University, Bartholins Allé 2, Aarhus DK-8000, Denmark
Research Centre for Cancer Diagnosis in Primary Care (CaP), Department of Public Health, Aarhus University, Bartholins Allé 2, Aarhus DK-8000, Denmark
Department of Clinical Medicine, University Clinic for Innovative Health Care Delivery, Silkeborg Hospital, Aarhus University, Aarhus DK-8000, Denmark

Flemming Bro
Research Unit for General Practice, Department of Public Health, Aarhus University, Bartholins Allé 2, Aarhus DK-8000, Denmark
Section for General Medical Practice, Department of Public Health, Aarhus University, Bartholins Allé 2, Aarhus DK-8000, Denmark

Greer Dawson
Sax Institute, Level 13, Building 10, 235 Jones Street, Ultimo, NSW, Australia 2007
School of Public Health and Community Medicine, Samuels Building, University of New South Wales, Sydney, NSW, Australia 2052

Daniel B. Nelson, Evan G. Martin and Rebecca Northway
University of Michigan Medical School, Ann Arbor, MI, USA

Berit Skjødeberg Toftegaard and Alina Zalounina Falborg
Research Unit for General Practice, Department of Public Health, Aarhus University, Bartholins Allé 2, Aarhus DK-8000, Denmark
Research Centre for Cancer Diagnosis in Primary Care (CaP), Department of Public Health, Aarhus University, Bartholins Allé 2, Aarhus DK-8000, Denmark

Melanie Crane
Prevention Research Collaboration, The Charles Perkins Centre, Level 6, The Hub, School of Public Health, University of Sydney, Sydney, NSW, Australia 2006

Anna Burnham, Tara Bowman and Donna Perez
Cancer Institute NSW, Australian Technology Park, Level 9, 8 Central Avenue, Sydney, NSW, Australia 2015

Joanne Travaglia
Faculty of Health, University of Technology Sydney, Level 7, 235 Jones Street, Sydney, NSW, Australia 2007

Claudine Lyons
NSW Department of Premier and Cabinet, 52 Martin Place, Sydney, NSW, Australia 2000

Dina Hafez
VA Ann Arbor Healthcare System, 2800 Plymouth Road, Building 14, Room G100-36, Ann Arbor, MI 48109-2800, USA
Robert Wood Johnson Foundation Clinical Scholars Program, University of Michigan, Ann Arbor, MI, USA
University of Michigan Medical School, Ann Arbor, MI, USA
University of Michigan Institute for Healthcare Policy and Innovation, Ann Arbor, MI, USA

Jeffrey T. Kullgren
VA Ann Arbor Healthcare System, 2800 Plymouth Road, Building 14, Room G100-36, Ann Arbor, MI 48109-2800, USA
University of Michigan Medical School, Ann Arbor, MI, USA
University of Michigan Institute for Healthcare Policy and Innovation, Ann Arbor, MI, USA

Alicia J. Cohen
Robert Wood Johnson Foundation Clinical Scholars Program, University of Michigan, Ann Arbor, MI, USA
University of Michigan Medical School, Ann Arbor, MI, USA
University of Michigan Institute for Healthcare Policy and Innovation, Ann Arbor, MI, USA

Index

www.ingramcontent.com/pod-product-compliance
Lightning Source LLC
LaVergne TN
LVHW080727210926
848485LV00003B/527